# NEPHROLOGY SECRETS

## Second Edition

# NEPHROLOGY SECRETS
## Second Edition

**DONALD E. HRICIK, MD**
Professor of Medicine
Chief, Division of Nephrology
Case Western Reserve University School of Medicine
Medical Director, Transplantation Services
University Hospitals of Cleveland
Cleveland, Ohio

**R. TYLER MILLER, MD**
Professor of Medicine and Physiology
Case Western Reserve University School of Medicine
Chief, Renal Section
Louis Stokes Veterans Affairs Medical Center
Cleveland, Ohio

**JOHN R. SEDOR, MD**
Professor of Medicine and Physiology and Biophysics
Case Western Reserve University School of Medicine
Director, Division of Nephrology and Hypertension
MetroHealth Medical System Campus
Cleveland, Ohio

HANLEY & BELFUS, INC. / Philadelphia

**HANLEY & BELFUS, INC.**
An *Imprint of Elsevier*

The Curtis Center
Independence Square West
Philadelphia, Pennsylvania 19106

Library of Congress Control Number: 2002114163

**NEPHROLOGY SECRETS, 2nd edition**                                    ISBN 1-56053-502-4

Printed in the United States of America

Last digit is the print number:    9    8    7    6    5    4    3    2

# CONTENTS

## I. PATIENT ASSESSMENT

## II. CLINICAL SYNDROMES

## III. PRIMARY GLOMERULAR DISEASE

## IV. SECONDARY GLOMERULAR DISEASE

## V. OTHER PARENCHYMAL RENAL DISEASES

# VI.  END-STAGE RENAL DISEASE: CAUSES AND CONSEQUENCES

# VII.  RENAL FAILURE: MANAGEMENT

# VIII.  HYPERTENSION

## IX.  ACID-BASE AND ELECTROLYTE DISORDERS

# CONTRIBUTORS

**Bruce E. Berger, M.D.**
Associate Professor, Department of Medicine, Case Western Reserve University School of Medicine; University Hospitals of Cleveland, Cleveland, Ohio

**Kenneth A. Bodziak, M.D.**
Assistant Professor, Department of Medicine, Case Western Reserve University School of Medicine; University Hospitals of Cleveland, Cleveland, Ohio

**Carolyn P. Cacho, M.D.**
Assistant Professor, Division of Nephrology, Department of Medicine, Case Western Reserve University School of Medicine; University Hospitals of Cleveland, Cleveland, Ohio

**Marigel Constantiner, R.Ph., M.Sc., BCPS**
Clinical Specialist in Adult Medicine, Pharmacy Department, MetroHealth Medical Center, Cleveland, Ohio

**Ira D. Davis, M.D., M.S.**
Associate Professor, Department of Pediatrics, Case Western Reserve University School of Medicine; Rainbow Babies and Children's Hospital, Cleveland, Ohio

**Katherine MacRae Dell, M.D.**
Assistant Professor, Department of Pediatrics, Case Western Reserve University School of Medicine; Rainbow Babies and Children's Hospital, Cleveland, Ohio

**Essam B. Elashi, M.D.**
Department of Nephrology, Firelands Regional Medical Center, Sandusky, Ohio

**Ronald Flauto, D.O.**
Division of Nephrology, Department of Medicine, Case Western Reserve University School of Medicine, Cleveland, Ohio

**Michael B. Ganz, M.D.**
Associate Professor, Department of Medicine, Case Western Reserve University School of Medicine; Louis Stokes Veterans Affairs Medical Center, Cleveland, Ohio

**Patrick S. T. Hayden, M.D.**
Department of Medicine, Case Western Reserve University School of Medicine; University Hospitals of Cleveland; MetroHealth Medical Center, Cleveland, Ohio

**Donald E. Hricik, M.D.**
Professor, Department of Medicine, and Chief, Division of Nephrology, Case Western Reserve University School of Medicine; University Hospitals of Cleveland, Cleveland, Ohio

**Thomas C. Knauss, M.D.**
Associate Professor, Department of Medicine, Case Western Reserve University School of Medicine; Louis Stokes Veterans Affairs Medical Center; University Hospitals of Cleveland, Cleveland, Ohio

**R. Tyler Miller, M.D.**
Professor, Departments of Medicine and Physiology, Case Western Reserve University School of Medicine; Chief, Renal Section, Louis Stokes Veterans Affairs Medical Center, Cleveland, Ohio

**Lavinia A. Negrea, M.D.**
Assistant Professor, Department of Medicine, Case Western Reserve University School of Medicine; University Hospitals of Cleveland; Louis Stokes Veterans Affairs Medical Center, Cleveland, Ohio

**Andrew S. O'Connor, D.O.**
Division of Nephrology, Department of Medicine, Case Western Reserve University School of Medicine; MetroHealth Medical Center, Cleveland, Ohio

**Mahboob Rahman, M.D., M.S.**
Assistant Professor, Division of Nephrology, Department of Medicine, Case Western Reserve University School of Medicine; Attending Physician, University Hospitals of Cleveland, Cleveland, Ohio

**Edmond Ricanati, M.D.**
Professor, Department of Medicine, Case Western Reserve University School of Medicine; Staff Physician, Division of Nephrology, MetroHealth Medical Center, Cleveland, Ohio

**Jeffrey R. Schelling, M.D.**
Associate Professor, Department of Medicine, Case Western Reserve University School of Medicine; MetroHealth Medical Center, Cleveland, Ohio

**John R. Sedor, M.D.**
Professor, Departments of Medicine and Physiology and Biophysics, Case Western Reserve University School of Medicine; Director, Division of Nephrology and Hypertension, MetroHealth Medical Center, Cleveland, Ohio

**Ashwini R. Sehgal, M.D.**
Associate Professor, Department of Medicine, Case Western Reserve University School of Medicine; Nephrologist, MetroHealth Medical Center, Cleveland, Ohio

**Marcia R. Silver, M.D.**
Associate Professor, Department of Medicine, Case Western Reserve University School of Medicine; Division of Nephrology and Hypertension, MetroHealth Medical Center, Cleveland, Ohio

**Michael S. Simonson**
Associate Professor, Department of Medicine, Case Western Reserve University School of Medicine, Cleveland, Ohio

**Michael C. Smith, M.D.**
Professor, Department of Medicine, Case Western Reserve University School of Medicine; University Hospitals of Cleveland, Cleveland, Ohio

**Stephen Tamarkin, M.D.**
Assistant Professor, Department of Radiology, Case Western Reserve University School of Medicine; Chief, Body Imaging, Department Of Radiology, MetroHealth Medical Center, Cleveland, Ohio

**Beth A. Vogt, M.D.**
Associate Professor, Department of Pediatrics, Case Western Reserve University School of Medicine; Rainbow Babies and Children's Hospital, Cleveland, Ohio

**Miriam F. Weiss, M.D.**
Associate Professor, Department of Medicine, Case Western Reserve University School of Medicine; University Hospitals of Cleveland, Cleveland, Ohio

**Jay B. Wish, M.D.**
Professor, Department of Medicine, Case Western Reserve University School of Medicine; Medical Director, Hemodialysis Services, University Hospitals of Cleveland, Cleveland, Ohio

**Linda Zarif, M.D.**
Department of Medicine, Case Western Reserve University School of Medicine; University Hospitals of Cleveland, Cleveland, Ohio

**Thomas Zipp, M.D., FACP**
Assistant Professor, Department of Medicine, Case Western Reserve University School of Medicine; MetroHealth Medical Center, Cleveland, Ohio

# PREFACE TO THE SECOND EDITION

Since publication of the first edition of *Nephrology Secrets* in 1999, there has been continued growth in the number of patients who require treatment with renal replacement therapy for end-stage renal disease. Research efforts have increasingly focused on early recognition of patients with renal disease, understanding the genetic factors and physiologic mechanisms favoring progression of renal disease, and treatment strategies to retard progression. In the past few years, major advances have been made in optimizing the management of patients who require chronic dialysis and continued improvements in the outcomes of kidney transplant recipients.

In the second edition of *Nephrology Secrets*, we have updated most of the chapters dealing with specific renal disorders, end-stage renal disease, hypertension, and electrolyte disturbances. Entirely revamped or new chapters have been included on drug therapy in renal disease, hepatorenal syndrome, renal disease in pregnancy, management of patients with progressive renal failure, nutrition in dialysis patients, and continuous renal replacement therapy. Using the informal question-and-answer format of the popular Secrets Series®, it is hoped that this second edition will once again provide an enjoyable learning experience for those who care for patients with renal disease.

Donald E. Hricik, M.D.
R. Tyler Miller, M.D.
John R. Sedor, M.D.

## DEDICATION

This book is dedicated to past and present faculty members and fellows
in the Division of Nephrology at Case Western Reserve University.

# PREFACE TO THE FIRST EDITION

The roots of the specialty of nephrology are firmly entrenched in disciplines such as histopathology, immunology, and physiology—the basic sciences that helped to elucidate both the pathogenesis of various renal diseases and the kidney's role in hypertension and common electrolyte and acid-base disturbances. With the availability of hemodialysis, peritoneal dialysis, and effective immunosuppressive therapy for kidney transplant recipients, however, the clinical practice of nephrology has centered increasingly on the management of patients with end-stage renal disease. Technological improvements in renal replacement therapies (i.e., dialysis and kidney transplantation) have resulted in a dramatic increase in the numbers of patients whose lives can be sustained despite end-stage renal disease. In the United States alone, more than 300,000 patients currently are receiving renal replacement therapy. A growth rate of 5–8% per year is anticipated for at least the next 5 years.

To the extent that renal disorders such as hypertension, electrolyte and acid-base disturbances, and various kidney diseases occur in patients cared for by virtually all medical and surgical specialists, students and house officers should regard basic concepts in nephrology as an essential element of training. *Nephrology Secrets* provides information about all aspects of nephrology that should be of value to trainees learning this specialty and to more advanced health care professionals who seek a review of essential topics in the field. Using the informal question-and-answer format of the popular Secrets Series®, it is hoped that the material presented here will provide an enjoyable learning experience and a foundation for excellent patient care.

Donald E. Hricik, M.D.
John R. Sedor, M.D.
Michael B. Ganz, M.D.

# I. Patient Assessment

## 1. PHYSICAL DIAGNOSIS

*Thomas C. Knauss, M.D.*

**1. What is the single most important question to ask a patient suspected of having renal disease?**

"Have you had this before?" A prior history of renal disease is important in constructing a differential diagnosis and assessing the acuity or chronicity of disease.

**2. What renal diseases should be considered when there is a strong family history of kidney problems?**

Polycystic kidney disease
Alport syndrome
Hypertensive nephrosclerosis
Diabetic nephropathy
Fabry's disease
Lupus nephritis
Focal segmental glomerulosclerosis (rarely familial)

**3. What features of the medical history should be elicited in hospitalized patients who develop acute renal failure?**

• Recent episodes of hypotension
• Exposure to intravenous contrast
• Treatment with nephrotoxic drugs
• Recent systemic infection
• Risk factors for volume depletion (e.g., gastrointestinal losses, diuretic therapy)

**4. Describe the physical exam findings that may be seen in patients with uremia.**

Hypertension
Signs of fluid overload
Pallor of skin and mucous membranes
Asterixis
Peripheral neuropathy
Pericardial friction rub
Uremic frost (in advanced uremia)

**5. What are the physical signs of fluid overload?**

Hypertension
Elevated jugular venous pressure
Hepatojugular reflux
S3 heart sound
Pulmonary crackles
Ascites
Edema

**6. What are the signs and symptoms of volume depletion?**
Postural hypotension
Dizziness
Dry mucous membranes
Skin tenting
Flat neck veins (low jugulovenous pressure)
Dark yellow urine
Decreased urine output

**7. Which kidney diseases are frequently associated with skin rashes?**

| RASH | ASSOCIATED KIDNEY DISEASE |
| --- | --- |
| Purpura | Idiopathic thrombocytopenic purpura (ITP)<br>Henoch-Schönlein purpura<br>Other forms of vasculitis |
| Petechiae | Hemolytic uremic syndrome<br>Focal glomerulonephritis secondary to subacute bacterial endocarditis<br>Acute interstitial nephritis |
| Hives | Henoch-Schönlein purpura<br>Acute interstitial nephritis |
| Discoid lupus | Systemic lupus erythematosus |
| Impetigo | Poststreptococcal glomerulonephritis |
| Angiokeratoma | Fabry's disease |

**8. Which kidney diseases are frequently associated with signs and symptoms of arthritis?**
Lupus nephritis
Amyloidosis
Henoch-Schönlein purpura
Cryoglobulinemia
Sarcoidosis

**9. What physical finding best characterizes the nephrotic syndrome?**
Edema.

**10. What happens to blood pressure in nephrotic syndrome?**
Blood pressure may be normal in patients with nephrotic syndrome, especially if renal function is well preserved. Nephrotic patients with severe hypoalbuminemia (< 2 gm/dl) sometimes exhibit a postural drop in blood pressure due to relative intravascular volume depletion.

**11. What physical finding in a patient with nephrotic syndrome and diabetes mellitus best correlates with diabetic nephropathy?**
Proliferative diabetic retinopathy. Forty-five percent of patients with biopsy-proven diabetic nephropathy will have retinopathy at the time they present with proteinuria. By the time these patients reach end-stage renal disease, 95% will have retinopathy.

**12. Peripheral neuropathy due to uremia can be seen in advanced azotemia. Which diseases can independently cause peripheral neuropathy and renal dysfunction?**

1. Diabetes mellitus can cause distal polyneuropathy.
2. Vasculitis can cause mononeuritis multiplex.
3. Fabry's disease can cause distal polyneuropathy.
4. Amyloidosis can result in bilateral carpal tunnel and distal neuropathy.

**13. Which renal diseases are associated with hemoptysis?**

- Pulmonary edema secondary to acute or chronic renal failure
- Goodpasture's syndrome
- Pulmonary embolus or infarct in a patient with glomerulonephritis and renal vein thrombosis
- Bacterial endocarditis

**14. What renal disease is associated with deafness?**

Alport syndrome.

**15. What are some renal causes of flank pain and gross hematuria?**

Renal stone disease
Renal neoplasms
Renal vein thrombosis
Papillary necrosis
Pyelonephritis

**16. What physical findings can be seen in patients with cholesterol atheroembolic disease?**

Cyanosis and microinfarcts in toes
Livedo reticularis on buttocks and thighs
Cholesterol plaques at branch points of retinal arteries

**17. List some of the extrarenal physical findings that may be seen in patients with systemic lupus erythematosus.**

Alopecia
Nasal or oral ulcerations
Pleural or pericardial effusion or rub
Hepatosplenomegaly
Ascites
Edema
Arthritis, fever

BIBLIOGRAPHY

1. Abuelo JG: Diagnosing vascular causes of renal failure. Ann Intern Med 123:601–614, 1995.
2. Breyer JA: Diabetic nephropathy in insulin-dependent patients. Am J Kidney Dis 6:533–547, 1992.
3. Cameron JS: The nephrotic syndrome and its complications. Am J Kidney Dis 10:157–171, 1987.
4. Fraser CL, Arieff A: Nervous system complications in uremia. Ann Intern Med 109:143–153, 1988.
5. Gleeson MJ: Alport's syndrome: Audiological manifestations and implications. J Laryngol Otol 98:449–465, 1984.
6. Kassirer JP: Atheroembolic renal disease. N Engl J Med 280:812–818, 1969.
7. Liano F, Pascual J: Epidemiology of acute renal failure: A prospective multicenter community-based study. Kidney Int 50:811–818, 1996.
8. Turner AN, Rees AJ: Goodpasture's disease and Alport's syndrome. Annu Rev Med 47:377–386, 1996.
9. Vanholder R: The uremic syndrome. In Greenberg A (ed): Primer on Kidney Diseases, 2nd ed. San Diego, Academic Press, 1998, pp 403–407.

# 2. URINALYSIS

*Michael B. Ganz, M.D.*

**1. What are the major determinants of urine color?**

The color of urine (usually yellow!) is determined predominantly by chemical content and concentration. Urine may be relatively colorless when volume is high and concentration is low. Cloudy urine may be the result of phosphates (usually normal) or white blood cells and bacteria (abnormal). Red urine reflects hemoglobin, while red urine without red blood cells indicates either free hemoglobin or myoglobin. Other colors can be seen. For instance, green urine may reflect exogenous chemicals (e.g., methylene blue) or *Pseudomonas* bacteriuria, whereas orange color may indicate the presence of bile pigments.

**2. What is the importance of the urine specific gravity?**

A standard part of the urinalysis, specific gravity reflects the concentration of dissolved solutes in urine. It is best measured using a hygrometer. Specific gravity normally ranges between 1.003 and 1.030. However, this range decreases as one ages, reflecting a decreased ability to dilute and concentrate urine. Urine osmolality, normally ranging between 50 and 1,200 mOsm/L also reflects the concentration of urine but is more cumbersome to measure and is not part of the routine urinalysis. Monitoring specific gravity or urine osmolality may aid in the management of stone-forming patients who should be encouraged to maintain a dilute urine. These measurements also provide a general sense of the patient's state of hydration and may provide clues in the differential diagnosis of patients with hypo- or hypernatremia (see Chapter 69, Hyponatremia and Hypernatremia).

**3. What is the significance of urine pH?**

Usually measured with a reagent strip, urine pH values in humans range from 4.5 to 7.8. Throughout the course of the day, urine pH is most often closer to the lower limit of this range, reflecting the renal hydrogen ion excretion that is necessary to maintain acid-base balance in the face of endogenous acid production of about 1 mEq/kg/day. The urine is transiently alkaline after meals or the ingestion of bicarbonate loads. Persistently alkaline urine (pH > 7.5) may aid in making a diagnosis of distal renal tubular acidosis (see Chapter 20, Disorders of Tubular Function). Infection with urea-splitting organisms such as Proteus also is associated with a high urine pH resulting from bacterial conversion of urea to ammonia.

**4. Can urine glucose be used to monitor glycemic control in patients with diabetes mellitus?**

Dipstick reagents generally detect concentrations of glucose as low as 50 mg/dl. The renal threshold for tubular reabsorption of glucose is approximately 180 mg/dl (i.e., with plasma glucose concentrations of 180 mg/dl or less, all of the glucose filtered by glomeruli is reabsorbed in the proximal tubules). Thus, detection of glucose in the urine crudely indicates a blood sugar of at least 230 mg/dl. Used as a screening test, this finding suggests the diagnosis of diabetes mellitus. However, glucosuria occasionally occurs when the blood sugar is normal, either as an isolated finding in patients with a defect in tubular glucose transport or in patients with more generalized tubular dysfunction (e.g., Fanconi syndrome) or tubulointerstitial disease. Furthermore, in diabetics, glucose may appear in the urine long after the blood sugar has normalized, rendering urine glucose measurements virtually worthless in the day-to-day management of diabetes.

**5. What is the significance of finding ketones in the urine?**

Ketones, generally detected with a nitroprusside assay, are detected in the urine of patients with diabetic, alcoholic, or starvation ketoacidosis. In patients with severe ketoacidosis and an altered redox state, urine ketones initially may be negative due to relative overproduction of beta-hydroxybutyrate but later become positive as the redox states return to normal.

**6. What is the meaning of a positive dipstick determination for "blood"?**

Reagent strips use peroxidase-like activity of hemoglobin to catalyze a reaction wherein both hemoglobin and myoglobin react positively. The major cause of a positive dipstick test for blood is the presence of hemoglobin-containing red blood cells. Free hemoglobin also can be filtered at the glomerulus and appears in the urine when the capacity for plasma protein binding with haptoglobin is exceeded. Some of the hemoglobin is catabolized by proximal tubules. The major cause for increased hemoglobin is hemolysis, while rhabdomyolysis gives rise to myoglobinuria.

**7. What is the significance of positive dipstick tests for leukocyte esterase and nitrites?**

The esterase assay relies on the fact that esterases are released from lysed white blood cells in the urine. Urinary bacteria convert nitrates to nitrites. Positive tests for leukocyte esterase or nitrites generally indicate leukocyturia and possible urinary tract infection.

**8. What urinary proteins are detected by the standard dipstick?**

Most dipstick reagents contain a pH-sensitive colorimetric indicator that changes color when bound to negatively charged proteins such as albumin. Positively charged proteins, such as immunoglobulin light chains, are less well detected even when large amounts are present (see Chapter 4, Measurement of Urinary Protein, and Chapter 14, Asymptomatic Proteinuria).

**9. Name the cellular elements from urinalysis depicted in the following figure.**

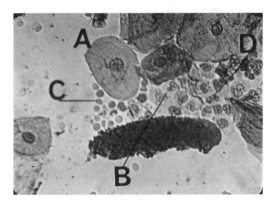

*A,* Squamous epithelial cell. *B* and *D,* White blood cells (polymorphonuclear cells). *C,* Red blood cells. Also shown in the lower center of the figure is a granular cast.

## 10. Name the urine crystals depicted in the following figure.

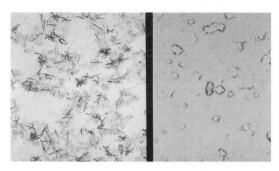

*Left,* Calcium phosphate crystals. *Right,* Calcium oxalate crystals.

## 11. What are red blood cell casts?

Red blood cell casts are formed elements that are excreted into the urine when an active glomerular lesion is present (i.e., acute glomerulonephritis) and red blood cells are extravasated through the glomerulus into the tubular lumen. In acute glomerular disease, there is usually urinary stasis. Proteins secreted from the tubules (e.g., Tamm-Horsfall glycoproteins) remain in the tubular lumen for a prolonged period of time, quite often in the presence of an acid urine, thereby forming a "cast" of the lumen. Any cell in the lumen will be trapped in that cast and excreted into the urine.

## 12. What are white blood cell casts?

Formed in the same manner as red blood cell casts (see question 11), white blood cell casts are indicative of some form of interstitial nephritis including suppurative pyelonephritis. Again, there is often urinary stasis allowing a cast to be formed that traps white blood cells (granulocytes) in the secreted glycoprotein material.

## 13. What are the causes of eosinophiluria?

Eosinophils are best detected with a Wright stain or Hansel stain. In the proper clinical setting, the presence of eosinophils in the urine suggests drug-induced acute interstitial nephritis. However, eosinophiluria is not specific for that disorder and can also be seen in acute prostatitis, other urinary tract infections, and renal transplant rejection.

## 14. What is the significance of lipiduria?

The presence of free lipid droplets or lipid droplets within tubular cells (oval fat bodies) is best detected with microscopy, using a polarizing lens. These droplets generally are found in the urine of patients with heavy proteinuria or nephrotic syndrome (see Chapter 17, Nephrotic Syndrome).

### BIBLIOGRAPHY

1. Kasiske BL, Keane WF: Laboratory assessment of renal disease: Clearance, urinalysis, and renal biopsy. In Brenner B (ed): The Kidney, 5th ed. Philadelphia, W.B. Saunders, 1996, pp 233–278.
2. McCormack M, Dessureault J, Guitard M: The urine specific gravity dipstick: A useful tool to increase fluid intake in stone forming patients. J Urol 146:1475–1482, 1991.
3. McNagny SE, Parker RM, Zenilman JM, Lewis JS: Urinary leukocyte esterase test: A screening test: A screening method for the detection of symptomatic chlamydial and gonococcal infections in men. J Infect Dis 165:573–577, 1992.
4. Schwab SJ, Dunn FL, Feinglos MN: Screening for microalbuminuria. Diabetes Care 15:1581–1587, 1992.

# 3. MEASUREMENT OF GLOMERULAR FILTRATION RATE

*Michael S. Simonson*

**1. What is the glomerular filtration rate (GFR)?**

GFR is the amount of plasma filtered through glomeruli per unit of time. Although the term can refer to the function of single nephrons, GFR most often refers to the sum filtration rate of all functioning nephrons.

**2. What is the clinical significance of the GFR?**

Early detection and management of patients with renal disease generally require an estimate of GFR, the single best index of functioning renal mass. Clinicians use serial measurements of GFR to monitor the severity and course of renal disease. In chronic kidney disease, estimates of GFR help determine appropriate dosages of drugs excreted by the kidney. Excretion of such drugs falls when GFR declines (see Chapter 8). Without lowering drug dosage accordingly, plasma drug concentrations can rapidly accumulate to toxic levels.

**3. What are normal values for GFR in adults?**

The range of normal values for GFR are:
    Men: 115–125 ml/min
    Women: 90–100 ml/min

**4. What is the relationship between GFR and renal function?**

Subnormal GFR signifies intrinsic renal disease (e.g., nephron injury) or a condition associated with decreased renal perfusion (e.g., volume depletion). In contrast, an increase in GFR usually indicates improvement of renal function. Stable but subnormal GFR suggests stable renal disease. Renal replacement therapy with dialysis or renal transplantation is generally necessary when GFR falls below 10–15 ml/min.

**5. How is GFR estimated in routine clinical practice?**

In most patients, it is unnecessary to determine an exact value for GFR. Instead, it is important to know whether GFR is declining (indicating renal disease), increasing, or stable. The most widely used clinical index of GFR is the serum concentration of creatinine. Creatinine is a by-product of the nonenzymatic conversion of creatine and phosphocreatine in skeletal muscle. Production of creatinine by skeletal muscle is proportional to muscle mass and remains relatively constant. These and other properties make creatinine a convenient, endogenous marker for GFR. Serum creatinine is determined in a routine panel of biochemical blood tests and can, therefore, be serially analyzed in the same patient to monitor renal function. Convenience, reproducibility, and low cost account for the popularity of serum creatinine as an index of GFR. Serum creatinine varies inversely with GFR.

**6. Why does serum creatinine correlate inversely with GFR?**

The amount of creatinine filtered at the glomerulus (GFR $\times$ plasma creatinine) approximates the amount excreted by the kidney, and the amount of creatinine produced by the muscle mass remains relatively constant. In the steady state, creatinine excretion equals creatinine production. Thus, the following relationship holds true:

Creatinine excretion (approximated by filtered creatinine) =
Muscle production of creatinine
*or*
GFR × Plasma creatinine = Constant
*or*
Plasma creatinine = Constant/GFR

It is apparent from this relationship that a decline in GFR increases serum creatinine.

**7. What are normal values for serum creatinine in adults?**
Men: 0.8–1.3 mg/dl (or 70–114 μmol/L)
Women: 0.6–1.0 mg/dl (or 53–88 μmol/L)
Reduced muscle mass and correspondingly lower rates of creatinine synthesis account for the slightly lower normal values of serum creatinine in women. To convert serum creatinine from mg/dl to Standard International units (mmol/L), multiply by 0.088.

**8. What are normal values for serum creatinine in children?**
Because growing children have an increasing muscle mass, serum creatinine increases somewhat with age. The following formulas estimate normal values for serum creatinine in children ages 1–20 years[5]:
Serum creatinine for boys = 0.35 + age in years/40
Serum creatinine for girls = 0.35 + age in years/55

**9. What are the major limitations of serum creatinine as a clinical index of renal disease?**
A low serum creatinine concentration may be misleading in patients with reduced muscle mass. In addition, serum creatinine is a somewhat insensitive index of renal function, especially in early and late stages of renal disease. As shown in the figure, serum creatinine does not increase (i.e., > 1.0 mg/dl) until major declines in GFR have occurred. Two mechanisms account for the relative insensitivity of serum creatinine as an indicator of renal disease. As part of the adaptation of the kidney to renal injury, uninjured nephrons undergo hypertrophy and hyperfiltration to compensate for the loss of functioning nephrons (compensatory hyperfiltration). Thus, total GFR and serum creatinine remain relatively normal despite a decrease in functioning nephrons. Another potential problem is that tubular secretion of creatinine, which normally contributes little to overall creatinine clearance, increases progressively as renal disease worsens. Thus, both the serum creatinine concentration and the creatinine clearance (see question 11) become increasingly unreliable as estimates of

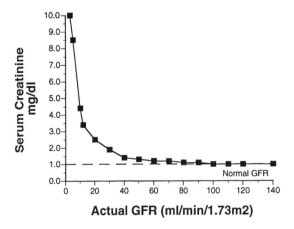

Relationship between serum creatinine and actual values for GFR in patients with renal failure. Normal value of serum creatinine is indicated by the dashed line. (Adapted from Shemesh O, Golbetz H, Kriss JP, Myers BD: Limitations of creatinine as a filtration marker in glomerulopathic patients. Kidney Int 28:830–838, 1985.)

GFR in patients with advanced renal disease. Finally, certain circumstances are associated with spurious elevations of serum creatinine independent of changes in GFR. Rhabdomyolysis or ingestion of cooked meat can transiently increase creatinine production and elevate serum creatinine, as can certain drugs (e.g., cimetidine, trimethoprim) that decrease tubular secretion of creatinine. High concentrations of certain exogenous compounds (e.g., flucytosine, cefoxitin, and other cephalosporin antibiotics) can be detected as creatinine. In patients with ketoacidosis, acetoacetic acid can be detected as creatinine leading to false elevations.

## 10. Can serum creatinine be used clinically to predict the course of renal disease in patients?

Some nephrologists use plots of the reciprocal of serum creatinine versus time (1/serum creatinine versus time) to predict the course of renal failure. Although this technique yields useful information in some patients (i.e., time to end-stage renal failure), in many patients, the decline in renal function is nonlinear and is therefore poorly modeled by such plots. Clinical predictions based on reciprocal plots should be interpreted with great care.

## 11. What other methods are available to measure GFR?

Effective management of patients with renal disease sometimes requires actual estimates of GFR, as opposed to the index of GFR provided by serum creatinine. To estimate GFR, one must measure the clearance of molecular markers that are (1) freely filtered at the glomerulus, (2) present at a stable plasma concentration, and (3) not reabsorbed, secreted, or metabolized by the kidney. Clearance is defined as the volume of plasma cleared of a specific compound (e.g., creatinine, glucose) per unit time. The clearance (C) of any compound X can be determined from the following formula:

$$C = ([U_X] \times V)/[P_X]$$

where $[U_X]$ is the concentration of X in urine, V is the volume of urine containing X, and $[P_X]$ is the plasma concentration of X.

The most common clinical method for directly estimating GFR consists of measuring the clearance of endogenous creatinine (see question 12). Variable tubular secretion of creatinine makes creatinine clearance an imperfect marker of GFR. Measurements of the clearance of the polysaccharide inulin or the radioisotope $^{125}$I-iothalamate are gold standards for estimates of GFR. However, the technical challenges and expense of inulin and $^{125}$I-iothalamate clearances render these tests impractical for clinical use except in research or therapeutic trials.

## 12. How is creatinine clearance measured?

Creatinine clearance is usually determined by using venous blood for serum creatinine and a 24-hour urine collection, using the following formula:

$$\text{Creatinine clearance} = ([U_{Cr}] \times V)/[\text{serum creatinine}]$$

where $[U_{Cr}]$ is the urine concentration of creatinine, and V is the 24-hour urine volume.

Normal values for creatinine clearance are 120 ± 25 ml/min in men and 95 ± 20 ml/min in women. In practice, several problems can severely compromise the utility of creatinine clearance. Because the renal tubules secrete creatinine, measurements of creatinine clearance can significantly overestimate true GFR, particularly in patients with renal disease. Accurate measurements of creatine clearance also require complete and carefully timed urine collections; inadequate urine collections yield spurious results.

## 13. What is a cimetidine-enhanced creatinine clearance?

One approach for enhancing the accuracy of creatinine clearance measurements is to assess clearance after oral administration of the histamine $H_2$-receptor antagonist cimetidine, which blocks tubular secretion of creatinine thereby improving its accuracy as a true marker of GFR. Creatinine clearance with cimetidine has been reported to be nearly identical to GFR, even in patients with mild or severe renal failure. A single dose of 1200 mg of cimetidine given 2 hours before starting the 24-hour urine collection has been proven effective.[8]

## 14. Can creatinine clearance and GFR be estimated from simple measurements of serum creatinine?

In an attempt to improve the accuracy of serum creatinine as a measure of GFR, variations in sex- and age-dependent differences in muscle mass have been incorporated into formulas that estimate GFR (in ml/min) from serum creatinine. The most widely used estimates are the Cockcroft-Gault and Levey formulas. The Cockcroft-Gault estimate is:

Creatinine clearance = [(140 – age) × body weight]/(72 × plasma creatinine)

where lean body weight is in kg, age is in years, and plasma creatinine is in mg/dl. For women, multiply the result by a factor of 0.85 to compensate for the lower average muscle mass. The utility of this formula is dramatically illustrated when one considers that a serum creatinine of 1.7 mg/dl corresponds to a creatinine clearance of 79 ml/min in an 80-kg, 20-year-old man but only a clearance of 36 ml/min in a 45-kg, 75-year-old woman.

For children older than 2 years, creatinine clearance is estimated as follows:

[0.55 × height (cm)]/[serum creatinine (mg/dl)]

The Levey formula, based on data generated from the Modification of Diet in Renal Disease (MDRD) study, is more complicated and difficult to calculate.[4] Programs are available on the Internet (www.calc.med.edu).

## 15. Can measurements of blood urea nitrogen (BUN) serve as an index of GFR?

BUN is not a reliable index of GFR. The renal tubules reabsorb urea in quantities that vary depending on the state of hydration, thus rendering the BUN an inaccurate marker for GFR. BUN concentration is also strongly affected by changes in catabolism and protein intake.

BIBLIOGRAPHY

1. Cockcroft DW, Gault MH: Prediction of creatinine clearance from serum creatinine. Nephron 16:31–39, 1976.
2. Kasiske BL, Keane WF: Laboratory assessment of renal disease: Clearance, unianalysis, and renal biopsy. In Brenner BM (ed): The Kidney, 5th ed. Philadelphia, W.B. Saunders, 1996, pp 1137–1174.
3. Levey AS: Measurement of renal function in chronic renal disease. Kidney Int 38:167–184, 1990.
4. Levey AS, Bosch JP, Lewis JB, et al: A more accurate method to estimate glomerular filtration rate from serum creatinine: A new prediction equation. Ann Intern Med 130:461–470, 1999.
5. Schwartz GJ, Haycock GB, Spitzer A: Plasma creatinine and urea concentration in children: Normal values for age and sex. J Pediatr 88:828–837, 1976.
6. Shemesh O, Golbetz H, Kriss JP, Myers BD: Limitations of creatinine as a filtration marker in glomerulopathic patients. Kidney Int 28:830–838, 1985.
7. Vander AJ: Renal clearance. In Vander AJ (ed): Renal Physiology, 5th ed. New York, McGraw-Hill, 1995, pp 51–61.
8. Walser M: Assessing renal function from creatinine measurements in adults with chronic renal failure. Am J Kidney Dis 32:23–31, 1998.

# 4. MEASUREMENT OF URINARY PROTEIN

*Michael S. Simonson*

**1. How does the kidney normally restrict the excretion of plasma proteins?**

The glomerulus functions as a size- and charge-selective ultrafilter that largely prevents filtration of plasma proteins into the tubules. As shown in the figure, glomerular capillaries comprise three distinct structures: a fenestrated endothelium, a glomerular basement membrane, and a lining of epithelial cells attached to the basement membrane by podocytes ("foot processes").

Size-selective properties reflect poorly characterized "pores" in the glomerular capillary wall structure that prevent filtration of proteins above a specific molecular radius. Charge-selective properties arise from the presence of negatively charged sialoproteins and proteoglycans in the endothelium, basement membrane, and epithelial podocytes. Because most plasma proteins including albumin are negatively charged, they are electrostatically repelled and fail to filter through the glomerulus. The glomerular capillary membrane is not a perfect filter. However, a large fraction of the plasma protein filtered through glomeruli is subsequently reabsorbed by renal tubular cells.

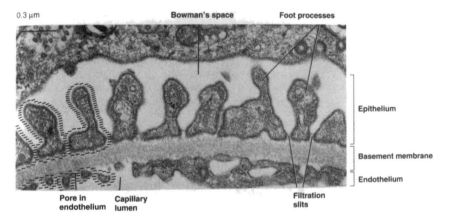

Ultrastructure of the glomerular capillary membrane as depicted by electron microscopy. Note the negataive charges illustrated on the fenestrated endothelium, basement membrane, and epithelial foot processes.

**2. What is the clinical significance of proteinuria?**

Proteinuria is often the first evidence of progressive kidney disease and is an important tool for early detection. In many patients with chronic kidney disease, proteinuria is a sensitive and independent predictor of the progression of renal disease and of cardiovascular disease. Urinary protein excretion exceeding 150 mg per day is often associated with renal disease and warrants further evaluation. Unlike measurements of glomerular filtration rate, which indicate the severity of renal dysfunction, proteinuria per se does not always correlate with the severity of renal disease. Some renal diseases cause heavy proteinuria (> 3.5 gm/24 hr), whereas others are associated with normal or only slightly elevated levels of urinary protein excretion. Furthermore, proteinuria is not always associated with renal disease

11

and can result from benign conditions (see Chapter 14, Asymptomatic Proteinuria and Hematuria). The degree of proteinuria can, however, strongly point to specific kinds of renal damage. Heavy proteinuria usually indicates the presence of glomerular disease.

### 3. What is the pathophysiology of proteinuria?

Glomerular proteinuria results from structural damage to any of the charge- or size-selective properties of the glomerular capillary. Tubular proteinuria results when the tubular absorption of the few normally filtered proteins is disrupted. The pathophysiology of these and other forms of proteinuria is discussed further in Chapters 14 and 17.

### 4. What proteins are present in normal urine?

The upper limit of total urinary protein excretion in normal individuals is 150 mg/day. A variety of proteins are excreted by the kidneys including small amounts of albumin (< 20 mg/day) and the Tamm-Horsfall mucoprotein (30–50 mg/day), also called uromodulin. Tamm-Horsfall protein, which is secreted by epithelial cells in the loop of Henle, is clinically important because it forms the matrix for most urinary casts (see Chapter 2, Urinalysis).

### 5. How is proteinuria measured?

Two methods are used clinically to estimate proteinuria semiquantitatively. In the most common procedure, a colorimetric analysis is performed using a dipstick (e.g., Albustix) impregnated with an indicator dye such as tetrabromophenol blue. The indicator color changes according to the amount of protein present; negative protein results in a yellow color, whereas increasing amounts of protein, 1+ to 4+, shift the color from green to blue. The dipstick method is rapid and easy to perform. Dipstick measurements of proteinuria are relatively insensitive (limit of detection of 10–30 mg/dl) and primarily detect albumin.

The second, less common procedure involves adding 5.0% sulfosalicylic acid to a urine sample to denature the urine proteins. Denatured urine proteins cause turbidity, and the amount of urine protein is proportional to the observed turbidity (1+ to 4+). The sulfosalicylic acid method is more sensitive (limit of detection 5–10 mg/dl) than the dipstick technique, and it measures all urine proteins.

### 6. How are these tests for proteinuria interpreted?

Semiquantitative tests for proteinuria are interpreted as follows:

| Dipstick Method | Sulfosalicylic Acid Method |
|---|---|
| Trace ≅ 10–30 mg/dl | Trace ≅ 20 mg/dl (slight turbidity) |
| 1+ ≅ 30 mg/dl | 1+ ≅ 50 mg/dl (print visible through specimen) |
| 2+ ≅ 100 mg/dl | 2+ ≅ 200 mg/dl (print invisible) |
| 3+ ≅ 500 mg/dl | 3+ ≅ 500 mg/dl (flocculation) |
| 4+ > 2000 mg/dl | 4+ > 1000 mg/dl (dense precipitate) |

Quantitative measurements of urinary protein excretion are usually obtained using timed urine collections (e.g., a 24-hour collection).

### 7. Can proteinuria be estimated without performing a 24-hour urine collection?

A newer method for estimating proteinuria involves extrapolation of 24-hour values from a single, randomly collected urine sample. This method is especially valuable for estimating proteinuria when accurate urine collections are inconvenient or impossible (e.g., incontinent patients or small children). Proteinuria is estimated by calculating the ratio of total urine protein to urine creatinine (in mg/mg) in a single urine sample. The ratio approximates 24-hour protein excretion in gm/day per 1.73 $m^2$ body surface area (see figure, top of next page).

The ratio of urine protein to creatinine in a single urine specimen closely approximates the actual 24-hour protein excretion. Patients with normal protein excretion have a ratio < 0.2. Patients with proteinuria can have ratios between 0.2 and 3.5 or higher. (Adapted from Ginsberg JSM, Chang BS, Maltarese RA, Garella S: Use of single voided urine samples to estimate quantitative proteinuria. N Engl J Med 309:1543–1546, 1983, with permission.)

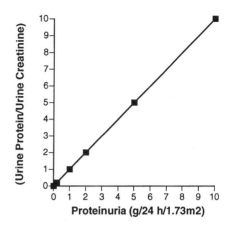

Using this approximation, normal individuals have a ratio less than 0.2, whereas patients with any type of renal disease can have values between 0.2 and 3.5. Patients with nephrotic syndrome (see Chapter 17, Nephrotic Syndrome) will have ratios greater than 3.5. Consider the following example: A patient with a single random urine specimen has a urine protein of 100 mg/dl (2+ dipstick) and a urine creatinine of 50 mg/dl. The patient's proteinuria would be approximately 2 gm/day per 1.73 $m^2$ (100/50 = 2).

## 8. How accurate and specific are clinical tests for proteinuria?

In most patients, the dipstick and sulfosalicylic acid techniques yield similar results that roughly correlate with exact measurements of urine proteins using more sophisticated techniques. Dipstick indicators are more sensitive to albumin whereas sulfosalicylic acid recognizes all proteins. Immunoglobulin light chains are detected by sulfosalicylic acid but not by dipstick. Thus, in patients with multiple myeloma, proteinuria can be missed unless the sulfosalicylic acid test is used. False-positive dipstick results can occur in highly alkaline urine and in highly concentrated or dilute urine. Occasionally, false-positive readings in the sulfosalicylic acid test can occur if large amounts of radiocontrast materials, tolbutamide, penicillin, or cephalosporin antibiotics are present.

## 9. What is microalbuminuria?

Normal individuals excrete extremely low levels of albumin, usually less than 20 mg/day and well below the limit of detection by dipstick (300–500 mg/day). In diabetics, even small increases in renal albumin excretion (> 30 mg/day) are highly predictive of subsequent overt diabetic nephropathy. By the time elevated albumin excretion is detected by dipstick, significant glomerular damage has already occurred. To improve early diagnosis of diabetic renal disease, sensitive tests (enzyme-linked immunosorbent assays) have been developed to specifically measure low levels of urine albumin (microalbuminuria). Detection of microalbuminuria can signal the need for therapeutic interventions such as the use of angiotensin-converting enzyme (ACE) inhibitors or strict glycemic control. Note that microalbuminuria can occur even when total protein excretion remains normal (< 150 mg/day). Many nephrologists and diabetologists recommend that patients with type 1 and type 2 diabetes be screened regularly for microalbuminuria.

Increasingly, evidence from clinical studies suggests that microalbuminuria is important to identify patients at increased risk for cardiovascular disease. Indeed, cardiovascular disease is the major cause of death in individuals with microalbuminuria. Although the mechanisms underlying this association are uncertain, accumulating evidence suggests that microalbuminuria reflects generalized endothelial dysfunction that may predispose to both cardiovascular disease and progression of kidney disease.

## BIBLIOGRAPHY

1. Anderson S: Proteinuria. In Greenberg A (ed): Primer on Kidney Diseases, 2nd ed. San Diego, Academic Press, 1998, pp 42–46.
2. Bernard DB, Salant DJ: Clinical approach to the patient with proteinuria and the nephrotic syndrome. In Jacobson HR, Striker GE, Klahr S (eds): The Principles and Practice of Nephrology, 2nd ed. St. Louis, Mosby, 1995, pp 110–121.
3. Brenner BM, Hostetter TH, Humes DH: Molecular basis of proteinuria of glomerular origin. N Engl J Med 298:826–833, 1978.
4. Ginsberg JSM, Chang BS, Maltarese RA, Garella S: Use of single voided urine samples to estimate quantitative proteinuria. N Engl J Med 309:1543–1546, 1983.
5. Keane WF, Eknoyan G: Proteinuria, albuminuria, risk, assessment, detection, and elimination (PARADE): A position paper of the National Kidney Foundation. Am J Kidney Dis 33:1004–1010, 1999.
6. Larson T: Evaluation of proteinuria. Mayo Clin Proc 69:1154–1159, 1994.

# 5. RENAL IMAGING TECHNIQUES

*Essam B. Elashi, M.D., and Mahboob Rahman, M.D., M.S.*

**1. List the most commonly used imaging modalities for the kidneys.**
- Urographic procedures (plain film, excretory urography, retrograde pyelography, and cystography)
- Ultrasonography
- Computed tomography (CT) scan and spiral CT scan
- Magnetic resonance imaging (MRI) and magnetic resonance angiography (MRA)
- Radionuclide imaging
- Renal angiography

**2. What factors determine the choice of imaging procedure?**
1. The information needed to guide further management of an individual patient
2. Accuracy and reliability of a given study
3. Invasiveness and the risk of the study
4. Cost of the study

In general, the simplest noninvasive studies are performed first as long as they provide the information needed. If the diagnostic yield is low, more invasive studies may be warranted.

**3. Name the different urographic procedures and the information they provide about the urinary tract.**

| Procedure | Information |
|---|---|
| Plain abdominal film (kidneys, ureters, bladder [KUB]) | Bone: Changes of renal osteodystrophy and either lytic or blastic metastases |
| | Soft tissue changes: Obliteration of psoas or renal outline may indicate inflammation or tumor |
| | Air: Air within or adjacent to the kidneys may be due to severe infection, especially in diabetics |
| | Calcifications: Renal calculus, calcified neoplasm, sloughed papilla, medullary or cortical nephrocalcinosis, ureteric or bladder calculus or tumor |
| Renal tomography | Renal calcification not observed on plain film especially when bowel gas or stool obscures the renal shadows |
| Excretory urography (intravenous pyelography) | Evaluation of the collecting structures, ureters, and bladder; provides the greatest spatial resolution of any imaging technique for evaluation of the urinary tract |
| Retrograde pyelography | Evaluation of possible filling defects not definite on excretory urography |
| | Selective cytological studies and cultures |
| | Additional delineation of an obstructed lesion, especially the length of the obstruction and the ureter distal to the obstruction |
| | Evaluation of ureteral trauma |

*Table continued on next page*

| Procedure | Information |
| --- | --- |
| Cystography | Evaluation of vesicoureteral reflux |
| | Anatomic delineation of the bladder in patients with reduced renal function |
| | Evaluation of urethra after pelvic trauma |
| | Evaluation of vesicovaginal or vesicoenteric fistulas |
| | Evaluation of urinary incontinence |
| Voiding cystourethrography | Evaluation of ureteral valve |
| | Evaluation of ureteral strictures |
| | Evaluation of incontinence |
| | Evaluation of vesicoureteral reflux |

4. **What are the relative contraindications to excretory urography?**
   1. Previous allergic reaction to contrast media
   2. Concern about contrast-induced nephrotoxicity in certain high-risk groups:
      - Preexisting renal insufficiency
      - Diabetic nephropathy
      - Multiple myeloma
      - Volume depletion
   3. Cardiac diseases (especially patients with arrhythmias and cardiac irritability)
   4. Pregnancy (radiation hazard)

5. **List the strengths and weaknesses of ultrasonography in the evaluation of renal disease.**

| Strengths | Weaknesses |
| --- | --- |
| Sensitive detector of intrarenal fluid collections, pelvicalyceal dilatation, and cysts | Does not show fine pelvicalyceal detail |
| | Does not show the normal ureter |
| Differentiates cortex and medulla | Shows the retroperitoneum poorly |
| Differentiates cystic and solid masses | Can miss small renal calculi and most ureteric calculi |
| Shows the whole renal contour and perinephric space | Gives no functional information |
| Demonstrates renal blood flow by Doppler technique | Operator dependent |
| Provides good renal imaging irrespective of renal function | |
| Portable—can be used at bedside in the intensive care unit | |
| Uses no irradiation or contrast medium | |

6. **What are the clinical circumstances in which ultrasound may be of value?**
   Ultrasonography is a good first-line diagnostic method for:
   - Estimating kidney size
   - Assessing the echogenicity of the kidney. Increased echogenicity may indicate chronic renal disease, but it can also be seen in other pathologic states.
   - Diagnosing collecting system dilatation, including possible obstruction in renal failure, pelvic neoplasm, renal transplants, and acute urinary tract infection with suspected pyonephrosis
   - Assessing renal blood flow by Doppler technique

- Diagnosing adult polycystic kidney disease and screening involved families
- Guiding interventional procedures such as renal biopsy and cyst aspiration
- Detecting perinephric fluid collections
- Evaluating a renal allograft to assess any suspected fluid collection in the pelvis such as lymphocele, hematoma, or urinoma. Obstruction also can be detected by ultrasound and differentiated from rejection and acute tubular necrosis. Moreover, Doppler ultrasound can be used in evaluating the blood flow to the transplanted kidney without the use of nephrotoxic contrast media.

### 7. When is a CT scan superior to ultrasound for evaluation of renal disease?
- For evaluation of a solid mass especially if a malignant neoplasm is suspected. CT can define the extent of the neoplasm and lymph node involvement and help in staging.
- For evaluation of perirenal and pararenal spaces and Gerota's fascia
- CT is the imaging method of choice in evaluation of suspected renal trauma. Nonexcretion, contusion, fracture, shattered kidney, and perirenal fluid collection are readily detected on CT. Additional information about other organ injuries can be obtained at the same time.
- CT and MRI are the most efficacious imaging modalities for visualizing retroperitoneal structures including the adrenal glands. CT is particularly helpful in excluding the presence of disease when unusual positions of the kidney or changes in the renal axes have suggested a retroperitoneal mass.

### 8. What is the role of MRI in evaluating renal disease?
Although most renal diseases can be adequately imaged with other modalities, MRI may be especially helpful in the evaluation of extension of renal cell carcinoma into the renal veins or inferior vena cava when equivocally demonstrated by CT or ultrasound. MRI may play a role in staging of transitional cell carcinoma involving the pelvic floor and evaluation of carcinoma of the prostate. MRI, like CT, is useful in evaluation of the retroperitoneum.

### 9. What are the indications for radionuclide renal imaging?
The most common uses of nuclear medicine studies are:
- Measurement of renal function including glomerular filtration rate and effective renal plasma flow even in cases of renal impairment
- Measurement of "split" renal function to determine whether nephrectomy is warranted or safe
- Diagnosis of renovascular hypertension by differential blood flow studies using 99m technetium diethylenetetraamionpentaacetic acid (99m Tc DTPA) or 99m technetium mercaptoacetyltriglycerine (99m Tc MAG3) pre- and postadministration of an angiotensin-converting enzyme (ACE) inhibitor such as captopril in appropriately screened hypertensive patients with intact renal function. The sensitivity and specificity approach 90%.
- Evaluation of renal transplants: Radionuclide imaging can detect impaired blood flow at renal arterial anastomotic site, urinary tract obstruction, and extravasation of the urine.
- Differentiation of obstructive from nonobstructive hydronephrosis

### 10. How can renal perfusion and excretion be evaluated by radionuclide scan?
After intravenous administration of 99m Tc DTPA, serial nuclear images are displayed pictorially, and corresponding radioactive counts from the kidneys are plotted over time in a graphic form. Early images and counts primarily reflect renal perfusion whereas later images and counts reflect renal excretion.

**11. How can a renal scan differentiate between obstructive and nonobstructive distention of the collecting system?**

In both obstructive and nonobstructive distention, the excretory phase of the renogram shows initially low but gradually increasing activity over time. Differentiation is possible based on the response to furosemide administration (Lasix renogram). In nonobstructive disease, the intravenous administration of furosemide results in prompt decrease of nuclear activity reflecting the diuresis, whereas, in obstruction, washout of the activity is limited.

**12. What is an ACE inhibitor–stimulated radionuclide renal scan?**

ACE inhibitor renal scanning is an imaging technique for diagnosis of renovascular hypertension. In the setting of renovascular hypertension, both glomerular filtration rate and renal plasma flow depend on angiotensin II–mediated constriction of the glomerular efferent arteriole. Treatment with ACE inhibitor antagonizes this vasoconstriction and decreases renal uptake and excretion of radioactive tracer. A renogram is considered abnormal if there is evidence of:

- Marked delay in the tracer uptake
- Decrease in the tracer count compared to the normal kidney
- Delay in the excretion of the tracer

Estimates of the sensitivity and specificity of ACE inhibitor–stimulated renography vary widely, but on average probably exceed 80%.

**13. What other modalities can be used for evaluation of renovascular hypertension?**

**Duplex ultrasound:** The use of color-flow Doppler in the diagnosis of renovascular hypertension combines anatomic information from ultrasound with hemodynamic information from Doppler. This technique is limited by the fact that the proximal main renal artery is not visualized in 25% of cases. Duplex ultrasound is highly operator-dependent and requires over 1 hour to perform correctly. In experienced hands, the sensitivity and specificity of the duplex ultrasonography are greater than 90%.

**MRA:** This is a noninvasive modality that can provide information about both anatomy and blood flow. Studies suggest that MRA can detect renal artery stenosis with 70–90% sensitivity and 78–94% specificity.

**14. List the indications for renal angiography.**

1. Evaluation of renovascular hypertension
2. Interventional angiography:
   - Use of special catheters and embolization technique to control hemorrhage or to occlude arteriovenous fistulas
   - Balloon angioplasty for management of renovascular hypertension and renal artery stenosis due to atherosclerosis
3. Preoperative evaluation of the donor kidney
4. Evaluation of the renal graft for renal artery occlusion or stenosis
5. Establishing the diagnosis of renal vein thrombosis
6. Complex renal masses or complications of polycystic disease or trauma may require angiography.

**15. What is a percutaneous nephrostomy?**

Percutaneous nephrostomy is the nonoperative placement of a catheter into the renal pelvis under imaging control for drainage of an obstructed kidney. It has largely replaced surgical nephrostomy and can be used for short- and long-term drainage.

## 16. What is antegrade pyelography?

Antegrade pyelography is a percutaneous injection of an iodinated contrast medium into the renal pelvis under ultrasound guidance of fluoroscopy. It is indicated when evaluation of the anatomy of the upper urinary tract is necessary but cannot be done with excretory urography or retrograde pyelography.

## 17. What imaging studies should be used to evaluate a renal mass?

The choice of imaging study for evaluation of a renal mass depends on the clinical situation. Although cystic or solid parenchymal masses may first be detected with excretory urography, they require ultrasound or CT for further differentiation, staging, and possible biopsy. Further testing depends on the findings:

- For a probable cystic mass, confirm it by ultrasound.
- For a probable solid mass, do a CT or MRI according to the clinical setting.
- To determine mass versus normal, evaluate by radionuclide renal scan.

## 18. What are the ultrasonographic features of a simple renal cyst?

Simple renal cysts occur in up to 30% of normal adults and can easily be differentiated from solid masses or tumor. Simple renal cysts:

- Are round and sharply demarcated with smooth borders
- Have no echoes within the mass

## 19. What imaging studies are needed for evaluating renal failure?

Generally, imaging is needed to define the size and shape of the kidneys and to exclude obstruction as the cause of renal failure. This can be done by:

1. Ultrasound:
   - Evaluates renal size. Generally, small atrophic kidneys are seen in chronic disease.
   - Calculi are shown as echogenic foci with shadowing.
2. CT: Provides additional information about extrinsic causes of ureteral obstruction.
3. Retrograde pyelography:
   - Demonstrates the presence of papillary necrosis and calyceal abnormalities
   - May help to determine the site and cause of obstruction. Bilateral peritoneal narrowing indicates retroperitoneal fibrosis.

## 20. Describe the radiologic evaluation of patients with suspected urinary tract obstruction.

The radiographic evaluation of suspected urinary tract obstruction should be guided by the results of the history, physical examination, and laboratory data. When an approach is chosen for a patient with renal insufficiency, the risk associated with the use of radiocontrast agents needs to be considered. The following are possible approaches:

**Ultrasonography** is the preferred screening modality for obstruction because of its high sensitivity for hydronephrosis (sensitivity and specificity about 90%), safety, low cost, and lack of radiation exposure. Moreover, it can be used in patients with elevated serum creatinine. Ultrasonography can determine renal size and reveal dilatation of calyces, the renal pelvis, and occasionally the proximal ureter. In addition, it may show the cortical thickness that may indicate longstanding obstruction.

**Abdominal film** is used for possible stones or masses.

**Excretory urography** can be used to identify the site of obstruction and detect associated conditions such as papillary necrosis; however, it is does require the administration of a contrast. It is performed when ultrasound or CT is unable to provide the necessary information, especially when acute calcular obstruction is suspected, because there will be no collecting system dilatation. In obstructive kidneys, the renal density (nephrogram) increases

with time after contrast injection. Visualization of the collecting system may be delayed for hours or may not be seen in cases of chronic obstruction. Signs of obstruction are:
- Abrupt termination of the contrast-filled pelvis or ureter
- Dilatation of the collecting system proximally
- Negative pyelogram effect sign, which represents the dilated collecting system seen as branching lucency against the background of density of the nephrogram
- Full-column ureter sign, which is the appearance of the ureter as a full column of contrast rather than the normally interrupted one caused by peristalsis of the normal ureter

**Retrograde pyelogram** may allow better delineation of the exact point of obstruction and the collecting system distal to the obstruction and may be used to relieve the obstruction

**CT** is most helpful in obstruction related to a mass and in evaluation of hydronephrosis if simpler methods of evaluation are unsuccessful.

**Antegrade studies** such as percutaneous antegrade pyelography may be used to delineate the point of obstruction and provide drainage from above. Pressure measurement can be done and may be helpful in separating nonobstructive from obstructive hydronephrosis.

**Radionuclide studies** are used primarily in the evaluation of the effect of chronic outflow disorders on renal function.

**21. What imaging studies are helpful in evaluation of hematuria?**

The choice of an imaging study depends on the age of the patient and the suspected cause of hematuria. Infection and calculi are common in young patients, whereas tumors are more common in older patients. The following is usually suggested:

1. **Excretory urography:** This is the primary study in most cases. It may demonstrate:
   - Parenchymal lesions (neoplasm, arteriovenous malformation, non-neoplastic mass, or papillary necrosis)
   - Collecting system tumors, stones, or medullary sponge kidney

2. **Cystoscopy:** This is the procedure of choice for evaluation of suspected mass in the bladder.

3. **CT:** With persistent hematuria and if the above studies are negative, it is reasonable to perform CT. CT is also used to evaluate solid masses and their extent before surgery.

4. **Renal biopsy:** This is used if clinical evidence suggests acute glomerulonephritis or other glomerular problems (proteinuria or red cell casts)

5. **Selective renal arteriography:** This is used for suspected arteriovenous malformation and small renal carcinomas.

BIBLIOGRAPHY

1. Blaufox MD (ed): Radionuclides in Nephro-urology, 2nd ed. Basel, Karger, 1990.
2. Greenberg A (ed): Primer on Kidney Diseases, 2nd ed. San Diego, Academic Press, 1998.
3. Pollack HM (ed): Clinical Urology. Philadelphia, W.B. Saunders, 1990.
4. Resnick MI, Rifkin MD: Ultrasonography for the Urinary Tract, 3rd ed. Baltimore, Williams & Wilkins, 1991.

# 6. RENAL BIOPSY

*Jeffrey R. Schelling, M.D., and Stephen Tamarkin, M.D.*

**1. What are some of the indications for renal biopsy?**
- Persistent hematuria (especially if accompanied by red blood cell casts)
- Persistent proteinuria (especially if greater than 3 gm/24 hr)
- Unexplained acute renal failure
- Renal transplant allograft dysfunction

**2. What are the benefits of a renal biopsy?**
A renal biopsy may:
- Help to establish the diagnosis of disease that is either limited to the kidney or part of a systemic disease complex
- Help to provide a prognosis regarding possible renal disease progression and subsequent need for renal replacement therapy
- Help to guide therapeutic options
- Help to limit the pursuit of additional diagnostic studies
- Be used as an investigational tool to better understand the pathophysiology of renal disease. Recent studies have suggested that it is possible to examine the gene expression profile from tissue samples as small as a renal biopsy specimen. Because there are few quantitative, histologic predictors of disease progression, these molecular techniques have the capacity to define signature mRNA patterns that could better guide therapy, either by identifying patients who are likely to respond or be resistant to existing therapies or by identifying new therapeutic targets.

**3. What are the risks of renal biopsy?**
Small perinephric hematomas are an inevitable complication of renal biopsies. Clinically significant bleeding requiring transfusion or intervention (embolization or surgery) for persistent gross hematuria is uncommon. Surgical intervention for intractable bleeding is required in approximately 0.3% of renal biopsies. The risk of introducing infection is very small, particularly when sterile technique is carefully practiced. Arteriovenous fistulas and aneurysms have been described as complications of renal biopsies, although both are rarely clinically significant. The fact that there are few reports of mortality from renal biopsies indicates that death is an extremely rare complication. Most sources cite a procedure-related mortality ranging from 1 in 800 to 1 in > 10,000.

**4. What are the contraindications to renal biopsy?**
Coagulation disorders and thrombocytopenia predispose to bleeding complications. Uremic platelet dysfunction is a relative contraindication to renal biopsy, but this can usually be controlled with dialysis or administration of desmopressin (DDAVP), a vasopressin analogue that stimulates platelet coagulation. Uncontrolled hypertension is a relative risk, and it is advisable to maintain blood pressure less than 140/90. Preexisting pyelonephritis may increase the risk of subsequent abscess development. Anatomic abnormalities, particularly the presence of a solitary kidney, are usually considered a contraindication to biopsy. This rationale is based on concerns that (1) uncontrolled bleeding from a solitary kidney may lead to nephrectomy and an anephric state and (2) urinary tract obstruction from a blood clot may result in renal failure. However, there are case series demonstrating the

safety of performing biopsy in patients with a solitary kidney. It remains unclear whether a laparoscopic or surgical wedge resection ("open biopsy") is associated with a lower morbidity in the setting of a solitary kidney. Patients with impaired mental status may not be candidates for renal biopsy if they are unable to follow the instructions required during the procedure, although heavy sedation or general anesthesia administered by an anesthesiologist may allow performance of a biopsy (see question 6).

### 5. What laboratory studies should be performed prior to a renal biopsy?

It is customary to obtain a baseline hematocrit, platelet count, prothrombin time (PT; INR), and partial thromboplastin time (PTT). Some nephrologists will request additional tests to assess the hemostasis adequacy in azotemic patients (e.g., bleeding time measurement), but there are no data indicating that bleeding time assays alter the morbidity and mortality associated with a renal biopsy.

### 6. How is a renal biopsy performed?

In general, intravenous conscious sedation or oral anxiolytic agents can be given, depending on physician and patient preferences. Renal biopsies are most commonly performed using ultrasound (US) or computed tomography (CT) as guidance at the discretion of the operator (see question 7). Laparoscopic or open surgical techniques are also possible. Following initial imaging, an appropriate biopsy site and approach are chosen (see below). Local anesthesia is applied to the skin and to deeper tissues along the expected biopsy needle path. The biopsy needle or gun is gradually directed into the lower pole cortex during suspended respiration and core biopsy samples are obtained. Once the needle tip is within the kidney, the needle will sway in a superior-inferior direction upon normal respiration.

Most renal biopsies are currently obtained using a *biopsy gun,* which obtains cylindrically shaped "core" samples using a rapid, spring-loaded cutting mechanism. Different cartridge gauge sizes and needle lengths are available from multiple manufacturers, with some variation in cartridge shape, deployment mechanisms, and other features. Samples of 14–18G typically are obtained, with two or more samples obtained as needed. The sample adequacy (acceptable number of glomeruli) can be assessed rapidly using a dissecting microscope, and some centers confirm adequacy prior to removing the patient from the biopsy suite. The sample should be sent immediately to the pathology laboratory on a saline-soaked, rather than formalin, pad.

If fresh, pulsatile blood returns through the guiding needle, or if there is evidence of significant immediate perinephric hematoma (e.g., large hematoma on imaging, accompanied by tachycardia or decreased blood pressure), consider immediate angiographic evaluation and possibly embolization.

### 7. What radiology procedures are used to aid in the renal biopsy?

**Ultrasound:** US-guided biopsies can be performed using a needle-guidance device or freehand technique. Needle-guidance devices have needle grooves fixed to the transducer, with a corresponding demonstration on the US monitor of the expected needle trajectory. The needle should be removed from the guiding slot quickly once the needle tip enters the kidney, before the patient resumes breathing. US-guided biopsies allow "real-time" visualization and can be performed portably if necessary.

**CT:** Nonenhanced images typically are obtained through the kidneys to assess renal anatomy, to exclude unexpected focal lesions, and for biopsy localization. The lower pole cortex of one of the kidneys is selected as the target based on favorable anatomy, such as relatively thick lower pole cortex and absence of closely related colon or other vital structures. A posterolateral approach typically is used. The position of the kidneys changes significantly with respiration, and the patient must be coached regarding the importance of consistent, reproducible inspirations for all scanning and needle manipulations.

CT guidance is advisable in larger or frankly obese patients, and some physicians prefer CT to US guidance for all biopsies.

### 8. What constitutes an adequate biopsy?

Because the most commonly suspected clinical diagnosis is usually a form of glomerular disease, a biopsy core from renal cortex containing a minimum of 6–8 glomeruli is preferable. Two such samples are usually necessary to provide enough tissue for light, immunofluorescence, and electron microscopy studies. Sample adequacy can be assessed in the biopsy suite by observation under a dissecting microscope, as described in question 6. It is advisable to consult with the renal pathologist prior to the biopsy to determine appropriate tissue fixation conditions and facilitate prompt sample processing.

### 9. How should the patient be monitored following a renal biopsy?

After a native kidney biopsy, the patient should be instructed to lie on his or her back for approximately 6 hours after the biopsy. Following a transplant biopsy, it is also advisable to maintain constant pressure over the biopsy site, for example, with weighted sandbags. Pulse and blood pressure should be checked every 15 minutes for the first 2 hours as an index of hemodynamically significant bleeding. If stable, vital signs can be checked less frequently thereafter. All urine specimens should be saved and observed for hematuria. Virtually all postbiopsy specimens will reveal microscopic hematuria, and gross hematuria occurs after approximately 10% of renal biopsies. Therefore, one should not be alarmed at the presence of initial gross hematuria, provided that subsequent specimens reveal resolution of the hematuria. A hematocrit should be measured 4–6 hours after the biopsy to assess change from the baseline value. If there is no evidence of complications at this point, further observation within the hospital generally is not necessary. Therefore, if procedures are performed early in the day, renal biopsies can be done safely on an outpatient basis. Particularly with active children, it is advisable to avoid contact sports for 2–4 weeks postbiopsy, to avoid the possibility of rupturing a renal hematoma.

### 10. Is it necessary to obtain diagnostic serologic studies prior to a renal biopsy?

The spectrum of serologic studies that may aid in a clinical diagnosis include complement levels (C3, C4, CH50), antinuclear antibodies (ANA), antineutrophil cytoplasmic antibodies (ANCA), antiglomerular basement membrane antibodies (anti-GBM), cryoglobulins, hepatitis B surface antigen, hepatitis C antibodies, and VDRL (Venereal Disease Research Laboratory) and anti-HIV antibodies. Many nephrologists will order some of these studies prior to a renal biopsy. However, a cogent argument can be made that it would be more cost-effective to obtain serologic studies after obtaining the biopsy, inasmuch as the biopsy results may dictate which tests are actually necessary.

### 11. Is it necessary for a patient with hematuria or proteinuria to undergo a renal biopsy?

The answer is variable and depends on the training of the nephrologist. The primary arguments for withholding or delaying a renal biopsy are (1) finite incidence of risks (see questions 2 and 3) and (2) the fact that there is no definitive therapy for many types of glomerular disease. Therefore, one approach, which has been advocated in patients with idiopathic proteinuria, is to biopsy only those patients who do not respond to empiric corticosteroid or antiplatelet therapy. However, because most regimens that have been shown to be effective for the treatment of glomerular disease contain potentially toxic immunosuppressive or cytotoxic drugs, many nephrologists would recommend a biopsy prior to institution of treatment.

BIBLIOGRAPHY

1. Falk RJ, Jennette JC: Renal biopsy and treatment of glomerular disease. In Humes HD (ed): Kelley's Textbook of Internal Medicine, 4th ed. Philadelphia, Lippincott Williams & Wilkins, 2000, pp 1273–1290.
2. Fraser IR, Fairley KF: Renal biopsy as an outpatient procedure. Am J Kidney Dis 25:876–878, 1995.
3. Kasiske BL, Keane WF: Laboratory assessment of renal disease: Clearance, urinalysis and renal biopsy. In Brenner BM (ed): The Kidney, 6th ed. Philadelphia, W.B. Saunders, 2000, pp 1153–1159.
4. Kretzler M, Cohen CD, Doran P, et al: Repuncturing the renal biopsy: Strategies for molecular diagnosis in nephrology. J Am Soc Nephrol 7:1961–1972, 2002.
5. Madaio MP: Clinical conference: Renal biopsy. Kidney Int 38:529–543, 1990.
6. Menon SK, Kirchner KA: The role of percutaneous renal biopsy in clinical nephrology. Curr Opin Nephrol Hypertens 2:968–973, 1993.
7. Parrish AE: Complications of percutaneous renal biopsy: A review of 37 years' experience. Clin Nephrol 38:135–141, 1992.
8. Tisher CC, Croker P: Indications for and interpretations of the renal biopsy: Evaluation by light, electron, and immunofluorescence microscopy. In Schrier RW, Gottschalk CW (eds): Diseases of the Kidney, 6th ed. Boston, Little, Brown, 1997, pp 435–461.

# 7. INDICATIONS FOR DIALYSIS

*Edmond Ricanati,* M.D.

### 1. What is dialysis?

Dialysis is a procedure that removes excess fluid and the toxic end products of metabolism. The major forms of dialysis are hemodialysis, continuous renal replacement therapy (CRRT), and peritoneal dialysis (see Chapter 46, Technical Aspects of Hemodialysis, Chapter 49, Continuous Renal Replacement Therapy, and Chapter 50, Technical Aspects of Peritoneal Dialysis). Dialysis is usually prescribed to patients with significant impairment of renal function resulting from acute or chronic renal failure. It is also used occasionally to remove ingested drugs and other toxins in patients who may have normal renal function.

### 2. What are the common indications for initiating dialysis in patients with acute renal failure?

- Uremic symptoms (e.g., anorexia, nausea, vomiting, encephalopathy)
- Electrolyte or acid-base abnormalities refractory to medical therapy, especially:
  Hyperkalemia
  Metabolic acidosis
  Hyponatremia
- Fluid overload or pulmonary edema refractory to diuretic therapy
- Uremic pericarditis

### 3. Is there a role for early, prophylactic dialysis in patients with acute renal failure?

There is no evidence that early dialysis improves morbidity or mortality in patients with acute renal failure. Indeed, early dialysis might even delay recovery of renal function. Initiation of dialysis in the setting of acute renal failure is sometimes associated with an abrupt decline in urine output. This phenomenon could be related to repeated episodes of dialysis-induced hypotension or to activation of vasoactive compounds as a consequence of blood-dialysis membrane interactions. In some centers, dialysis is instituted only if the blood urea nitrogen (BUN) exceeds 140 mg/dl and is rising rapidly.

### 4. What are the common indications for initiating dialysis in patients with chronic renal failure?

In the United States, there are few obstacles to providing dialysis for the treatment of end-stage renal disease (ESRD). The main barriers to hemodialysis are hemodynamic instability; an inability to establish vascular access; end-stage cardiac, hepatic, or respiratory failure; and metastatic tumors. Patients are disqualified from peritoneal dialysis if a peritoneal access is not possible or if they are unable to participate in the treatment procedure and plan. Absolute indications are:

- Persistent nausea, vomiting, and weight loss. Patients with these symptoms are at increased risk for malnutrition and uremic complications. This is of concern especially when there is a progressive decrease in serum albumin concentration.
- Uremic pericarditis
- Fluid overload and pulmonary edema refractory to diuretic therapy
- Uremic neuropathy, especially when associated with uremic encephalopathy (restlessness, insomnia, anxiety, difficulty with memory, confusion, asterixis)

- Uncontrolled hypertension, especially when associated with fluid overload
- Significant bleeding attributed to uremia
- Glomerular filtration rate (GFR) of less than 10 ml/min (usually estimated either by cre-
atinine clearance or, more accurately, by the mean of the creatinine and urea clearances)

It is not appropriate to wait until the patient becomes severely ill before initiating dialysis. However, neither is it advisable to start dialysis in a patient who is asymptomatic and
who has no uremic complications, such as hyperkalemia, metabolic acidosis, fluid overload,
or malnutrition. There are wide variations in GFR at the initiation of dialysis in the U.S.
ESRD population. Data from the U.S. Renal Data System indicate that the mean GFR at the
start of dialysis was 7.1 ml/min/1.73 m$^2$ with a range from 1 to 42 ml/min/1.73 m$^2$. The mean
serum creatinine at initiation of dialysis was 8.5 mg/dl.

### 5. Is there a role for early, prophylactic dialysis in patients with chronic renal failure?

Some studies suggest that long-term patient survival is enhanced when dialysis is initiated "early," that is, before patients have developed significant symptoms of uremia. Other
studies indicate better long-term outcomes in patients who are referred to a nephrologist
early in the course of their renal disease.

### 6. How important is the assessment of the nutritional state of the patient as an indi-
cator for early initiation of chronic maintenance dialysis?

According to the Dialysis Outcomes Quality Initiative (DOQI) guidelines, which were
based on an extensive and critical review of the literature, dialysis should be initiated when
evidence of malnutrition develops in a patient with advanced chronic renal failure. Patients
with chronic progressive renal failure develop anorexia, and their protein intake gradually
diminishes with progressive drops in creatinine clearance despite efforts to increase nutrition.
The long-term survival and the potential for rehabilitation of patients on dialysis are significantly decreased when patients develop malnutrition prior to initiating chronic dialysis.

### 7. What markers are commonly used in clinical practice for the detection of malnu-
trition in advanced chronic renal failure?

1. **Anorexia, nausea, vomiting, weight loss**
2. **Low plasma albumin and prealbumin concentrations**. The plasma albumin concentration correlates quite well with body protein stores. Plasma prealbumin has a shorter
half-life than albumin and changes rapidly when there are changes in nutritional status. A
value below 13 mg/dl is indicative of malnutrition.
3. **Diminished dietary protein intake**. A protein intake of less than 0.8 gm/kg/day or
nPNA (protein equivalent of nitrogen appearance normalized using ideal body weight) less
than 0.8 gm/kg/day is strongly suggestive of malnutrition.
4. **Subjective global assessment.**
5. **Abnormal anthropometric measurements**. This is a rapid and reproducible method
for evaluating body fat and muscle mass. Values obtained below reference standards for
healthy adults are suggestive of malnutrition.
6. **Abnormally low plasma creatinine concentration**. The blood level of plasma creatinine reflects muscle mass. Patients with a plasma creatinine concentration of less than 10
mg/dl at the start of dialysis are considered to be malnourished. This is substantiated by data
from the United States Renal Data Systems (USRDS) that revealed that later mortality rate
is higher in patients with a plasma creatinine concentration below 10 mg/dl at the time of
initiation of dialysis.
7. Other markers of malnutrition are **decreased plasma concentrations of cholesterol,
transferrin**, and **somatomedin C.**

Malnutrition should be considered a strong indication for starting dialysis in chronic renal failure.

## BIBLIOGRAPHY

1. CANUSA Peritoneal Dialysis Study Group: Adequacy of dialysis and nutrition in continuous peritoneal dialysis: Association with clinical outcomes. J Am Soc Nephrol 7:198–207, 1995.
2. Chertow GM, Miller SB: Intensity of dialysis in established renal failure. Semin Nephrol 9:476–481, 1996.
3. Conger JD: Does hemodialysis delay the recovery from acute renal failure? Semin Dial 3:146–154, 1990.
4. Hamel MB, Phillip RS, Davis RB, et al: Outcomes and cost-effectiveness of initiating dialysis and continuing aggressive care in seriously ill hospitalized adults. Ann Intern Med 127:195–202, 1997.
5. Lazarus JM, Hakim RM: Timing the initiation of dialysis. J Am Soc Nephrol 6:1319–1326, 1996.
6. Obredor GT, Arora P, Kaersz AT, et al: Level of renal function at the initiation of dialysis in the U.S. end-stage renal disease population. Kidney Int 56:2227–2235, 1999.
7. US Renal Data System: Patient mortality and survival. In USRDS 1996 Annual Report. Bethesda, MD, National Institutes of Health, National Institutes of Diabetes and Digestive and Kidney Diseases, 1996, pp 68–84.

# 8. DRUG DOSING IN PATIENTS WITH RENAL DISEASE

*Marigel Constantiner, R.Ph., M.Sc., BCPS*

**1. How can drug pharmacokinetics be altered in patients with renal failure?**
Alterations of drug pharmacokinetics in patients with renal failure are based on changes in absorption, distribution, metabolism, or elimination.

|  |  |  |  | Metabolites |
|---|---|---|---|---|
| Drug at | *Absorption* | Drug | *Metabolism* ↗ | |
| Absorption | →→→→ | in the body | | |
| Site | | | *Excretion* ↘ | Excreted Drug |

1. **Absorption and bioavailability.** The effect of renal failure on bioavailability has been evaluated for only a few drugs. *Decreased* drug absorption may be due to:
- Changes in gastric pH induced by commonly used drugs (e.g., calcium carbonate, $H_2$ receptor antagonists, proton pump inhibitors)
- Altered gastrointestinal (GI) emptying time (e.g., diabetic gastroparesis)
- Edema of the GI tract
- Drug interactions (e.g., phosphate binders and iron supplements when given together decrease the absorption of iron)

*Increased* drug bioavailability may result from reduction in the "first-pass" metabolism which is the removal of drug during absorption by metabolism in the gut wall, portal circulation, or liver before appearance in the systemic circulation.

2. **Distribution.** Volume of distribution is not an actual volume but rather represents the size of a compartment for the total amount of the drug in the body if it were present throughout the body in the same concentration found in the plasma. When a drug has a large volume of distribution, it is distributed widely throughout the tissues and is present in relatively small amounts in the blood. High tissue binding, high lipid solubility, and low plasma protein binding cause a large volume of distribution. The proportion of free drug that would be pharmacologically active will increase when the protein binding is decreased. Changes in drug distribution in patients with renal impairment may arise from either fluid retention that may change the volume of distribution of water-soluble drugs (e.g., aminoglycosides) or changes in the extent of protein binding in tissue and plasma.

In patients with renal disease, the presence of malnutrition and proteinuria reduces the amount of protein available for protein binding. Uremia also may have an effect on protein binding of some drugs. The extent of protein binding of acidic drugs is decreased in renal failure patients. This may be due to qualitative changes in binding sites, accumulation of other organic acids that may compete for the same binding sites, or decreased concentrations of albumin caused by malnutrition or proteinuria. The amount of free drug will increase when there is a decrease of the drug from its binding sites, resulting in increased drug availability and possibly toxic effects.

If an assay is available, it is important to monitor for free or unbound drug levels in patients with renal insufficiency or heavy proteinuria (e.g., free phenytoin levels). It is

28

important to understand the clinical implications of altered protein binding for highly protein-bound drugs in patients with renal insufficiency.

3. **Metabolism.** Although renal elimination may be minimal for a drug, dosing may still be difficult in patients with renal impairment. Renal disease reduces the activity of a number of enzymes in the P450 system in the liver and kidneys, thereby reducing drug metabolism. Renal failure may increase, decrease, or have no effect on nonrenal clearance. The mechanism of action for reduced hepatic clearance in renal disease is unclear but may be related to an inhibitory factor present in uremic blood.

In addition, some drugs are metabolized to active metabolites, which are excreted by the kidney (e.g., morphine, procainamide, propoxyphene, and meperidine). Accumulation of the active metabolites may cause serious adverse events in patients with chronic renal disease.

4. **Elimination.** Drug elimination in chronic renal disease depends on the fraction of drug normally eliminated unchanged in the urine and the degree of renal impairment. Overall renal clearance is determined by the contribution of glomerular filtration plus tubular secretion minus tubular reabsorption. The renal disease process (glomerular versus tubular disease) may affect how much of a specific drug may be eliminated. For example, tubular secretion of drugs (e.g., ampicillin, cephalexin) may be affected when tubulointerstitial disease is present.

### 2. What characteristics determine whether a drug is removed by dialysis?

Dialysis clearance must increase total clearance by at least 30% to be considered clinically significant and to require a replacement dose after hemodialysis. The following physicochemical characteristics determine the extent that a drug may be affected by dialysis.

**Molecular size.** As a general rule, smaller molecular weight substances pass through the membrane much easier compared to larger size molecules. In general, free drug molecules with a molecular weight of less than 500 D are removed efficiently by hemodialysis.

**Protein binding.** When decreased, protein binding may increase free drug available for removal during dialysis. When overdoses occur, the amount of ingested drug may exceed protein-binding capacity, allowing removal of the drug by hemodialysis even though dialysis has a minimal effect on drug removal when it is used at normal doses.

**Volume of distribution.** Drugs with large volumes of distribution are not removed effectively by dialysis. Lipid-soluble drugs usually have large volumes of distribution, making significant removal from the plasma volume by dialysis less likely.

**Water solubility.** Drugs with high water solubility will be dialyzed to a greater extent than those with high lipid solubility.

**Dialysis membrane.** The pore size, surface area, and geometry are the primary factors in determining whether a dialysis membrane will clear a specific drug. For example, standard dialysis membranes do not effectively remove the antibiotic vancomycin (molecular weight, 3300 D). In contrast, high-flux membranes will remove larger molecular weight molecules compared with conventional membranes. Therefore, vancomycin needs to be dosed after each hemodialysis session when high-flux membranes are used but not when patients are dialyzed with standard membranes. Published literature on drug removal by dialysis needs to reviewed carefully because newer membranes may have different clearance characteristics.

**Blood and dialysate flow rates.** Increased flow rates during hemodialysis will increase drug clearance. Patients who cannot tolerate standard blood flow rates will require less replacement dosing of a drug after hemodialysis.

### 3. How is renal function assessed for drug dosing determination?

The most common glomerular filtration rate assessment continues to involve the measurement of creatinine. Before interpreting serum creatinine values, it is important to assess potential analytic interferences based on the assay used or concurrent drug therapy. Some commonly used drugs may artifactually increase or decrease the measured serum creatinine concentration without directly influencing glomerular filtration rate. Drugs that inhibit the tubular secretion of creatinine and increase serum creatinine include trimethoprim, cimetidine, and probenecid.

## 4. What commonly prescribed drugs require dose adjustment in hemodialysis patients?

Many drugs require dosing adjustments in patients who have creatinine clearance < 50 ml/min. Notable examples include aminoglycosides, vancomycin, 5-flucytosine, procainamide, and digoxin. Dosing adjustments can be modified either by decreasing the dose and keeping the same interval or by keeping the same dose but extending the interval. In many instances, a combination of both approaches makes the dosing adjustment more practical for the patient. It is important to remember that a loading dose may be indicated to generate a steady-state level within a short period if the drug's half-life is increased in the presence of renal failure. The loading dose required depends on the pharmacokinetic characteristics of each drug but in general does not differ from normal. Drug concentrations should be measured whenever possible.

## 5. Which antimicrobials should be avoided on days that hemodialysis is delivered?

The administration of various antimicrobials can be made easier compared to normal patients because of the altered pharmacokinetics in patients with renal failure. Although penicillin and its derivatives (e.g., nafcillin) are not therapeutic options for outpatient administration on hemodialysis days because of short half-lives, even in presence of renal failure, some of the cephalosporins can be given every 48–72 hours. These cephalosporins include cefazolin, ceftazidime, and ceftizoxime, all of which have longer half-lives. Cefuroxime, ceftriaxone and cefotetan should not be dosed on dialysis days only.

## 6. How should aminoglycosides be adjusted for hemodialysis?

Aminoglycosides distribute into the extracellular fluid compartment. The volume of distribution is increased as the patient reaches end-stage renal disease (ESRD) because of an increased percentage of total body weight. The average volume of distribution of aminoglycosides in ESRD patients is between 0.30 and 0.35 L/kg. In addition, the drug distribution after an intravenous dose is prolonged (approximately 2 hours) compared to normal patients (0.5–1 hr). If a peak concentration measurement is checked, the level should be drawn after the drug distribution phase is completed. It is incorrect to draw a peak level half an hour after the intravenous dose in patients with ESRD. An aminoglycoside rebound phenomenon also occurs after hemodialysis. Posthemodialysis levels should be assessed after the redistribution is completed. Some experts recommend drawing aminoglycosides levels 1 or 2 hours posthemodialysis. Dosing guidelines have been developed at different institutions based on the 1 or 2 hours posthemodialysis aminoglycosides levels to maintain the patient at the target therapeutic range. If obtaining a drug level 1 or 2 hours after hemodialysis is not feasible, aminoglycosides also can be redosed using the prehemodialysis aminoglycoside level, the elimination rate for the specific aminoglycoside in ESRD patients, and specific dialysis membrane.

## 7. What is rebound phenomenon?

Rebound phenomenon is defined as the rate of transport of the drug from plasma during hemodialysis exceeding the rate of transport from the peripheral compartment(s) into the central compartment or if the tissue clearance is decreased during hemodialysis. As an example, gentamicin concentrations will increase by about 26% 1 hour after completion of hemodialysis because of the rebound phenomenon.

**8. What adjustments should be made for administering vancomycin to patients receiving hemodialysis?**

The volume of distribution for vancomycin is increased as the patient reaches ESRD because of increased total body weight. The average ESRD population volume of distribution for vancomycin is 0.92 L/kg. It is important to load these patients adequately to achieve therapeutic concentrations. An initial load of vancomycin between 20 and 25 mg/kg should be given to ESRD patients. Maintenance doses will depend on the dialysis membrane used during hemodialysis. High-flux membranes will remove vancomycin significantly compared with conventional membranes. Also, a rebound phenomenon occurs after hemodialysis is completed with vancomycin when patients are dialyzed with high-flux membranes. The average vancomycin level 6 hours posthemodialysis will increase approximately 30% compared with the prehemodialysis vancomycin level. This increase should be accounted for when dosing recommendations are designed for patients dialyzed with high-flux membranes. The target prehemodialysis vancomycin level in ESRD patients is between 10 and 15 mg/L. Some dialysis units are dosing vancomycin during the last hour of hemodialysis to avoid having patients stay for an additional time at the dialysis unit for the antibiotic administration. The maintenance dose should be adjusted based on the prehemodialysis vancomycin levels to maintain patients within the target range. Individual institutions can develop their own vancomycin dosing nomograms for how the maintenance dose should be adjusted based on these levels.

**9. What adjustments should be made for patients with diabetes?**

Insulin metabolism is decreased when kidney function deteriorates. Diabetic patients must be monitored for symptoms of hypoglycemia as their requirement of insulin decreases. Oral hypoglycemics that are excreted by the kidneys also may have prolonged hypoglycemic effect in the presence of kidney disease. One example is glyburide. Metformin should not be used in the presence of renal disease or renal dysfunction (serum creatinine $\geq$ 1.5 mg/dl in males or $\geq$ 1.4 mg/dl in females or abnormal clearance).

**10. How does narcotic pain management differ in patients with renal failure?**

**Meperidine.** Avoid meperidine in patients with renal failure due to metabolite accumulation (normeperidine); normeperidine has less analgesic efficacy than the parent compound and undergoes renal elimination. Normeperidine also has an excitatory effect on the central nervous system (CNS) and causes seizures if it accumulates. The opioid antagonist naloxone will reverse the CNS depressant effect of meperidine but not the excitatory effect of normeperidine. As a result, naloxone use is this setting may result in unopposed excitatory stimulation and thus worsen possible adverse effects.

**Propoxyphene.** Accumulation of norpropoxyphene occurs in patients with renal failure. Both propoxyphene and norpropoxyphene have class IA antiarrhythmic properties that can cause ventricular arrhythmias. Another complication of therapy is propoxyphene-induced hypoglycemia in patients with renal insufficiency. The exact mechanism is unknown but may involve inhibition of gluconeogenesis. Neither substance is removed by dialysis.

**Morphine.** Morphine undergoes glucuronidation to morphine-6-glucuronide (M6G) and morphine-3-glucuronide (M3G). M6G accumulates in renal failure and is a more potent analgesic than the parent compound. In patients with ESRD, the half-life of M6G is estimated to be 38–103 hours. The overall consensus is that morphine should be used with caution in patients with renal failure.

**Codeine.** Codeine is metabolized in the liver to codeine-6-glucuronide, norcodeine, and morphine.

**Hydromorphone.** It is metabolized in the liver to hydromorphone-3-glucuronide (H3G) followed by a reduction to 6-$\alpha$-hydroxyhydromorphone and 6-$\beta$-hydroxyhydromorphone, both of which are less potent analgesics than the parent drug. Neuroexcitation with seizure activity and cognitive impairment have been reported in patients with renal failure receiving high-dose hydromorphone therapy. However, hydromorphone is generally considered to be relatively safe and effective in patients with renal failure.

**Buprenorphine.** This drug undergoes metabolism to an inactive metabolite, buprenorphine-3-glucuronide (B3G), and a much less potent metabolite, norbuprenorphine. This agent is relatively safe in renal failure patients, but there is a ceiling effect on the analgesia.

**Fentanyl.** This is another good option for pain management in renal failure patients, even though the kidneys eliminate both the parent drug and its metabolites.

## BIBLIOGRAPHY

1. Barth RH, DeVincenzo N: Use of vancomycin in high-flux hemodialysis: Experience with 130 courses of therapy. Kidney Int 50:929–936, 1996.
2. Bohler J, Reetze-Bonorden P, Keller E, et al: Rebound of plasma vancomycin levels after hemodialysis with highly permeable membranes. Eur J Clin Pharmacol 42:635–640, 1992.
3. DeSoi CA, Sahm DF, Umans JG: Vancomycin elimination during high-flux hemodialysis: Kinetic model and comparison of four membranes. Am J Kidney Dis 20:354–360, 1992.
4. Halstenson CE, Berkseth RO, Mann HJ, Matzke GR: Aminoglycoside redistribution phenomenon after hemodialysis: Netilmicin and tobramycin. J Clin Pharmacol 25:50–55, 1987.
5. Lam YW, Banerji S, Hatfield C, Talbert RL: Principles of drug administration in renal insufficiency. Clin Pharmacokinet 32:30–57, 1997.
6. Lanese DM, Alfrey PS, Molitoris BA: Markedly increased clearance of vancomycin during hemodialysis using polysulfone dialyzers. Kidney Int 35:1409–1412, 1989.
7. Lewis MJ, Swan SK: A potpourri of drug idiosyncrasies in ESRD. Semin Dial 10:278–281, 1997.
8. Matzke GR, Frye RF: Drug administration in patients with renal insufficiency: Minimising renal and extrarenal toxicity. Drug Saf 16:205–231, 1997.
9. Matzke GR, Millikin SP: Influence of renal function and dialysis on drug disposition. In Evans WE, Schentag JJ, Jusko WJ (eds): Applied Pharmacokinetics: Principles of Therapeutic Drug Monitoring, 3rd ed. Vancouver, WA, Applied Therapeutics, 1992, pp 1–43.
10. Quale JM, O'Halloran JJ, DeVincenzo N, Barth RH: Removal of vancomycin by high-flux hemodialysis membranes. Antimicrob Agents Chemother 36:1424–1426, 1992.
11. St. Peter WL, Redic-Kill KA, et al: Clinical pharmacokinetics of antibiotics in patients with impaired renal function. Clin Pharmacokinet 22:169–210, 1992.
12. Talbert RL: Drug dosing in renal insufficiency. J Clin Pharmacol 34:99–110, 1994.
13. Touchette MA, et al: Vancomycin removal by high-flux polysulfone hemodialysis membranes in critically ill patients with end-stage renal disease. Am J Kidney Dis 26:469–474, 1995.

# II.  Clinical Syndromes

# 9.  ETIOLOGY, PATHOPHYSIOLOGY, AND DIAGNOSIS OF ACUTE RENAL FAILURE

*Miriam F. Weiss, M.D.*

**1.  What is acute renal failure?**
Acute renal failure is a sudden decrease in renal function usually manifested by azotemia (increase in blood urea nitrogen [BUN] and serum creatinine concentration) and sometimes associated with oliguria.

**2.  Define oliguria.**
Oliguria is defined as urine volumes less than 400 ml/day or 20 ml/hour.

**3.  What is the difference between acute renal failure and acute tubular necrosis?**
Acute renal failure (ARF) refers to any condition characterized by decreased renal excretory capacity. The differential diagnosis of ARF includes prerenal azotemia (about 70% of cases) and obstructive uropathy (5% of cases) (see Chapter 11, Prerenal Azotemia, and Chapter 12, Obstructive Uropathy). Renal parenchymal disease is the cause of ARF in about 25% of patients. Renal diseases associated with ARF include acute glomerulonephritis, acute interstitial nephritis, and rapidly progressive glomerulonephritis. The vast majority of patients with parenchymal renal disease and ARF have acute tubular necrosis (ATN). Thus, the two terms often are used synonymously even though patients with ATN represent only a subset of patients with ARF.

**4.  How common is acute renal failure?**
ARF develops in up to 5% of patients admitted to medical or surgical services and as many as 15% of critically ill patients.

**5.  Has there been an improvement in incidence or outcome of ARF?**
No. Neither the incidence nor the morbidity and mortality rates have changed, even with improvements in renal replacement therapies (see Chapter 10). The mortality is high, with overall rates between 50% and 70%.

**6.  Why does ARF continue to be such a big problem for hospitalized patients?**
The severity of underlying diseases that can cause ARF is increasing, particularly in the ICU setting, where ATN often develops in the context of multiple organ failure.

**7.  What laboratory parameters help to differentiate prerenal azotemia from ATN?**

|  | PRERENAL AZOTEMIA | ACUTE TUBULAR NECROSIS |
|---|---|---|
| Urine specific gravity | > 1.018 | ~ 1.010 |
| Urine sodium | < 10 mEq/L | > 20 mEq/L |
| Fractional excretion of sodium | < 1% | > 2% |
| Urine osmolality | > 500 mOsm/L | ~ 280 mOsm/L |
| Urine sediment | Normal, or clear hyaline casts | Renal tubular cells and "muddy-brown" granular casts |

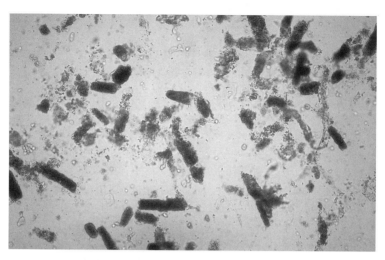

Light microscopic view of unstained urinary sediment from patient with acute tubular necrosis (ATN). Note multiple granular casts, typical of the "dirty brown" urine of ATN. (Original magnification ×40.)

### 8. Calculate the fractional excretion of sodium (FENa, %).

$$FENa = \frac{Na^+\ excreted}{Na^+\ filtered} \cdot 100 = \frac{U\ Na^+ \cdot V}{P\ Na^+ \cdot \dfrac{U\ creat \cdot V}{P\ Creat}} \cdot 100 = \frac{U/P\ Na^+}{U/P\ creatinine} \cdot 100$$

where U = urine, P = plasma, and V = volume.

### 9. What are the major categories of ATN?
1. Ischemic
2. Nephrotoxic

However, in up to 50% of patients with ATN, the etiology is multifactorial, and both ischemic and nephrotoxic etiologies can exist in the same severely ill patient.

### 10. What is ischemic acute tubular necrosis?

Ischemic ATN results from hypoperfusion of the kidneys and can occur in any of the conditions associated with prerenal azotemia (see Chapter 11, Prerenal Azotemia) when the hypoperfusion is sustained and severe. Ischemic ATN is often more severe than ATN caused by nephrotoxins, which can be self-limited (see question 16). Ischemia is followed by **reperfusion injury**, which is characterized by the generation of oxygen radicals, disruption of cell membranes, leak of calcium and other cations into the cell, depletion of high-energy phosphate compounds, and mitochondrial dysfunction leading to cell death.

### 11. What are the causes of nephrotoxic acute tubular necrosis?
**Exogenous toxins**
    Radiocontrast agents
    Nephrotoxic antibiotics (e.g., aminoglycosides)
    Nephrotoxic anticancer agents (e.g., cisplatin)
    Heavy metals (lead, mercury)
    Lithium
    Fluorinated anesthetics (methoxyflurane, halothane)
    Organic solvents (e.g., ethylene glycol)

**Endogenous toxins**
　　Rhabdomyolysis (myoglobin)
　　Hemolysis (hemoglobin)
　　Tumor lysis syndrome
　　Myeloma
　　Hypercalcemia

### 12. Why aren't nonsteroidal anti-inflammatory drugs (NSAIDs) and cyclooxygenase-2 (COX-2) inhibitors on the list above?

They should be! These agents always have some effect on the kidney. Renal prostaglandins (i.e., $PGE_2$ and $PGI_2$) play critical roles in normal renal function. Inhibition of $PGE_2$ explains sodium retention, edema, and increase in blood pressure caused by these agents. Because $PGI_2$ is a potent renal vasodilator and keeps blood flow to the kidney constant in conditions of ischemia, its inhibition increases the risk of nephrotoxic or ischemic ATN.

Whether selective (e.g., COX-2 inhibitors such as celecoxib or rofecoxib) or nonselective (e.g., NSAIDs such as indomethacin, ibuprofen, or naproxen), the effect of these agents on renal function is comparable at comparable doses. The risk of renal impairment associated with these agents is increased in patients with underlying renal disease and in those with conditions in which preservation of renal function is dependent on the compensatory effects of prostaglandins (e.g., volume depletion or congestive heart failure).

### 13. What is the pathophysiology of ATN?

ATN is characterized by a decrease in glomerular filtration. The connection between tubular damage and loss of glomerular function is not immediately apparent. Experimental evidence can be boiled down to four major pathophysiologic mechanisms. The interplay of these four mechanisms forms the basis for the drop in glomerular filtration that characterizes ATN.

1. **Intratubular obstruction:** Following an ischemic or nephrotoxic insult, tubular cells, cellular debris (brush border membranes), crystals (e.g., uric acid), or casts formed from myoglobin, hemoglobin, or protein slough into the tubular lumen and occlude the flow of filtrate by increasing intratubular pressure. (See figure of granular casts in urine in question 7.)

2. **Tubular back leak:** Disruption in tubular basement membranes leads to abnormal reabsorption of filtrate and decreased urine flow through the tubule.

3. **Vasoconstriction:** Damage to tubules causes vasoconstriction mediated through the renin-angiotensin system, endothelin, and the decreased production of vasodilatory substances such as $PGI_2$ and nitrous oxide (NO).

4. **Changes in glomerular permeability:** The ischemic or nephrotoxic insult directly alters the intrinsic permeability of glomerular capillary membrane.

These mechanisms are not mutually exclusive; some combination of mechanisms is likely involved in humans with ATN.

### 14. Which underlying conditions increase the risk of developing ATN after exposure to radiocontrast agents?

　　Chronic renal insufficiency
　　Diabetes mellitus
　　Dehydration

### 15. Characterize the course of ATN.

The **initiation phase** is the period of time during which exposure to a nephrotoxic agent or ischemia takes place. In clinical practice, it is common for there to be more than one cause of ATN; ischemic and nephrotoxic insults often coexist.

The **maintenance phase** may last from days to as long as 6 weeks. This period of time is characterized by persistent oliguria. During the maintenance phase, patients are often dependent on some form of renal replacement therapy (dialysis or continuous hemofiltration).

With stabilization of other underlying disease processes and nutritional support, the patient may enter the **recovery phase** of ATN. This period, also called the **diuretic phase**, is characterized by increasing urine output and the gradual recovery of renal function. BUN and creatinine levels generally return to normal. However, evidence of tubular dysfunction (e.g., failure to maximally concentrate the urine in response to water deprivation) may persist for months to years after recovery from ATN.

### 16. How do nephrotoxic and ischemic ATN differ from each other?

Nephrotoxic ATN is more likely to be associated with a nonoliguric presentation. The increase in BUN and creatinine may be relatively gradual. ATN caused by nephrotoxins also is more likely to fit the criteria for the **intermediate syndrome**. Patients with intermediate syndrome show some characteristics of reversible prerenal azotemia, such as a relatively low urine sodium, a partial response to fluid challenge, and a shorter maintenance phase.

### 17. Describe the pathologic lesion of ATN.

Whether ATN follows ischemia or toxic injury, renal parenchymal changes are patchy and irregular. There is tubular cell necrosis with varying degrees of regeneration. Reflecting the findings on urinalysis, loss of tubular brush border membranes and renal tubular cell casts are frequent findings. Interstitial edema and interstitial inflammation may be present. The findings are relatively nonspecific and may persist even during the recovery phase.

### 18. How do proteins such as myoglobin and hemoglobin cause tubular toxicity?

Iron released from these proteins generates free radicals. Free radicals attack cell membranes, oxidizing cell membranes and causing cell-death. Markedly elevated levels of oxidized lipids such as $F_2$-isoprostanes lead to renal vasoconstriction. In addition, free radicals consume endogenous vasodilatory substances such as NO, resulting in even more renal ischemia.

### 19. What are the common causes of death in patients with ARF?

1. Infections (30–70%)
2. Cardiovascular events (5–30%)
3. Gastrointestinal, pulmonary, or neurologic complications (7–30%)
4. Hyperkalemia or technical issues related to dialytic therapy (1–2%)

### BIBLIOGRAPHY

1. Brady HR, Brenner BM, Clarkson MR, Lieberthal W: Acute renal failure. In Brenner BM (ed): The Kidney, 6th ed. Philadelphia, W.B. Saunders, 2000, pp 1201–1222.
2. Brivet FG, Kleinknecht DJ, Loirat P, Landais PJM, on behalf of the French Study Group on Acute renal Failure: Acute renal failure in intensive care units—causes, outcomes and prognostic factors of hospital mortality: A prospective multicenter study. Crit Care Med 24:192–198, 1996.
3. Harris RC: Cyclooxygenase-2 inhibition and renal physiology. Am J Cardiol 89:10–17, 2002.
4. Holt SG, Moore KP: Pathogenesis and treatment of renal dysfunction in rhabdomyolysis. Intens Care Med 27:803–811, 2001.
5. Klahr S, Miller SB: Acute oliguria. N Engl J Med 338:671–675, 1998.
6. Weisberg LS, Kurnik PB, Kurnik BRC: Risk of radiocontrast nephropathy in patients with and without diabetes mellitus. Kidney Int 45:259–265, 1994.

# 10. MANAGEMENT OF ACUTE RENAL FAILURE

*Miriam F. Weiss, M.D.*

**1. What are the principles of managing patients with acute tubular necrosis?**

To date, there is no evidence that any therapeutic approach will alter the development or course of acute tubular necrosis (ATN). Usually, recovery from ATN is spontaneous. Therefore, the principles of management are to provide support.

- Restrict fluid, sodium, potassium, and phosphate intake.
- Restrict protein intake to reduce the generation of urea.
- Use diuretics to control hypervolemia.
- Administer $NaHCO_3$ to correct acidemia.
- Adjust the dosage of medications that rely on the kidney for clearance or metabolism.
- Provide renal replacement therapy to the patient when conservative management is not sufficient to maintain solute and water balance.

**2. Can fluid administration prevent ATN?**

Hypovolemia is a risk factor for the development of ATN. Therefore, adequate fluid replacement is important, and fluid loading to maintain urine output may reduce the transit time of nephrotoxins. A clear role for aggressive fluid resuscitation has been shown in cases of ATN resulting from rhabdomyolysis.

**3. Can diuretics prevent ATN?**

It has become routine to administer IV fluids and diuretics *together* under certain circumstances. For example, IV fluids and mannitol are administered routinely prior to cross-clamping of the aorta in patients undergoing repair of abdominal aortic aneurysms. Aggressive hydration and forced alkaline-osmotic diuresis using $NaHCO_3$ and mannitol have been demonstrated to be effective in patients with rhabdomyolysis to maintain a high-output state and minimize the risk of developing acute renal failure (ARF). In addition, in patients at high risk for the development of radiocontrast-induced renal failure, administration of IV fluids (0.45% saline) before the imaging procedure has been found to be more effective in preventing ARF than the combination of IV fluids and diuretics (either furosemide or mannitol). However, recent randomized trials show that loop diuretics may *cause harm—* increasing the risk of ARF after cardiac surgery or coronary angiography.

**4. Can diuretics convert oliguric to nonoliguric ATN?**

It is widely believed that the prognosis of patients with nonoliguric renal failure is better than those with oliguria. Consequently, high doses of loop diuretics often are administered to patients in the early phase of ATN to promote urine flow. The results of recent randomized, controlled studies suggest that this practice should be considered with caution.

**5. What is the downside of using diuretics in ARF?**

Excessive diuresis may lead to volume depletion and renal hypoperfusion, adding insult to injury.

**6. Why do some practitioners infuse diuretics and albumin together in oliguric patients?**

Furosemide and other loop diuretics act on the luminal side of tubular cells in the ascending limb of the loop of Henle. They arrive there following active secretion into the tubular lumen by proximal tubular cells. In patients with tubular necrosis, the latter process is impaired so that large doses or continuous infusions often are needed to achieve a diuretic effect. The addition of albumin to loop diuretics increases urine output in patients with nephrotic syndrome (who have low serum albumin levels and central volume contraction). No benefit has been demonstrated in any other setting.

### 7. How does "renal-dose" dopamine improve urine output in ARF?

Administration of renal-dose (1–3 µg/kg/min) dopamine is a widespread practice in the management of oliguric patients. Renal-dose dopamine is thought to increase urine output through direct tubular effects, by increasing the tubular delivery of diuretics and by blocking aldosterone's salt-retaining effect in the distal tubule. Theoretically, renal-dose dopamine increases renal blood flow through specific renal dopaminergic receptors. Finally, dopamine may increase urine output through increased cardiac output as a result of beta-adrenergic stimulation of the heart. However, several large studies have found no evidence of benefit from this practice.

### 8. What are the risks of administering renal-dose dopamine?

Even low-dose dopamine can induce tachycardia, cardiac arrhythmia, or myocardial ischemia. Dopamine also blunts hypoxemic ventilatory drive and can decrease minute ventilation. Because of its alpha-adrenergic effect, ischemia of the digits can occur. Bowel ischemia, although uncommon, can result in translocation of bacteria or bacterial products across the intestine. This is a particularly important risk in the face of increased susceptibility to infection seen in patients with ARF.

### 9. Are there any promising new therapeutic approaches for preventing ARF?

Low-osmolality contrast media reduces the risk of ARF in patients with baseline chronic renal disease, but has no benefit in patients with normal renal function. Atrial natriuretic peptide, theophylline (an inhibitor of the renal vasoconstrictor adenosine), and calcium channel blockers have all been tried without any evidence of benefit. The jury is still out on the antioxidant compound acetylcysteine and on whether the use of single versus multiple doses of aminoglycosides will reduce the risk of ARF. At present it is not clear that lipid formulations of amphotericin improve the risk of renal damage compared to standard formulations of this nephrotoxic agent.

To date, anabolic factors such as thyroxine, insulin-like growth factor-1 (IGF-1), and growth hormone (GH) have proven unsuccessful or harmful in patients with critical illnesses at high risk of ARF. Overall survival in critically ill patients is improved with continuous insulin infusion whether or not diabetes is present. Other antioxidant compounds, such as vitamin E or glutathione, have shown promise in animal models but have not been tested in human beings.

### 10. What are the goals of renal replacement therapy (dialysis or continuous hemofiltration) in ARF?

When conservative therapy fails to maintain fluid and electrolyte balance within safe ranges, or when uremic symptoms (including pericarditis) develop, renal replacement therapy is initiated. The goal of renal replacement therapy is to normalize the fluid-volume status, correct electrolyte balance, and control uremia. This simple statement masks the complexity of the decision making involved in starting renal replacement therapy. The exact method chosen, whether to start dialysis early or late in the course of ARF, and the intensity of the renal replacement therapy are areas of controversy.

**11. What are the advantages and disadvantages of intermittent versus continuous renal replacement therapies?**

| | ADVANTAGES | DISADVANTAGES |
|---|---|---|
| Intermittent hemodialysis | Efficient and rapid removal of volume and small molecules<br>Cost effective<br>Readily available | Central venous access required<br>Anticoagulation may be required<br>May not be tolerated by hemo-dynamically unstable patients |
| Continuous hemofiltration | Excellent control of volume enabling liberal use of hyperalimentation, blood products, etc.<br>Good removal of larger molecules<br>Can be used in relatively hypotensive patients | Central venous access required<br>Anticoagulation may be required<br>Labor intensive and expensive |
| Peritoneal dialysis | No need for anticoagulation<br>Cost-effective | Slow removal of uremic toxins<br>Risk of peritonitis<br>May be tolerated poorly in patients with splanchnic hypoperfusion |

**12. Are there any differences in survival among the different renal replacement therapies?**

No good studies directly compare continuous hemofiltration to intermittent hemodialysis. However, daily hemodialysis improves survival compared with alternate-day therapy. In addition, higher doses of continuous hemofiltration can improve outcome compared with lower dose therapy (see Chapter 49).

**13. What about nutritional support for patients with ARF?**

ARF results in insulin resistance, changes in nitrogen balance due to increased protein turnover, exhaustion of antioxidant defenses, and hormonal alterations. Current recommendations for enteral or parenteral nutrition during ARF are to give ~35 kcal/kg body weight/day, ~1.2 gm protein/kg body weight/day, and a ratio between glucose and lipid in the nonprotein part of energy of ~70/30. There is no proven difference between essential amino acid–enriched and routine formulas for hyperalimentation.

**14. Does appropriate nutritional support result in improved morbidity and mortality?**

Because of the severity of illness, complexity of care, and high incidence of comorbid conditions, the efficacy of nutritional therapy has *not* been demonstrated in patients with ARF. Administration of large volumes of enteral nutrition to patients with renal failure can result in volume overload, more rapid increases in BUN, and alterations in critical plasma electrolyte levels. Careful attention must be given to controlling these factors when nutritional support is prescribed.

**15. What is the importance of "biocompatible" hemodialysis?**

An inflammatory response can be induced when cellular and chemical components of blood come in contact with an artificial dialysis membrane. The less biocompatible the membrane, the more likely it is to activate white blood cells or the complement cascade. In several studies, dialyzing patients with ARF using older style nonbiocompatible (cellulose-based) dialysis membranes has been associated with excess mortality (25% or more) compared with dialysis with synthetic membranes. This interesting observation suggests that external sources of inflammation may exacerbate underlying disease processes and interfere with normal renal recovery.

### BIBLIOGRAPHY

1. Australian and New Zealand Intensive Care Society (ANZICS) Clinical Trials Group: Low dose dopamine in patients with early renal dysfunction: A placebo-controlled, randomized trial. Lancet 356:2139–2143, 2000.
2. Hatala R, Dinh TT, Cook DJ: Single daily dosing of aminoglycosides in immunocompromised adults: A systematic review. Clin Infect Dis 24:810–815, 1997.
3. Himmelfarb J, Tolkoff RN, Chandran P, et al: A multicenter comparisons of dialysis membranes in the treatment of acute renal failure requiring dialysis. J Am Soc Nephrol 9:257–266, 1998.
4. Kellum JA: The use of diuretics and dopamine in acute renal failure: A systematic review of the evidence. Crit Care 1:53–59, 1997.
5. Lameire N, Vanholder R: Pathophysiologic features and prevention of human and experimental acute tubular necrosis. J Am Soc Nephrol 12:20–32, 2001.
6. Ronco C, Bellomo R, Homel P, et al: Effects of different doses in continuous veno-venous hemofiltration on outcomes of acute renal failure: A prospective, randomized trial. Lancet 356:26–30, 2000.
7. Solomon R, Werner C, Mann D, et al: Effects of saline, mannitol and furosemide on acute decreases in renal function induced by radiocontrast agents. N Engl J Med 331:1416–1420, 1994.
8. Schiffl H, Lang SM, Fischer R: Daily hemodialysis and the outcome of acute renal failure. N Engl J Med 346:305–310, 2002.

# 11. PRERENAL AZOTEMIA

*Edmond Ricanati*, M.D.

**1. What is prerenal azotemia?**

Prerenal azotemia is an elevation of the serum creatinine concentration and blood urea nitrogen (BUN) due to "effective" volume depletion resulting in diminished renal perfusion. Impaired renal perfusion will reduce renal blood flow and glomerular filtration rate (GFR), resulting in the retention of creatinine and urea nitrogen. The kidney's intrinsic ability to function remains intact. Prerenal azotemia is the most common cause of acute renal failure and is potentially reversible when diagnosed early and treated effectively. Patients with established chronic renal failure with diminished GFR can develop superimposed prerenal azotemia.

**2. What are the most common pathologic causes of prerenal azotemia?**

Hypovolemia
    Dehydration
    Hemorrhage
    Renal fluid losses (diuretics)
    Gastrointestinal losses (vomiting, diarrhea)
    "Third spacing"
Low cardiac output (e.g., congestive heart failure)
Conditions associated with systemic vasodilatation
    Sepsis
    Neurogenic shock

**3. Which medications can cause prerenal azotemia? Explain the mechanism(s) responsible for their adverse effects.**

1. **Nonsteroidal anti-inflammatory drugs that inhibit renal prostaglandin biosynthesis** can trigger prerenal azotemia, particularly in patients with volume depletion. They act by interfering with the renal afferent arteriolar adaptive response to hypovolemia, namely afferent arteriolar vasodilation mediated by increased synthesis of prostaglandins ($PGE_2$ and $PGI_2$) in volume-depleted states.

2. **Angiotensin-converting enzyme (ACE) inhibitors or angiotensin II receptor blockers**. Angiotensin II maintains glomerular filtration pressure in renal hypoperfusion by preferentially constricting the efferent arterioles. Angiotensin inhibitors blunt this response and can result in a dissociation of the autoregulation of renal blood flow and glomerular filtration rate, leading to a significant reduction in glomerular filtration rate. This is a problem particularly in patients with bilateral renal artery stenosis but sometimes can be seen in volume-depleted patients.

3. **Other antihypertensive drugs** can cause prerenal azotemia if blood pressure is lowered excessively.

4. **Cyclosporine** causes intrarenal vasoconstriction that may be related to release of endothelin, a potent vasoconstrictor peptide released from the endothelial cells in the walls of the arterioles.

5. **Amphotericin B** causes intrarenal vasoconstriction and can lead to renal ischemia and prerenal azotemia with increasing doses of the drug. Amphotericin B is also directly toxic to the proximal epithelial cells.

**4. What drugs elevate the plasma creatinine concentration in the absence of a reduction of GFR?**

The drugs that elevate plasma creatinine without a change in GFR either interfere with secretion of creatinine in the proximal tubule or interfere with the plasma assay of creatinine:

- The drugs that commonly decrease proximal tubular secretion of creatinine are cimetidine ($H_2$-blocker) and trimethoprim. By inhibiting creatinine secretion, cimetidine was used clinically to measure the GFR more accurately. Normally, the creatinine clearance overestimates the GFR by as much as 15%.
- Drugs that are recognized as creatinine chromogens and falsely raise the plasma creatinine concentration are fluoxytosine and cefoxitin.

Note that in the above instances the elevation in serum creatinine concentration is not associated with a concomitant elevation in the BUN.

**5. What renal hemodynamic changes in states of diminished "effective" volume preserve glomerular perfusion and filtration rate? How are they altered in prerenal azotemia?**

When effective volume is diminished, several compensatory mechanisms are invoked to preserve glomerular filtration:

- Diminished glomerular perfusion stimulates stretch receptors in the afferent arterioles resulting in vasodilatation through a local myogenic response.
- Increased production of vasodilator substances (vasodilator prostaglandins such as $PGE_2$ and $PGI_2$ and possibly nitric oxide) maximally dilate the afferent arterioles.
- Increased intrarenal production of angiotensin II from renin causes a preferential constriction of the efferent arterioles resulting in increased filtration pressure.

Preglomerular arteriolar dilatation and postglomerular arteriolar constriction preserve glomerular perfusion and, by increasing filtration pressure, maintain a normal GFR. In prerenal azotemia, renal perfusion is significantly compromised, and the above autoregulatory mechanisms fail to maintain adequate glomerular perfusion and filtration pressure, resulting in the retention of creatinine and urea.

**6. What clinical and laboratory findings distinguish prerenal azotemia from acute tubular necrosis?**

In acute tubular necrosis (ATN), there is significant renal parenchymal damage due to severe renal ischemia or the administration of a nephrotoxic agent. Renal perfusion and tubular function are disrupted. In prerenal azotemia, renal tubular function is preserved. The major laboratory findings that distinguish prerenal azotemia from acute tubular necrosis are:

1. **Urine sediment**. Urine sediment, which is normal in prerenal azotemia, reveals renal epithelial cells, renal epithelial cell casts, and muddy brown granular casts when examined at the time of the acute injury.

2. **Fractional excretion of sodium** (FENa; the percentage of filtered sodium that is excreted in the urine). In prerenal azotemia, there is intense retention of sodium, and the FENa is less than 1%. It is above 2% in ATN, an indication that there is tubular injury. The FENa is the most reliable index for the diagnosis of ATN (see Chapter 9, Etiology, Pathophysiology, and Diagnosis of Acute Renal Failure, for calculation of the FENa).

3. **Urine osmolality**. In ATN, there is early loss of concentrating ability. The urine osmolality is usually below 350 mOsm/kg. In prerenal azotemia, urine osmolality is usually above 500 mOsm/kg and reflects normal tubular function.

4. **BUN-to-plasma creatinine ratio**. This is in the normal range in ATN (10–15 to 1). In prerenal azotemia, it is usually greater than 20 to 1 and reflects the increase in urea absorption that follows the enhanced proximal reabsorption of sodium and water. This parameter is less reliable than the FENa and urine osmolality determinations.

None of the above criteria is helpful when prerenal azotemia is superimposed on underlying chronic renal disease. In chronic renal disease, sodium conservation and urine concentration are impaired, and the urine sediment may be abnormal.

## 7. When is the diagnostic utility of FENa of limited value?

The FENa is of limited value when prerenal azotemia is associated with:

- Chronic renal failure in which high fractional excretion of sodium is required to maintain sodium balance
- Use of diuretics, which results in excessive urinary sodium loss
- Acute volume expansion, which promotes increased sodium excretion

There are a number of cases of acute renal failure other than prerenal azotemia in which fractional excretion of sodium may be less than 1%:

- Acute glomerulonephritis or vasculitis. In these conditions, GFR is reduced, but tubular function is preserved.
- Some cases of acute interstitial nephritis
- Some cases of acute renal failure due to radiocontrast media or heme pigments
- When prerenal azotemia is changing to ATN. This usually occurs within the first 48 hours of the ischemic event. Under these conditions, GFR is reduced, but tubular function is largely preserved.

## 8. What are the guidelines for treatment of prerenal azotemia?

1. Restore the normal circulating blood volume. In the absence of congestive heart failure, administration of fluids (usually normal saline) at a rate of 75–100 ml/hr is adequate. Hypovolemia due to hemorrhage or the presence of severe anemia should be corrected with blood transfusions.

2. The types of fluid administered and the rate at which replacement fluids are given will depend on the serum electrolytes (especially serum sodium, potassium, and the acid-base status of the patient) and the clinical status of the patient.

3. Monitor the adequacy of fluid replacement by the clinical examination of the patient and by the serial determinations of serum creatinine concentrations, which reflect renal function. Follow daily weights, fluid intake, and urine output, as well as urine sodium excretion and serial measurements of the serum creatinine, BUN, serum electrolytes, and acid-base parameters. Hemodynamic monitoring may be necessary if clinical assessment of cardiovascular function and fluid status is difficult. Response to proper fluid replacement in prerenal azotemia is rapid; renal function usually returns to the previous baseline within 3–4 days.

### BIBLIOGRAPHY

1. Hricik DE, Dunn MJ: Angiotensin-converting enzyme inhibitor–induced renal failure: Causes, consequences, and diagnostic uses. J Am Soc Nephrol 1:845–858, 1990.
2. Klahr S, Miller SB: Acute oliguria. N Engl J Med 338:671–675, 1998.
3. Miller TR, Anderson RJ, Linas SL, et al: Urinary diagnostic indices in acute renal failure: A prospective study. Ann Intern Med 47:89–96, 1978.

# 12. HEPATORENAL SYNDROME

*Jeffrey R. Schelling, M.D.*

**1. Define clinical features of the hepatorenal syndrome.**

The hepatorenal syndrome (HRS) is defined as unexplained acute renal failure in the context of severe hepatic dysfunction. Oliguria is present in about 90% of HRS cases. Commonly observed physical examination findings include low blood pressure (although generally not overt hypotension), jaundice, ascites, and metabolic encephalopathy, which is characterized by somnolence, confusion, and asterixis. Results from a recent consensus conference have established criteria for type I and type II forms of HRS. **Type I HRS** is characterized by a rapid decline in glomerular filtration rate (GFR), as defined by doubling of serum creatinine to > 2.5 mg/dl or 50% reduction in creatinine clearance to < 20 ml/min within 2 weeks. **Type II HRS** is defined by a more protracted course and a better prognosis (see below). It is unclear whether types I and II HRS represent different diseases or a continuum of the same disease process.

**2. Who is at risk of developing HRS?**

HRS can occur in patients with any underlying etiology of hepatic failure, including viral hepatitis, biliary tract obstruction, primary biliary cirrhosis, hepatic resection, or fatty liver of pregnancy. However, in the United States, the most common liver disorder associated with HRS is alcoholic cirrhosis. In many cases, HRS is preceded by a catastrophic precipitating event, such as a serious infection or gastrointestinal bleeding. Often, however, an underlying problem in addition to hepatic dysfunction cannot be identified. Because the HRS is usually diagnosed in the inpatient setting, it has been suggested that it may sometimes be an iatrogenic disorder, such as a complication of large-volume paracentesis with inadequate concomitant extracellular fluid volume replacement or aggressive diuresis. Therefore, to avoid precipitation of the HRS, one should exercise caution to avoid large extracellular fluid volume shifts or prescription of potentially nephrotoxic medications (e.g., nonsteroidal anti-inflammatory medications) in patients with hepatic dysfunction.

**3. What is the differential diagnosis of acute renal failure in patients with hepatic dysfunction?**

With a few exceptions, the differential diagnosis of acute renal failure in patients with and without hepatic failure is similar. Prerenal azotemia due to intravascular volume depletion or congestive heart failure, acute tubular necrosis due to ischemia or sepsis, and urinary tract obstruction, in conjunction with a separate cause for hepatic dysfunction, are the most common scenarios. In particular, intravascular volume depletion and acute tubular necrosis are more common diagnoses than HRS in cirrhotics. Although it is rarely encountered, one should also consider parsimonious diagnoses that explain both renal and hepatic dysfunction, such as autoimmune diseases (systemic lupus erythematosus, polyarteritis nodosa, hepatitis B- and C-associated glomerulonephritides), infiltrating diseases (amyloidosis, sarcoidosis, lymphoma), toxins (carbon tetrachloride, *Amanita phalloides*), and genetic diseases (autosomal dominant and recessive forms of polycystic kidney diseases, hereditary oxalosis).

**4. What is the pathophysiology of the HRS?**

The actual cause of HRS is unclear. However, based on the characteristic hemodynamic features, which include systemic vasodilatation and renal vasoconstriction, the prevailing theory is that the combination of the underfilled arterial vasculature and renal vasoconstriction results in renal hypoperfusion. Multiple vasoactive substances have been implicated as potential etiologic factors. Candidate systemic vasodilators have included nitric oxide, atrial natriuretic peptide, intestinal-derived bacterial endotoxin, which evades hepatic catabolism, false neurotransmitters (octopamine and phenoethanolamine), vasoactive intestinal peptide, and substance P. Candidate renal vasoconstrictors include endothelin, catecholamines, angiotensin II, diminished bradykinin, and an imbalance between vasodilator and vasoconstrictor prostaglandins, which favors vasoconstriction. However, none of these substances completely accounts for the cause of HRS, suggesting that multiple factors may be involved.

### 5. What are characteristic laboratory features in the HRS?

By definition, the serum creatinine and blood urea nitrogen (BUN) are elevated in the HRS due to diminished GFR. However, it should be recognized that cirrhotics characteristically have decreased muscle mass from malnutrition. Because of the associated decrease in muscle creatinine mobilization, the serum creatinine corresponding to a normal GFR is usually much lower than 1.0 mg/dl. Therefore, the serum creatinine rarely rises above 4.0–5.0 mg/dl in the HRS, and values in the range of 1.0–2.0 mg/dl are likely to represent significantly decreased GFR. The serum sodium concentration is often low in HRS because of nonosmotic vasopressin release, which acts both as a vasoconstrictor and as a stimulus for $H_2O$ reabsorption at the collecting duct. Assays for liver function, such as serum bilirubin, serum albumin, and INR, are almost always abnormal in HRS. The urinalysis generally reveals concentrated urine (specific gravity > 1.025; urine osmolality > 500 mOsm/L), but is otherwise unremarkable. The presence of hematuria or proteinuria should raise suspicions about diagnoses other than HRS. As discussed in detail below, HRS is viewed as an extreme form of prerenal azotemia, with the kidneys avidly reabsorbing NaCl in response to a decrease in *effective arterial blood volume* associated with hepatic dysfunction. Consistent with this model, the urine Na and fractional excretion of Na (FENa = [urine Na × serum creatinine]/[serum Na × urine creatinine]) are characteristically very low in HRS: < 10 mEq/L and < 0.5%, respectively.

### 6. How can HRS be distinguished from other causes of acute renal failure?

Urinary tract obstruction initially should be excluded with an appropriate radiologic technique, such as renal ultrasound, magnetic resonance imaging (MRI), or a noncontrasted computed tomography (CT) scan. In patients with oliguric acute renal failure, either measurement of urine Na from a spot sample or calculation of the FENa is an effective means of differentiating between prerenal and intrarenal causes of acute renal failure. Urine Na and FENa are extremely low in HRS.

If these criteria are satisfied, the differential diagnosis can then be narrowed to HRS versus other causes of prerenal azotemia. If clinical diagnoses of congestive heart failure and glomerulonephritis can be ruled out, the major distinction is between HRS and intravascular volume depletion. The most definitive way to distinguish these two possibilities is by central hemodynamic monitoring with a Swan-Ganz catheter. It should be recognized, however, that the risk of placing a central venous catheter in patients with cirrhosis is associated with increased risk of bleeding. In volume-depleted patients, the systemic vascular resistance (SVR) is elevated, and the cardiac output may be somewhat diminished. In contrast, the SVR is generally very low and the cardiac output elevated in patients with the HRS. Because this hemodynamic pattern of HRS is identical in sepsis, systemic infections should be ruled out.

If a Swan-Ganz catheter is not placed, a less acceptable, but alternative approach, is to administer intravenous fluids empirically and then remeasure serum and urine chemistry values. Because of the propensity for fluid transudation in cirrhotics, intravenous colloids are preferable to crystalloid fluids. In volume-depleted patients, 2 L of intravenous fluid is generally sufficient to restore intravascular volume and should result in a prompt decrease in serum creatinine, and increases in urine Na, FENa, and urine volume. The response to an intravenous fluid challenge in HRS can be difficult to interpret because fluid administration may result in a transient increase in renal blood flow. However, sustained improvement in GFR, urinary Na retention, or urine volume is generally inconsistent with a diagnosis of the HRS.

### 7. What are characteristic histopathologic findings in HRS kidneys?

HRS is a diagnosis based on clinical criteria, so a renal biopsy generally is not necessary. Furthermore, the risk of biopsy-associated bleeding complications is increased because of the prevalence of coagulopathies in HRS subjects. However, if a biopsy were performed, the kidney histology should be normal, supporting the position that the kidney is simply an "innocent bystander" in HRS, with the pathogenesis of decreased GFR due to hemodynamic alterations that are caused by the diseased liver. This view is further supported by remote studies that demonstrate that HRS donor kidneys function well when transplanted into chronic renal disease recipients.

### 8. What is the prognosis for HRS?

In type I HRS, GFR deteriorates rapidly, with mean survival measured in weeks. Type II HRS patients, by contrast, have a more protracted course, with gradual declines in GFR and somewhat longer survival, usually on the order of months. However, the mortality associated with either type of HRS is nearly 100% unless liver function improves, either spontaneously or from liver transplantation. Because of the grim prognosis, it is critical to exclude other reversible causes of acute renal failure, as described above.

### 9. What is the treatment for HRS?

There is presently no definitive therapy, other than liver transplantation, for HRS. Many therapeutic protocols have been developed for HRS, most of which have targeted correction of the hemodynamic abnormalities, either through administration of vasoactive agents or creation of a form of portosystemic shunt. Although some case series demonstrate successful GFR, or more rarely, patient survival outcomes, most of the studies were small and none was a randomized, controlled trial. Therefore, the therapy for HRS is largely supportive and should obviously include avoidance of nephrotoxic medications, such as aminoglycoside antibiotics or nonsteroidal anti-inflammatory agents.

### 10. Is hemodialysis an effective therapy for HRS?

Hemodialysis as a therapy for HRS is somewhat controversial. In the few cases in which spontaneous liver function recovery is anticipated or a liver transplant is imminent, it is quite reasonable to support HRS patients with hemodialysis therapy. In the absence of liver improvement or anticipated transplantation, however, many nephrologists would not favor institution of dialysis because dialysis does not alter mortality in HRS. This is consistent with the concept that renal dysfunction is a manifestation of the kidney as an innocent bystander, and mortality is due to hepatic or multiorgan failure rather than renal failure.

### BIBLIOGRAPHY

1. Brensing KA, Textor J, Perz J, et al: Long-term outcome after transjugular intrahepatic portosystemic stent-shunt in non-transplant cirrhotics with hepatorenal syndrome: A phase II study. Gut 47:288–295, 2000.
2. Gines A, Escorsell A, Gines P, et al: Incidence, predictive factors, and prognosis of the hepatorenal syndrome in cirrhosis with ascites. Gastroenterology 105:229–236, 1993.

3. Gines P, Arroyo V, Vargas V, et al: Paracentesis with intravenous infusion of albumin as compared with peritoneovenous shunting in cirrhosis with refractory ascites. N Engl J Med 325:829–835, 1991.
4. Gonwa TA, Morris CA, Goldstein RM, et al: Long-term survival and renal function following liver transplantation in patients with and without hepatorenal syndrome-experience in 300 patients. Transplantation 51:428–430, 1991.
5. Iwatsuki S, Popovtzer MM, Corman JL, et al: Recovery from "hepatorenal syndrome" after orthotopic liver transplantation. N Engl J Med 289:1155–1159, 1973.
6. Koppel MH, Coburn JW, Mims MM, et al: Transplantation of cadaveric kidneys from patients with hepatorenal syndrome. Evidence for the functional nature of renal failure in advanced liver disease. N Engl J Med 280:1367–1371, 1969.
7. Papadakis MA, Arieff AI: Unpredictability of clinical evaluation of renal function in cirrhosis. Prospective study. Am J Med 82:945–952, 1987.
8. Schelling JR, Linas SL: Hepatorenal syndrome. Semin Nephrol 10:565–570, 1990.
9. Suzuki H, Stanley AJ: Current management and novel therapeutic strategies for refractory ascites and hepatorenal syndrome. Q J Med 94:293–300, 2001.
10. Wong F, Blendis L: New challenge of hepatorenal syndrome: Prevention and treatment. Hepatology 34:1242–1251, 2001.

# 13. OBSTRUCTIVE UROPATHY

*Lavinia A. Negrea, M.D.*

### 1. What is obstructive uropathy?

Obstructive uropathy refers to structural or functional interference with normal urine flow anywhere along the urinary tract from the renal tubule to the urethra. Depending on the underlying disease process, obstruction may involve one or both kidneys. Obstruction of both kidneys generally results in some degree of renal failure.

### 2. What are the most common causes of obstructive uropathy?

The causes of obstructive uropathy vary with age and gender. In children, congenital abnormalities such as ureteropelvic junction obstruction (both sexes) and posterior urethral valves (boys) are the most common causes. Nephrolithiasis is the most common cause of obstructive uropathy in young men. In young women, the most common cause of obstruction is pregnancy, although this form of obstructive uropathy is rarely clinically significant. In the elderly, benign and malignant tumors emerge as important causes of obstructive uropathy, especially benign hypertrophy and carcinoma of the prostate in men and ovarian cancer in women.

### 3. How does pregnancy cause obstructive uropathy?

Ureteral dilatation may be seen as early as the first trimester and probably reflects the hormonal effect of progesterone on ureteral peristalsis. In late pregnancy, ureteral dilatation has been attributed to pressure by the gravid uterus on the pelvic brim. The right ureter is more often affected than the left.

### 4. What is functional obstructive uropathy?

This term generally refers to neurologic disorders that affect the neuromuscular activity of the urinary tract. Functional disorders include adynamic ureteral segments, vesicoureteric reflux., spastic bladder (upper motor neuron lesion), and atonic bladder (lower motor neuron lesions). Bladder dysfunction is very common in multiple sclerosis, spinal cord injuries, diabetes mellitus, and cerebrovascular accidents. These conditions lead to impaired bladder emptying and functional obstruction. Medications such as levodopa and anticholinergics also can cause decreased bladder tone and contractility.

### 5. What changes in renal blood flow occur during obstruction?

An increase in renal blood flow to more than 40% above normal occurs within a few minutes of ureteral occlusion and is due to a decrease in renal vascular resistance. This effect is mediated by the local production of prostacyclin and prostaglandin $E_2$. In later stages of obstruction, renal blood flow decreases sharply below normal. Angiotensin II and thromboxane mediate this vasoconstrictive phase.

### 6. Why does the GFR decrease during obstruction?

Early in obstruction, intrarenal tubular pressure proximal to the obstruction increases. The net glomerular filtration pressure (which equals glomerular filtration pressure minus intratubular pressure) then decreases, and GFR subsequently decreases. In later stages of obstruction, the GFR decreases because of the decrease in renal blood flow.

### 7. Does the GFR improve after the relief of obstruction?

The degree of improvement in GFR is influenced by the duration of obstruction. Normal renal function can be restored if the obstruction is corrected within 1 week. Approximately 20% of the GFR can be recovered after 4 weeks. Little or no recovery is expected after 6–8 weeks of continuous and complete obstruction.

### 8. What happens to urine output in obstructive uropathy?

Urine output varies from anuria (in complete obstruction) to significant degrees of polyuria. Polyuria is sometimes observed in patients with partial or incomplete obstruction. It represents a form of nephrogenic diabetes insipidus resulting from a concentrating defect that may be mediated by the direct effects of increased tubular pressure on the function of distal renal tubular cells.

### 9. Is pain always present in obstructive uropathy?

Pain due to obstruction is caused by distention of the collecting system. Its intensity is a reflection of the rapidity rather than the degree of obstruction. Acute blockage of the ureter may be associated with excruciating pain, whereas slowly developing obstruction may be completely painless.

### 10. What electrolyte abnormalities are associated with obstructive uropathy?

Obstructive uropathy often is associated with hyperkalemia and metabolic acidosis. Defects in the excretion of potassium or hydrogen sometimes reflect a state of resistance to mineralocorticoids such as aldosterone.

### 11. What is the most common complication of obstructive uropathy?

Urinary tract infection is by far the most common complication and results, at least partly, from decreased bacterial washout in the face of reduced urine flow. Eradication of infection is difficult as long as obstruction persists. As a corollary, relief of obstruction is critical to management of an infection.

### 12. What mechanisms account for hypertension in obstructive uropathy?

In chronic bilateral ureteral obstruction, hypertension is generally secondary to renal failure and extracellular fluid volume expansion. In acute unilateral obstruction, increased renin secretion is usually responsible for the hypertension.

### 13. What is postobstructive diuresis?

Postobstructive diuresis may occur from 2 to 8 days following relief of obstruction. It usually occurs after one has relieved sudden, complete obstruction and is often brief in duration. The diuresis is caused by an expanded extracellular fluid volume, an osmotic diuresis resulting from rapid elimination of retained solutes, and a transient concentrating defect in the distal nephron resulting from the mechanical effects of high intratubular pressure. Iatrogenic contributions include excessive volume replacement, particularly with isotonic solutions containing glucose or NaCl.

### 14. What are the merits and the limitations of the renal ultrasound in diagnosing obstruction?

Ultrasound is a noninvasive diagnostic test used initially in suspected obstruction. The main findings vary depending on the site of obstruction but can include dilation of the ureters or renal collecting systems. False-negative tests can occur, rarely, as a consequence of dehydration, recent onset of obstruction (within the first 1–3 days, when the collecting system is relatively noncompliant), encasement of the collecting system by retroperitoneal fibrosis (idiopathic, drug-related, postradiation), or tumors.

**15. What are the advantages and disadvantages of an intravenous pyelogram in diagnosing obstructive uropathy?**

Intravenous pyelography can identify both the presence and the location of obstruction. It is considered the procedure of choice in acute obstruction due to kidney stones. In patients with multiple renal cysts, it is superior to ultrasound in distinguishing hydronephrosis from parapelvic renal cysts. With increasing degrees of azotemia, the ability of intravenous pyelography to delineate the collecting system diminishes, and the risk of acute renal failure from exposure to radiocontrast increases.

**16. What is the role of computed tomography (CT) scans in diagnosing obstruction?**

The CT scan is an accurate technique for detection of urinary tract dilatation and is particularly helpful in identifying lesions extrinsic to the collecting system. However, administration of intravenous contrast often is required. The value of noncontrast helical (spiral) CT in the evaluation of obstruction is currently being investigated.

**17. When is retrograde pyelography indicated in the diagnosis of obstructive uropathy?**

Retrograde pyelography is used to diagnose an obstruction when other imaging techniques yield equivocal results, in patients with poor renal function, and in patients who are allergic to radiocontrast dye.

**18. What is a "furosemide renogram"?**

A furosemide renogram is a radionuclide study in which images of the kidney are obtained before and after administration of the diuretic. By exaggerating urine flow, the study may demonstrate obstructive uropathy when other studies are equivocal. Loop diuretics other than furosemide can probably be employed with comparable results.

**19. What percentage of end-stage renal disease is due to obstructive nephropathy?**

Obstructive nephropathy accounts for approximately 2% of all of the patients with end-stage renal disease.

BIBLIOGRAPHY

1. Klahr S: Obstructive nephropathy. Kidney Int 54:286–300, 1998.
2. Klahr S: Obstructive nephropathy. In Jacobson HR, Striker GE, Klahr S (eds): The Principles and Practice of Nephrology. St. Louis, Mosby, 1991, pp 432–457.
3. Korbet SM: Obstructive uropathy. In Greenberg A (ed): Primer on Kidney Diseases, 2nd ed. San Diego, Academic Press, 1998, pp 348–356.
4. Schlueter W, Battle DC: Chronic obstructive nephropathy. Semin Nephrol 8:17–28, 1988.
5. Yarger WE, Harris RH: Urinary tract obstruction. In Seldin DW, Giebisch G (eds): The Kidney: Physiology and Pathophysiology. New York, Raven Press, 1985, pp 1963–1978.

# 14. ASYMPTOMATIC PROTEINURIA AND HEMATURIA

*Jeffrey R. Schelling, M.D.*

### 1. How is asymptomatic proteinuria defined?

Urine protein excretion usually ranges between 40 and 80 mg per day, but most laboratories define 150 mg per day as the upper limit of normal. Asymptomatic proteinuria is urinary protein excretion greater than 150 mg, but less than 3.5 gm per day, not associated with symptoms or signs of the nephrotic syndrome (edema, hypoalbuminemia, hyperlipidemia, thrombotic complications). Despite the broad range of urinary protein excretion included in this definition, patients with asymptomatic proteinuria characteristically excrete less than 1 gm of protein per day. In general, the clinical conditions associated with asymptomatic proteinuria are of less serious consequence than those associated with the nephrotic syndrome.

### 2. Is the dipstick examination a reliable measurement of urine protein excretion?

Under most circumstances, it is. However, there are certain exceptions that should be considered. First, urine dipsticks most reliably measure albumin, but even albumin is not consistently detectable until the concentration exceeds 20–30 mg/dl. Second, the dipstick exam is not useful for the detection of globulins, mucoproteins, and Bence Jones proteins. Finally, dipstick detection of protein provides only a semiquantitative assessment of proteinuria. A given protein concentration in a dilute urine reflects much greater protein excretion than does the same protein concentration in a concentrated urine. Therefore, the dipstick protein concentration should be assessed in the context of the urine specific gravity, which can be measured simultaneously during a routine urinalysis. Even normal amounts of urinary protein can register as 1+ on a dipstick if the urine is highly concentrated (specific gravity > 1.025).

### 3. What are the most reliable methods for quantitative measurement of urinary protein excretion?

The traditional method is a 24-hour urine collection for measurement of total protein. This assay should always be accompanied by measurement of the urine creatinine concentration to assess the adequacy of the urine collection. Women with normal muscle mass excrete approximately 15–20 mg creatinine/kg body weight/day, whereas men with normal muscle mass excrete about 20–25 mg creatinine/kg body weight/day. Because elderly patient have decreased muscle mass and creatinine excretion, normal age-adjusted creatinine excretion values are 23 – (age/6) mg creatinine/kg body weight/day for women and 28 – (age/6) mg creatinine/kg body weight/day for men. Values significantly less than these, regardless of the urine volume, indicate an inadequate urine collection, which will result in spuriously depressed estimates of urine protein excretion. Urine protein excretion can also be reliably estimated from a spot urine sample by determining the ratio of urine protein (mg/dl) to urine creatinine (mg/dl) (see Chapter 4, Measurement of Urinary Protein).

### 4. What is glomerular permselectivity?

Glomerular permselectivity refers to a property of the glomerular capillary membrane whereby solutes, including proteins, are restricted from passage across the capillary wall into the urinary space. Exclusion of a protein from Bowman's space is based to some extent on its molecular size and conformation, but mostly results from its net negative charge. Negatively charged proteins are excluded from the glomerular ultrafiltrate due to their inability to pass through the negatively charged endothelial cells, glomerular capillary basement membrane, and surrounding endothelial cells, as well as epithelial structures that comprise the slit diaphragm.

### 5. What are the common causes of asymptomatic proteinuria?

In contrast to nephrotic-range proteinuria, which is almost invariably due to glomerular disease, asymptomatic proteinuria may result from glomerular or tubular disorders. Glomerular proteinuria tends to be associated with excretion of high–molecular weight proteins, such as albumin and globulins, whereas tubular proteinuria characteristically involves excretion of smaller proteins as well. Some of the most common causes of each type of asymptomatic proteinuria are listed below:

| GLOMERULAR | TUBULAR |
| --- | --- |
| Functional proteinuria | Hereditary (Fanconi syndrome, Wilson's disease) |
| Orthostatic proteinuria | Chronic $K^+$ depletion |
| Early glomerular disease | Acute tubular necrosis |
| | Analgesic nephropathy |
| | Heavy metal toxicity (e.g., cadmium) |
| | Pyelonephritis |
| | Overflow proteinuria |

### 6. What is functional proteinuria?

Functional proteinuria is transient protein excretion that is associated with a number of clinical conditions including fever, strenuous exercise, emotional stress, and congestive heart failure. The mechanism of increased protein excretion in these conditions is related, in part, to decreased renal plasma flow, which has been shown to facilitate albumin excretion. In conditions associated with high circulating levels of angiotensin II (e.g., heart failure, renovascular hypertension), proteinuria may be mediated by direct effects of angiotensin II on glomerular permselectivity.

### 7. What is orthostatic proteinuria?

Orthostatic or postural proteinuria is a condition in which patients excrete excess urine protein only when in the upright position. Orthostatic proteinuria occurs almost exclusively in young men and usually does not exceed 1 gm per 24 hours. To make a diagnosis, patients should be instructed to collect urine beginning in the morning and ending at bedtime (~ 16-hour collection). A second collection is then started at night and continued until the following morning (~ 8-hour collection). Both samples are then assayed for total protein, and values are extrapolated to 24 hours. A diagnosis of orthostatic proteinuria is made if the daytime (upright) protein excretion is elevated and the nighttime (recumbent) protein excretion is normal. If the protein content in both collections is increased, the patient has *persistent proteinuria,* which usually indicates the presence of structural glomerular or tubular renal disease. Long-term follow-up studies have revealed that the majority of patients with orthostatic proteinuria do not have associated glomerular pathology and exhibit spontaneous resolution of proteinuria over 5–10 years.

### 8. What is overflow proteinuria?

Overflow or overproduction proteinuria is a clinical condition in which the plasma concentration of filtered protein exceeds tubular reabsorptive capacity. Overflow proteinuria is most commonly associated with paraproteinemias, such as multiple myeloma, monoclonal gammopathy, or light chain disease. Although the mechanism of proteinuria is primarily increased filtration rather than a specific glomerular defect, paraproteinemias can be associated with glomerular diseases such as light chain nephropathy or amyloidosis, which can then lead to subsequent glomerular proteinuria.

### 9. How does tubular disease lead to abnormal proteinuria?

Despite glomerular permselectivity, small amounts of protein normally are filtered at the glomerulus. However, most of the filtered protein is subsequently reabsorbed and catabolized by proximal tubular epithelial cells. In the presence of injured or diseased tubules, the capacity for protein reabsorption may be compromised, and much of the filtered protein load is excreted, rather than reabsorbed. Furthermore, some proteins, such as Tamm-Horsfall proteins, are actually produced by tubular epithelial cells.

### 10. Define asymptomatic hematuria.

Hematuria can be either gross (obvious by visual inspection) or microscopic (detectable only by dipstick or microscopic examination) and may be associated with pain (e.g., in patients with infections, stones, or neoplasms). The term *asymptomatic hematuria* generally refers to painless hematuria that is usually, but not always, microscopic. In large cross-sectional studies, the prevalence of asymptomatic hematuria ranges from 2.5% to 13%.

### 11. How is a urinalysis performed to optimize detection of hematuria?

First, the voided specimen should be analyzed relatively soon after collection.
- A dipstick examination is conducted prior to centrifugation of the sample. The threshold for detection of red blood cells by dipstick is 3–5 cells per high-power (40X magnification) field.
- At least 10 ml is mildly centrifuged (1000–2000 rpm, 2–5 min) to avoid destruction of casts.
- The supernatant is then poured off, and the pellet is resuspended in the remaining ~ 0.5 ml of urine.
- A drop of this suspension is then placed on a glass microscope slide and covered with a glass coverslip.
- A thorough search for red blood cells is then made using the 40X magnification objective lens.

Under normal circumstances, there should be fewer than 3–5 red blood cells per field. Discovery of more than 3–5 cells per field on at least two separate examinations warrants further investigation.

### 12. What are some causes of a false-positive dipstick reading for blood in the urine?

One should be suspicious of a false-positive dipstick for hematuria whenever the dipstick is positive and red blood cells are not visualized on microscopic examination. Conditions that lead to a false-positive dipstick for blood include exposure to certain:
- Foods: beets, food dyes, high concentrations of vitamin C
- Drugs: ibuprofen, sulfamethoxazole, nitrofurantoin, rifampin, phenytoin, L-dopa, quinine, phenazopyridine (Pyridium)
- Red blood cell components: bile pigments, myoglobin, hemoglobin, porphyrins

Although not technically a false-positive result, a urinalysis performed on a specimen obtained during menstruation may lead to the false conclusion that hematuria is present. Therefore, vigilance is required in the interpretation of urinalyses in women of childbearing age.

## 13. What are the common causes of asymptomatic hematuria?

*Differential Diagnosis of Asymptomatic Hematuria*

| SYSTEMIC CAUSES | UPPER TRACT (KIDNEY) DISORDERS | LOWER TRACT DISORDERS |
|---|---|---|
| Fever | Vascular: infarction, embolism, venous | Stones |
| Strenuous exercise | thrombosis, arteriovenous malformation, | Tumors |
| Coagulopathies | vasculitis | Infections |
| Hemolytic disorders | Glomerular: IgA nephropathy, post- | Trauma |
| Factitious (e.g., | infectious glomerulonephritis, proliferative | Vascular |
| menstrual blood) | glomerulonephritis, thin basement | malformations |
| | membrane disease, lupus nephritis, | Endometriosis |
| | Henoch-Schönlein purpura, Goodpasture's | |
| | syndrome, Alport syndrome, Fabry's | |
| | disease | |
| | Tubulointerstitial: acute interstitial nephritis, | |
| | pyelonephritis, cystic diseases, sickle cell | |
| | nephropathy | |

## 14. What diagnostic clues help to differentiate upper and lower tract disease?

Upper tract disease is usually asymptomatic, but associated respiratory, gastrointestinal, or skin infections may suggest IgA nephropathy or postinfectious or proliferative glomerulonephritis. Infectious or toxic exposures have been associated with glomerular and interstitial inflammation. A family history of hematuria is suggestive for Alport syndrome (particularly if accompanied by neurosensory deafness and ocular defects) or polycystic kidney disease. In patients who have asymptomatic *gross* hematuria, the portion of the urinary stream in which hematuria is observed may provide a clue to the site of lower tract disease. Blood in the initial stream is characteristic of urethral or male genital lesions. Blood at the end of the stream is most commonly observed with bladder pathology.

## 15. What is the significance of blood clots within the urinary tract?

A blood clot within the urinary tract is merely a sign of large amounts of bleeding. In general, urinary blood clots are observed with lower tract disease and are exceedingly rare with glomerular diseases. The presence of blood clots is not dangerous unless they obstruct urinary outflow.

## 16. What is the appropriate work-up for a patient with asymptomatic hematuria?

As previously mentioned, hematuria should be confirmed by at least two separate urinalyses. Although infectious causes generally present as symptomatic hematuria, a urine culture should be performed routinely to rule out an infectious etiology. If the urine culture is negative and the presence of red blood cell casts, proteinuria, or dysmorphic red cells is noted, a diagnosis of glomerular disease is suggested, and a renal biopsy should be considered (see below). In the absence of such findings, a reasonable approach would include renal ultrasound to evaluate for tumors and cysts and urologic consultation for cystoscopy. Positive findings from these examinations would dictate further work-up, which might include additional radiologic imaging. In the setting of negative renal ultrasound and cystoscopic examinations, an argument could be made to proceed with a renal biopsy.

## 17. Should patients be routinely screened for hematuria?

Several large cross-sectional studies demonstrate a finite yield of urinary tract diseases from urine dipstick screening for hematuria. In particular, cases of urinary tract malignancies have been detected by such screening. For this reason, some studies recommend dip-stick screening for patients older than 60 years of age. However, the cost-effectiveness of this screening strategy has not been determined. There are no data regarding the value of screening for hematuria to detect occult renal disease.

## 18. Should a patient with asymptomatic proteinuria or hematuria undergo a diagnostic renal biopsy?

Under most circumstances, a renal biopsy is not necessary. However, if the proteinuria is persistent, a biopsy may be warranted, particularly (1) if the glomerular filtration rate is decreased, (2) if there is some clinical suspicion that the patient may have an undiagnosed systemic disease that may be causing the proteinuria (e.g., multiple myeloma, systemic lupus erythematosus), (3) if there is reasonable evidence that the biopsy will yield a diagnosis for which there is definitive treatment, or (4) to reassure the patient that the anticipated clinical course is benign. Asymptomatic hematuria is also not an absolute indication for a diagnostic renal biopsy, particularly because risk/benefit and cost-effectiveness studies have not been conducted. However, most nephrologists would probably recommend a renal biopsy in patients with persistent hematuria, particularly in the setting of declining glomerular filtration rate or concomitant proteinuria.

### BIBLIOGRAPHY

1. Ahmed Z, Lee J: Asymptomatic urinary abnormalities: Hematuria and proteinuria. Med Clin North Am 81:641–652, 1997.
2. Britton JP, Dowell AC, Whelan P, Harris CM: A community study of bladder cancer screening by the detection of occult urinary bleeding. J Urol 148:788–790, 1992.
3. Corwin HL: Urinalysis. In Schrier RW, Gottschalk CW (eds): Diseases of the Kidney, 6th ed. Boston, Little, Brown, 1997, pp 298–299.
4. Galla JH: Approach to the patient with hematuria. In Kelley WN (ed): Textbook of Internal Medicine, 4th ed. Philadelphia, Lippincott Williams & Wilkins, 2000, pp 1095–1098.
5. Ginsberg JM, Chang BS, Matarese RA, Garella S: Use of single voided urine samples to estimate quantitative proteinuria. N Engl J Med 309:1543–1546, 1983.
6. Kasiske BL, Keane WF: Laboratory assessment of renal disease: Clearance, urinalysis, and renal biopsy. In Brenner BM (ed): The Kidney, 6th ed. Philadelphia, W.B. Saunders, 2000, pp 1129–1170.
7. Kaysen GA: Proteinuria and the nephrotic syndrome. In Schrier RW (ed): Renal and Electrolyte Disorders, 5th ed. Boston, Little, Brown, 1997, pp 640–684.
8. Oberhauer R, Haas M, Mayer G: Proteinuria as a consequence of altered glomerular permselectivity: Clinical implications. Clin Nephrol 46:357–361, 1996.
9. Ritchie CD, Bevan EA, Collier SJ: Importance of occult hematuria found at screening. Br Med J 292:681–683, 1986.
10. Schelling JR, Sedor JR: Approach to the patient with proteinuria and nephrotic syndrome. In Kelley WN (ed): Textbook of Internal Medicine, 4th ed. Philadelphia, Lippincott Williams & Wilkins, 2000, pp 1098–1104.
11. Topham PS, Harper SJ, Furness PN, et al: Glomerular disease as a cause of isolated microscopic haematuria. Q J Med 87:329–335, 1994.
12. Wingo CS, Clapp WL: Proteinuria: Potential causes and approach to evaluation. Am J Med Sci 320:188–194, 2000.

# 15.  ACUTE GLOMERULONEPHRITIS

*Ronald Flauto*, D.O.

### 1. What are the clinical characteristics of acute glomerulonephritis?

Classically, the clinical syndrome of acute glomerulonephritis is characterized by the presence of hematuria, hypertension, edema, azotemia, and non–nephrotic-range proteinuria (< 3.0 gm of proteinuria per day). In severe cases, patients present with acute renal failure manifested by oliguria or severe renal insufficiency. Patients with acute glomerulonephritis are usually asymptomatic at presentation. However, those with severe cases may present with edema, signs or symptoms of uremia, or malignant hypertension.

### 2. What is clinically significant hematuria?

On microscopic examination of a centrifuged urine specimen, the finding of more than three red blood cells per high power field is considered to be clinically significant (see Chapter 14, Asymptomatic Proteinuria and Hematuria).

### 3. What criteria aid in differentiating glomerular hematuria from hematuria of non-glomerular origin?
- Red blood cell casts in the urine
- Dysmorphic red blood cells in the urine
- Proteinuria associated with red cells in the urine

### 4. Can the urinary sediment be helpful in diagnosing acute glomerulonephritis?

Yes. The urine sediment of patients with acute glomerulonephritis generally contains dysmorphic (crenated) red blood cells, red cell casts, or heme-pigmented casts. Urinary casts are detectable in 50–80% of cases. In contrast, the urine from patients with nephrotic syndrome rarely contains casts.

### 5. What laboratory tests aid in the diagnosis of glomerulonephritis?

Laboratory tests can aid in classifying the underlying condition, occasionally obviating the need for a biopsy. However, the sensitivity, specificity, and predictive value of such laboratory tests must always be kept in mind. Some commonly ordered tests are shown in the table.

| TEST | COMMENT |
| --- | --- |
| Antinuclear antibody | If positive, should confirm SLE with anti-dsDNA antibody or anti-Smith antibody |
| ANCA | c-ANCA more often positive in Wegener's granulomatosis; p-ANCA more often positive in microscopic polyarteritis |
| Anti-GBM antibody | Directed at the Goodpasture antigen within type IV collagen of the basement membrane |
| Complement levels | See question 11 |
| Blood cultures | To rule out infectious diseases such as endocarditis |
| Hepatitis B and C serologies | May be positive even with normal liver function tests |
| Cryoglobulins | Most often present in association with hepatitis C |

SLE = systemic lupus erythematosus; ANCA = antineutrophilic cytoplasmic antibody; GBM = glomerular basement membrane.

**6. What are the histologic features of acute glomerulonephritis?**

The hallmarks of acute glomerulonephritis are glomerular inflammation mediated by infiltrating inflammatory cells and proliferation of resident mesangial, epithelial, or endothelial cells. In severe cases, extensive inflammation and proliferation can cause rupture of the glomerulus into Bowman's space resulting in crescent formation. Renal prognosis is poor when more than 50% of glomeruli are affected by crescent formation (see Chapter 16, Rapidly Progressive Glomerulonephritis).

Most renal pathology associated with acute glomerulonephritis is proliferative in character. In contrast, nonproliferative renal lesions tend to present clinically as nephrotic syndrome. Cellular proliferation within the kidney can be classified as either **focal** (involving a small percentage of glomeruli) or **diffuse** (involving the majority of glomeruli). As might be suspected, diffuse proliferative glomerulonephritis is associated with a poor renal prognosis when compared to focal glomerulonephritis.

**7. What causes inflammation within the glomerulus?**

Both humoral and cell-mediated immunity play a role in the pathogenesis of glomerular inflammation. In humoral immunity, antibodies can bind to glomerular antigens within the glomerular basement membrane (as in Goodpasture's syndrome) or to circulating antigens that become trapped within the glomerulus. In addition, circulating antigen-antibody complexes can become deposited within the glomerulus. T lymphocytes have been identified in the renal parenchyma of patients with glomerulonephritis and support a role for cell-mediated immunity. Inflammatory mediators from infiltrating inflammatory cells or from resident glomerular cells also play a role in the pathogenesis of acute glomerulonephritis.

**8. What are the primary causes of acute proliferative glomerulonephritis?**

Mesangioproliferative glomerulonephritis
    IgA (immunoglobulin A) nephropathy
    IgM nephropathy
    Idiopathic
Membranoproliferative glomerulonephritis

**9. List the secondary causes of proliferative glomerulonephritis.**

- Postinfectious glomerulonephritis
- Lupus nephritis
- Glomerulonephritis secondary to hepatitis B or C
- Vasculitis (Wegener's granulomatosis, polyarteritis nodosa, Henoch-Schönlein purpura)

**10. What is the most common cause of glomerulonephritis worldwide?**

IgA nephropathy.

**11. What is the role of complement in the pathogenesis and diagnosis of glomerulonephritis?**

Many of the glomerulonephritides are associated with complement activation and hypocomplementemia. Activation of the alternative complement pathway results in low levels of circulating C3 and normal levels of C4. Activation of the classic pathway yields low levels of both C3 and C4. Activation of either pathway may lead to recruitment of inflammatory cells or to direct tissue injury. The glomerular diseases most commonly associated with complement abnormalities are shown in the table.

| DISEASE | C3 | C4 |
|---|---|---|
| Postinfectious glomerulonephritis | Low | Low or normal |
| Membranoproliferative glomerulonephritis | Low | Low or normal |
| Lupus nephritis | Low | Low |
| Cryoglobulinemia | Low | Low |
| Subacute bacterial endocarditis | Low or normal | Low |

## 12. What is the treatment for acute glomerulonephritis?

The treatment for acute glomerulonephritis depends on the underlying etiology of the renal disease. In some cases (e.g., poststreptococcal glomerulonephritis), therapy is supportive and focuses on management of the accompanying edema and hypertension. In contrast, patients with diffuse proliferative glomerulonephritis secondary to lupus may require aggressive treatment with steroids and cytotoxic drugs to prolong renal survival. For most of the mesangioproliferative glomerulonephritides, curative therapies are lacking.

### BIBLIOGRAPHY

1. Cibrik DM, Sedor JR: Immunopathogenesis of renal disease. In Greenberg A (ed): Primer on Kidney Diseases, 2nd ed. San Diego, Academic Press, 1998, pp 141–149.
2. Couser WG: Glomerulonephritis. Lancet 353:1509–1515, 1999.
3. Glassock RJ, Cohen AH: The primary glomerulonephropathies. Dis Mon 42:329–383, 1996.
4. Hricik DE, Chung-Park M, Sedor JR: Glomerulonephritis. N Engl J Med 339:888–899, 1998.
5. Jennette JC, Falk RJ: Glomerular clinicopathologic syndromes. In Greenberg A (ed): Primer on Kidney Diseases, 2nd ed. San Diego, Academic Press, 1998, pp 127–141.
6. Madaio MP, Harrington JT: The diagnosis of glomerular disease: Acute glomerulonephritis and the nephrotic syndrome. Arch Intern Med 161:25–34, 2001.

# 16. RAPIDLY PROGRESSIVE GLOMERULONEPHRITIS

*John R. Sedor, M.D.*

### 1. Define rapidly progressive glomerulonephritis (RPGN).

Patients with RPGN have evidence of glomerular disease (proteinuria, hematuria, and red cell casts) accompanied by rapid loss of renal function over days to weeks. If untreated, RPGN often results in renal failure. The pathologic hallmark of RPGN is the presence of crescents on kidney biopsy. Fortunately, the disorders associated with this syndrome are rare, so that rapidly progressive glomerulonephritis makes up only 2–4% of all cases of glomerulonephritis.

### 2. What are crescents?

Crescent formation is a nonspecific response to severe injury of the glomerular capillary wall. As a result, fibrin leaks into Bowman's space, causing parietal epithelial cells to proliferate and mononuclear phagocytes to migrate into the glomerular tuft from the circulation (see figure). Large crescents can compress glomerular capillaries and impair filtration. Although crescent formation can resolve, other chemotactic signals recruit fibroblasts, which ultimately may cause both the crescents and entire glomeruli to scar. Extensive scarring results in end-stage renal disease.

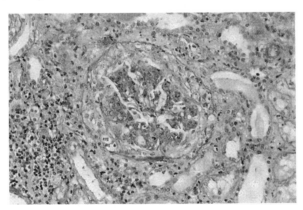

Micrograph from a patient with rapidly progressive glomerulonephritis showing a large crescent with a compressed glomerular capillary tuft. (From Hricik DE, Chung-Park M, Sedor JR: Glomerulonephritis. N Engl J Med 339:888–899, 1998, with permission.)

### 3. Do crescentic nephritis and RPGN describe the same disease process?

Although the terms *crescentic nephritis* and *RPGN* are used interchangeably, these diagnoses are not synonymous. RPGN describes a *clinical* syndrome of rapid loss of renal function over days to weeks in patients with evidence of glomerulonephritis. In contrast, crescentic nephritis is a *histopathologic* description of kidney biopsy specimens that demonstrate the presence of crescents in more than 50% of glomeruli. Biopsies of patients with RPGN very commonly reveal crescentic nephritis. However, RPGN can occur in the absence of crescentic nephritis, and extensive glomerular crescent formation rarely is identified in kidney biopsy specimens from patients without the clinical syndrome of RPGN.

### 4. How is primary RPGN classified?

RPGN can occur as a primary disorder in the absence of other glomerular or systemic diseases and is classified pathologically into three types using immunofluorescence microscopy to describe the presence or absence of immune deposits and their character. **Type I RPGN** is characterized by linear deposition of immunoglobulin along the glomerular basement membrane (GBM) and is found in approximately 20% of patients with primary RPGN without pulmonary hemorrhage. Granular immune complex deposition is detected in an additional 30% of patients with **type II RPGN**. The remaining patients have **type III RPGN** and no immune deposits (pauci-immune) are detectable in glomeruli.

### 5. What diseases are associated with RPGN ("secondary RPGN")?

RPGN can complicate the clinical course of some primary glomerular diseases such as IgA nephropathy, membranous nephropathy, membranoproliferative glomerulonephritis, and hereditary nephritis (Alport syndrome). In addition, RPGN is associated with infectious and multisystem diseases including systemic lupus erythematosus, cryoglobulinemia, and system vasculitides. The table below provides an overview of the classification of RPGN but is not intended to be exhaustive.

*Classification of RPGN*

| PRIMARY | SECONDARY |
|---|---|
| **Type I**: Anti-GBM antibody disease (Goodpasture's disease) | Superimposed on a primary glomerular disease |
| | Postinfectious |
| **Type II**: Granular glomerular immune complex association |     Poststreptococcal glomerulonephritis |
| |     Visceral abscess |
| **Type III**: Pauci-immune glomerulonephritis | Vasculitic |
| |     Small vessel |
| |         Microscopic polyangiitis |
| |         Wegener's granulomatosis |
| |         Churg-Strauss syndrome |
| |         Systemic lupus erythematosus |
| |         Henoch-Schönlein purpura |
| |         Cryoglobulinemia |
| |     Medium vessel |
| |         Polyarteritis nodosa |
| | Goodpasture's syndrome |
| | Carcinoma |
| | Medication-associated |
| |     Allopurinol |
| |     Penicillamine |

### 6. Describe the clinical manifestations of RPGN.

Unless complicated by systemic disease, RPGN is characterized by an insidious onset of generalized fatigue and malaise. Hematuria with dysmorphic red blood cells and red cell casts is usually detected on urinalysis. Moderate proteinuria, usually in the non-nephrotic range, is typical. Nephrotic-range proteinuria occurs in less than 30% of patients. Mild to severe azotemia is universally present.

**7. Aside from urinalysis, which other laboratory tests are useful in defining the etiology of RPGN?**

Certain serologic studies may be useful in narrowing the differential diagnosis. Complement levels (C3, C4) are usually normal in patients with either primary RPGN or RPGN associated with systemic disease, although patients with underlying systemic lupus erythematosus have depressed circulating C3 and C4 levels. In almost all patients, an antinuclear antibody level is a useful screen for lupus or other connective tissue diseases. Identification of circulating anti-GBM antibodies and antineutrophil cytoplasmic antibody (ANCA) can be useful in establishing a diagnosis in patients who present with RPGN. ANCA-positive patients frequently have a primary small-vessel vasculitis, although disease may be kidney-limited. The patient's clinical presentation also determines the predictive value of ANCA testing. For example, the predictive value of a positive ANCA test is considerably less significant in a patient who presents with hematuria, proteinuria, and a normal creatinine than in a patient with similar urinalysis findings in the presence of azotemia (see Chapter 37, Renal Vasculitis).

**8. What are anti-GBM antibodies?**

Anti-GBM antibodies are targeted toward the NC1 domain of the $\alpha$3 chain of type IV collagen, which is a component of the GBM. Formation of the type IV collagen network in normal GBM sequesters these epitopes from the immune system, preventing development of tolerance during development. Anti-GBM–associated disease probably occurs after the kidney is injured in some manner that exposes regions of the collagen molecule. These cryptic epitopes are not recognized as "self" and generate an immune response. Anti-GBM antibodies are found in approximately 90–95% of patients with Goodpasture's disease. On kidney biopsy, they form linear deposits of immunoglobulin along basement membranes detected by immunofluorescence (see figure).

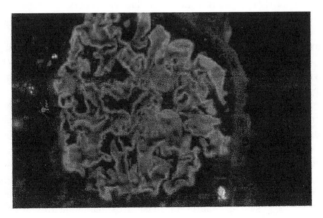

Linear deposition of IgG along the glomerular basement membrane on immunofluorescence microscopy in a patient with circulating antibodies to glomerular basement membrane. (From Hricik DE, Chung-Park M, Sedor JR: Glomerulonephritis. N Engl J Med 339:888–899, with permission.)

**9. Are Goodpasture's syndrome and anti-GBM glomerulonephritis (Goodpasture's disease) the same?**

No. Although both disease entities result from circulating anti-GBM antibodies, **Goodpasture's syndrome** describes a systemic disease with a clinical constellation of pulmonary hemorrhage, circulating anti-GBM antibodies, and glomerulonephritis. Anti-GBM glomerulonephritis, or **Goodpasture's disease**, is kidney-limited and describes a proliferative glomerulonephritis, which results from deposition of anti-GBM antibodies. Anti-GBM antibodies are the same in patients with Goodpasture's syndrome and Goodpasture's disease. Because alveolar basement membrane contains the epitope of type IV collagen that is recognized by anti-GBM antibodies, the variable presence of pulmonary disease seems to reflect whether alveolar basement membrane is accessible to the circulating anti-GBM antibodies. Alveolar injury from infections, smoking, toxins, or other underlying lung disease may predispose the lungs to deposition of anti-GBM antibodies.

**10. What are antineutrophil cytoplasmic antibodies (ANCAs)?**

Renal biopsies from patients with type III RPGN have no immune deposits, but type III RPGN usually results from small-vessel vasculitides associated with circulating ANCA. The ANCA-associated small-vessel vasculitides are Wegener's granulomatosis, microscopic polyangiitis (systemic and renal-limited), and Churg-Strauss syndrome. These are often systemic diseases but can be kidney-limited. ANCAs are directed against neutrophil proteinase 3 (PR3) and myeloperoxidase (MPO). Screening for ANCAs uses an indirect immunofluorescence examination of normal neutrophils, which, if positive, demonstrates a staining pattern characteristic of the target antigen (cytoplasmic for ANCA against PR3 and perinuclear for anti-MPO ANCA). This screening test has low specificity and needs confirmation by enzyme-linked immunosorbent assay (ELISA) for anti-PR3 and anti-MPO antibodies.

**11. What are the treatment options for patients with RPGN?**

RPGN needs to be treated aggressively and early in its course to reduce the likelihood of end-stage renal failure. Glucocorticoids and cyclophosphamide are the mainstays of treatment. The benefit of these agents is particularly great in patients with ANCA-associated vasculitis. The most common complications of therapy for patients with Wegener's granulomatosis or microscopic polyangiitis, who are treated with regimens developed at the National Institutes of Health, are infection and bladder cancers.

**12. Is there any role for plasma exchange in the therapy for RPGN?**

Plasma exchange is thought to remove circulating pathogenic autoantibodies from the circulation. Trials evaluating efficacy of plasma exchange for all causes of RPGN have been small. However, plasma exchange is a safe procedure in experienced centers and may be an appropriate therapeutic modality for subsets of patients with RPGN, in view of the high risk of renal failure with this syndrome. Plasma exchange and immunosuppressive therapy are standard treatments for patients with anti-GBM antibody disease. Most of the evidence supporting the use of plasma exchange in anti-GBM–associated diseases are case reports, although one small randomized, controlled trial demonstrated a nonsignificant trend toward improved outcome in patients treated with plasma exchange. More recently, use of plasma exchange has been included in the therapy of patients with both type 2 and type 3 (ANCA-associated) glomerulonephritis who have presented with renal failure and require dialysis. Case series have suggested a benefit for plasma exchange in this subgroup of RPGN patients, but a small, prospective, multicenter study failed to demonstrate that plasma exchange added any benefit to standard immunosuppressive therapy.

**13. What is the prognosis of RPGN?**

Prognosis and response to treatment in patients with anti-GBM antibody or Goodpasture's disease have not been studied in large trials. Data from a number of small case series with similar, but not identical, treatment strategies suggest that patient survivals are high (70–90%). Overall, only 40% of patients remain off dialysis at 1 year from presentation. However, patients who do not require dialysis at presentation and who are treated with immunosuppression and plasma exchange have 1-year renal survivals of approximately

70–75%, even if renal failure is severe. In contrast, renal survival is poor in patients with anti-GBM antibody–associated disease who require dialysis within 72 hours of presentation. Aggressive therapy with immunosuppressive drugs and plasma exchange may not be appropriate in this subgroup of anti-GBM–antibody patients unless significant acute tubular necrosis in addition to crescentic nephritis is demonstrated on renal biopsy. Clinical, laboratory, and pathologic parameters do not have sufficient predictive value for renal outcome to be used in an individual patient.

Although data on patients with kidney-limited, ANCA-positive RPGN are limited, treatment responses have been reported recently in several cohorts of patients with ANCA-associated necrotizing glomerulonephritis and either Wegener's granulomatosis or microscopic polyangiitis. Many patients (approximately 75%) achieve remission after induction therapy, but only 40–50% remain in long-term remission after 4–10 years. Entry serum creatinine is the strongest predictor of renal survival in ANCA-positive patients. In contrast to patients with anti-GBM glomerulonephritis, patients with ANCA-associated glomerulonephritis can respond to therapy even if they have already required initiation of dialysis.

## BIBLIOGRAPHY

1. Bolton WK: Rapidly progressive glomerulonephritis. Semin Nephrol 16:517–526, 1996.
2. Cibrik DM, Sedor JR: Immunopathogenesis of renal disease. In Greenberg A (ed): Primer on Kidney Diseases, 2nd ed. San Diego, Academic Press, 1998, pp 141–149.
3. Falk RJ, Jennette JC: Anti-neutrophil cytoplasmic autoantibodies with specificity for myeloperoxidase in patients with systemic vasculitis and idiopathic necrotizing and crescentic glomerulonephritis. N Engl J Med 318:1651–1657, 1988.
4. Franssen CF, Stegeman CA, Oost-Kort WW, et al: Determinants of renal outcome in anti-myeloperoxidase-associated necrotizing crescentic glomerulonephritis. J Am Soc Nephrol 9:1915–1923, 1998.
5. Heilman RL, Offord KP, Holley KE, Velosa JA: Analysis of risk factors for patient and renal survival in crescentic glomerulonephritis. Am J Kidney Dis 9:98–107, 1987.
6. Hricik DE, Chung-Park M, Sedor JR: Glomerulonephritis. N Engl J Med 339:888–899, 1998.
7. Jennette JC, Wilkman AS, Falk RJ: Diagnostic predictive value of ANCA serology [editorial; comment]. Kidney Int 53:796–798, 1998
8. Kalluri R, Sun MJ, Hudson BG, Neilson EG: The Goodpasture autoantigen: Structural delineation of two immunologically privileged epitopes of alpha3 (IV) chain of type IV collagen. J Biol Chem 271:9062–9068, 1996.
9. Kerr PG, Lan HY, Atkins RC: Rapidly progressive glomerulonephritis. In Schrier RW, Gottschalk CW (eds): Diseases of the Kidney, 6th ed. Vol. 2. Boston, Little, Brown, 1997, pp 1619–1644.
10. Lal DPSS, O'Donoghue DJ, Haeney M: Effect of diagnostic delay on disease severity and outcome in glomerulonephritis caused by anti-neutrophil cytoplasmic antibodies. J Clin Pathol 49:942–944, 1996.
11. Levy JB, Turner AN, Rees AJ, Pusey CD: Long-term outcome of anti-glomerular basement membrane antibody disease treated with plasma exchange and immunosuppression. Ann Intern Med 134:1033–1042, 2001.
12. Mokrzycki MH, Kaplan AA: Therapeutic plasma exchange: Complications and management. Am J Kidney Dis 23:817–827, 1994.
13. Savige J, Davies D, Falk RJ, Jennette JC, Wiik A: Antineutrophil cytoplasmic antibodies and associated diseases: A review of the clinical and laboratory features. Kidney Int 57:846-862, 2000.
14. Zäner I, Bach D, Braun N, et al: Predictive value of initial histology and effect of plasmapheresis on long-term prognosis of rapidly progressive glomerulonephritis. Am J Kidney Dis 39:28–35, 2002.

# 17. NEPHROTIC SYNDROME

*Ronald Flauto, D.O.*

### 1. What is nephrotic syndrome?

The nephrotic syndrome is characterized by heavy proteinuria (> 3.5 gm per day) and varying degrees of hypoalbuminemia, edema, hyperlipidemia, and lipiduria. Proteinuria develops because the charge or size selectivity of the glomerular capillary wall becomes altered by an underlying glomerular disease (see Chapter 4, Measurement of Urinary Protein). In some cases, humoral and cellular immune responses are involved in altering glomerular permselectivity; in others, degenerative and sclerosing processes are responsible for the proteinuria.

### 2. What is the clinical presentation of patients with nephrotic syndrome?

Some patients are asymptomatic and are diagnosed only when proteinuria is discovered on routine urinalysis. The most common presenting symptom is edema, which can be severe (anasarca). In nephrotic patients, edema tends to be most noticeable in bodily areas where intravascular hydrostatic pressure is highest (e.g., ankles and feet) and where tissue hydrostatic pressure is lowest (e.g., genital tissues and periorbital area). Rarely, patients first present with thromboembolic events such as a pulmonary embolus or renal vein thrombosis. The presence of hypertension, azotemia, and hematuria at the time of presentation is variable and depends greatly on the underlying glomerular histology.

### 3. How does excessive proteinuria cause other features of the nephrotic syndrome?

**Hypoalbuminemia:** Urine protein losses together with tubular absorption and catabolism of filtered plasma proteins combine to overwhelm the synthetic capacity of the liver.

**Edema:** In the "underfill" theory, hypoalbuminemia leads to a reduction in intracapillary oncotic pressure resulting in net movement of fluid into the interstitial space. The subsequent decrease in plasma volume activates the release of renin and aldosterone leading to renal sodium retention that worsens the edema. Recent observations cast doubt on the validity of the underfill hypothesis. In most patients with nephrotic syndrome, plasma volume is normal or elevated. Moreover, renin and aldosterone levels are not uniformly increased. Results of some studies suggest that a defect in renal sodium excretion (overfill theory) is the primary cause of edema in nephrotic syndrome while the reduction in intravascular oncotic pressure promotes edema secondarily.

**Hyperlipidemia:** In response to a decrease in intravascular oncotic pressure, the liver nonspecifically increases its synthesis of a number of proteins including lipoproteins.

**Lipiduria:** Like other proteins, lipoproteins are filtered on the basis of defects in size or charge selectivity of the glomerular capillary membrane.

**Thromboembolism:** The nephrotic syndrome often is associated with a hypercoagulable state that has been attributed to a number of factors including platelet hyperaggregability, increased hepatic synthesis of procoagulant proteins, and urinary losses of anticoagulant factors such as protein S, protein C, and antithrombin III.

### 4. What is an oval fat body?

Oval fat bodies are sometimes seen on microscopic examination of urine from nephrotic patients. They are thought to be sloughed renal tubular cells that are filled with refractile fat droplets that have been reabsorbed from the glomerular filtrate.

## 5. What are the causes of nephrotic syndrome?

The glomerular diseases associated with nephrotic syndrome are generally categorized as either **primary** (idiopathic) or **secondary** to some systemic condition or disease. In children, minimal change disease (see Chapter 22, Minimal Change Disease) accounts for more than 80% of cases of nephrotic syndrome. In adults, the most common causes of idiopathic nephrotic syndrome are shown in the table:

*Idiopathic Nephrotic Syndrome in Adults*

| COMMON CAUSES | SOMETIMES ASSOCIATED WITH NEPHROTIC SYNDROME |
|---|---|
| Membranous nephropathy | IgA (immunoglobulin A) nephropathy |
| Focal segmental glomerulosclerosis | Mesangioproliferative glomerulonephritis |
| Membranoproliferative glomerulonephritis | Fibrillary and immunotactoid glomerulonephritis |
| Minimal change disease | Crescentic glomerulonephritis |

The frequency of the entities listed above is dependent on age and race. In adults over the age of 50 years, membranous nephropathy is the most common cause of idiopathic nephrotic syndrome. African Americans with nephrotic syndrome are more likely to have focal segmental glomerulosclerosis.

## 6. What are the most common causes of secondary nephrotic syndrome?
- Diabetic nephropathy
- Systemic lupus erythematosus
- Amyloidosis
- Human immunodeficiency virus (HIV) infection
- Malignancy (especially lymphoproliferative disorders and cancers of the breast, lung, stomach, and colon)
- Drugs (gold, penicillamine, nonsteroidal anti-inflammatory drugs)

At least 50% of patients with nephrotic syndrome have an identifiable secondary cause. Overall, diabetic nephropathy is the most common cause of nephrotic syndrome.

## 7. What are some pearls to keep in mind regarding the various causes of nephrotic syndrome?

| DISEASE | PEARL |
|---|---|
| Membranous nephropathy | Most common cause of idiopathic nephrotic syndrome in adults |
| Focal segmental glomerulosclerosis | Most common cause of idiopathic nephrotic syndrome in African Americans |
| Minimal change disease | Most common cause of idiopathic nephrotic syndrome in children |
| IgA nephropathy | Most common cause of glomerulonephritis worldwide |
| Diabetic nephropathy | Most common cause of nephrotic syndrome overall |

## 8. What are the key elements of the history to obtain in a patient with nephrotic syndrome?

The history should focus on the presence or absence of a systemic disease. For patients with type 1 diabetes mellitus, eliciting a history of retinopathy is crucial because microvascular disease of the retina often accompanies diabetic nephropathy. The correlation is not as strong in type 2 diabetes, but the absence of retinopathy increases the possibility of a disease other than diabetic nephropathy. Symptoms associated with systemic lupus erythematosus should be investigated, especially in women. Risk factors for infectious diseases such as hepatitis B, hepatitis C, and HIV should be obtained. A complete drug history (including over-the-counter drugs) is mandatory. Finally, appropriate questions regarding symptoms associated with solid tumors should be included.

## 9. Is a detailed laboratory evaluation necessary in all patients with nephrotic syndrome?

In patients with an obvious systemic cause such as diabetes mellitus, a detailed laboratory evaluation is not necessary. In patients without an identifiable cause of nephrotic syndrome, diagnostic studies are often performed to identify a possible systemic disease. These tests often include a complete blood count, antitreponemal antibodies, antinuclear antibodies, complement levels, serum immunoelectrophoresis, urine immunoelectrophoresis, chest x-ray, stool for occult blood, mammogram, and serologic studies for hepatitis B, hepatitis C, and HIV. As noted in Chapter 14, cost-benefit analyses have not been performed to determine whether a wiser strategy might consist of performing a renal biopsy first, followed by a tailored laboratory evaluation based on the observed histology.

## 10. Is renal biopsy necessary in the management of patients with nephrotic syndrome?

In children, renal biopsy is not performed routinely because minimal change disease is the likely diagnosis. Instead, children more often are treated empirically with corticosteroids. Biopsy is reserved for those who do not respond to steroids or who present with atypical clinical features (see Chapter 22, Minimal Change Disease).

In adults, clinical findings alone are frequently inadequate to diagnose the cause of nephrotic syndrome. Although the indications for renal biopsy in nephrotic patients have been the subject of some debate, most nephrologists recommend biopsy for patients with idiopathic nephrotic syndrome. Biopsy usually is not performed when the underlying cause is clinically obvious (e.g., diabetes mellitus, systemic amyloidosis).

## 11. How is the nephrotic syndrome treated?
1. Treatment of the underlying disease (or the secondary cause)
2. Treatment of complications (e.g., edema, hyperlipidemia)
3. Nonspecific treatment of proteinuria

## 12. What are the treatment options for reducing proteinuria in nephrotic patients?

Persistence of heavy proteinuria is a predictor of progression to renal failure; conversely, reduction of urinary protein excretion may improve long-term prognosis. Antiproteinuric measures include:
1. Treatment with angiotensin-converting enzyme (ACE) inhibitors or angiotensin II receptor antagonists
2. Cautious treatment with nonsteroidal anti-inflammatory drugs
3. Dietary protein restriction

The benefit of a low-protein diet is paradoxical. Some patients with nephrotic proteinuria may become frankly catabolic when dietary protein is restricted so this treatment modality also should be employed with caution.

## 13. How are thromboembolic complications treated in patients with nephrotic syndrome?

Anticoagulation (usually a short course of heparin followed by treatment with warfarin [Coumadin]) is recommended for patients with documented thromboembolic events and should be continued for as long as the patient has heavy proteinuria. The benefit of prophylactic anticoagulant or antiplatelet therapy remains controversial.

**14. What diuretics should be used to treat edema in patients with nephrotic syndrome?**

Nephrotic patients sometimes exhibit resistance to commonly available diuretics and frequently require treatment with high doses of loop diuretics (e.g., furosemide, torsemide, bumetanide). Resistance to loop diuretics can be explained by their binding to albumin and other proteins. These drugs enter the lumen of the nephron through active secretion by proximal tubular cells. When heavy proteinuria exists, the secreted drug is bound to protein in the tubular lumen, limiting its availability to bind with receptors in more distant portions of the nephron. Such resistance can be overcome by increasing the dose of the drug. Combinations of loop diuretics and thiazide-like diuretics are often needed to achieve adequate diuresis.

Excessive diuresis may precipitate volume depletion and acute renal failure—a phenomenon most commonly observed in patients with minimal change disease. Combined infusions of albumin and loop diuretics may be required to achieve diuresis in patients with severe hypoalbuminemia.

BIBLIOGRAPHY

1. Brater DC: Diuretic therapy. N Engl J Med 339:387–395, 1998.
2. Cibrik DM, Sedor JR: Immunopathogenesis of renal disease. In Greenberg A (ed): Primer on Kidney Diseases, 2nd ed. San Diego, Academic Press, 1998, pp 141–149.
3. Glassock RJ, Cohen AH: The primary glomerulopathies. Dis Mon 42:329–383, 1996.
4. Hricik DE, Smith MC: Proteinuria and the Nephrotic Syndrome. Chicago, Year Book, 1986.
5. Larson T: Evaluation of proteinuria. Mayo Clin Proc 69:1154–1158, 1994.
6. Madaio MP, Harrington JT: The diagnosis of glomerular disease: Acute glomerulonephritis and the nephrotic syndrome. Arch Intern Med 161:25–34, 2001.
7. Orth SR, Ritz E: The nephrotic syndrome. N Engl J Med 338:1202–1211, 1998.
8. Palmer BF, Alpern RJ: Pathogenesis of edema formation in the nephrotic syndrome. Kidney Int 51(suppl 59):S21–S27, 1997.
9. Schelling JR, Sedor JR: Approach to the patient with proteinuria and nephrotic syndrome. In Kelley WN (ed): Textbook of Internal Medicine, 4th ed. Philadelphia, Lippincott-Raven, 2000, pp 1098–1105.

# 18. NEPHROLITHIASIS

*Miriam F. Weiss, M.D.*

### 1. How common is nephrolithiasis?

Kidney stones are one of the most common medical problems. Renal colic is a frequent cause of hospitalization. In Western countries, 4–10 men and 1–5 women per 1000 people per year will have a symptomatic episode relating to passing a stone. In men, the lifetime prevalence of nephrolithiasis is 10%. The chance of a second stone occurring within 5 years of the first one is 50%.

### 2. What is the chemical composition of kidney stones?

X-ray crystallography and infrared spectrometry can be used to determine the precise composition of a renal stone or fragment. Calcium is the primary ion in 70–80% of renal stones, either as calcium oxalate (~ 60%), calcium phosphate (~ 10%), or a mixture of calcium oxalate and calcium phosphate (~ 10%). Infection or struvite stones are also known as triple phosphate stones. These stones occur in about 10% of cases and contain calcium, magnesium, ammonium, and phosphate. Infection stones often grow to a large size and assume a "staghorn" or antler-like configuration as they fill the renal pelvis. They seldom pass spontaneously. Uric acid is the main constituent of about 10% of stones. Cystine and other substances make up less than 1% of stones.

### 3. How do stones form?

Urine is a complex mixture of many salts in solution. When urine is supersaturated with dissolved ions that can crystallize, nucleation occurs. Often nucleation and growth of the stone take place on the surface of another crystal, such as uric acid—a process known as *epitaxy* (see figure). The nuclei can aggregate into clumps that may adhere to the surface of the urothelium, particularly if there is inflammation or scarring in the urinary collecting system. Reducing the concentration of salts in the urine is the basis of many current medical treatments for nephrolithiasis.

In the majority of the population, stones do not form because of the presence of urinary inhibitor substances, a diverse group of molecules that prevent nucleation even in supersat-

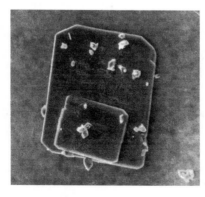

An example of stone growth by epitaxy. Microscopic calcium oxalate crystals have become adherent to the surface of a uric acid crystal. (Scanning electron microscopy X200.)

urated urine. A partial list of these substances includes Tamm-Horsfall protein, uropontin, nephrocalcin, prothrombin F1 peptide, uronic acid-rich proteins, glycosaminoglycans, and citrate. Eventually, medical therapy for nephrolithiasis may focus on enhancing or replacing the function of these molecules.

### 4. Name the disease processes that can result in calcium stone formation.

| DISEASE | MECHANISM |
| --- | --- |
| Primary hyperparathyroidism | ↑ parathyroid hormone (PTH) causes hypercalciuria by ↑ bone resorption and stimulating ↑ renal synthesis of 1,25 dihydroxyvitamin $D_3$ [$1,25(OH)_2D_3$], which results in ↑ gut absorption of calcium |
| Renal tubular acidosis | Acidemia causes release of bone buffers (calcium) and is associated with decreased urinary excretion of citrate<br>Renal tubular acidosis associated with phosphate wasting can result in hypophosphatemia, which is a major stimulus to the ↑ synthesis of $1,25(OH)_2D_3$ |
| Granulomatous disease (e.g., sarcoidosis, tuberculosis) | ↑ extrarenal synthesis of $1,25 (OH)_2D_3$, which results in ↑ gut absorption of calcium |
| Milk-alkali syndrome | ↑ oral intake of calcium-containing antacids |
| Primary/enteric hyperoxaluria secondary to chronic bowel disease | Primary disease or ↑ gut oxalate absorption due to ↑ intestinal permeability to oxalate induced by steatorrhea or bile acids |
| Gout with hyperuricemia | Uric acid crystals precipitate in an acid urine; calcium oxalate crystals nucleate and aggregate on the surface of the uric acid crystals |

### 5. What are the pathophysiologic mechanisms underlying "idiopathic" hypercalciuria?
- Increased intestinal absorption of calcium. The etiology of increased intestinal absorption of calcium may be genetic. Several families with this disorder have been identified. Transient increases in serum calcium after a meal tend to suppress parathyroid hormone (PTH) levels in these patients.
- Increased renal excretion of calcium (renal leak). The renal defect results in a decrease in serum calcium. Eventually secondary hyperparathyroidism develops, which stimulates the renal synthesis of $1,25 (OH)_2D_3$ and causes increased intestinal calcium absorption.

### 6. Which type of stone is radiolucent?
Uric acid stones (see figure at top of next page). Uric acid stones will not be visible on a plain film of the abdomen.

### 7. Do all patients with renal colic require urologic intervention?
Stones smaller than 5 mm in diameter may pass with hydration and medical management of pain. Up to 30% of stones require cystoscopy, extracorporeal shock wave lithotripsy, or surgery.

### 8. List the key aspects of the medical management of acute renal colic.
- Most patients require narcotic analgesia. Passing a kidney stone hurts!
- Use appropriate radiologic procedures to rule out ureteral obstruction. Prolonged obstruction can lead to kidney damage and may require urologic intervention.
- Treat concurrent urinary infection.

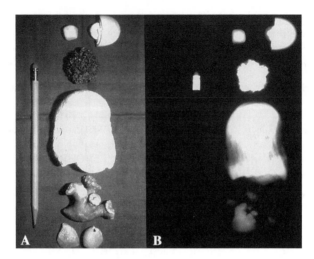

*A*, Recovered renal stones (from top to bottom): cystine, calcium oxalate, struvite, calcium phosphate, uric acid. Note the "staghorn" appearance of the calcium phosphate stone. Pencil provides size comparison. *B*, X-ray of *A*. All of the stones except the uric acid stone are radiopaque. The wood and graphite of the pencil, like the uric acid stones, are radiolucent. Note the lamellations present in the struvite stone.

- Save the stone or its fragments for subsequent analysis of stone composition (strain all urine during an episode of renal colic).

### 9. What is the role for medical intervention in nephrolithiasis?

In patients with recurrent nephrolithiasis and in all children who have passed a kidney stone, medical management is recommended. The goal of medical therapy is to prevent the formation of new stones and to reduce the rate of growth of existing stones. Medical management includes the use of allopurinol to decrease urinary uric acid, antibiotics to reduce infection, and potassium citrate to increase urinary inhibitor substances. Thiazide diuretics have unique efficacy. The costs of medical work-up and treatment (testing, follow-up, and medications) have been shown to be less than the cost of hospitalization and procedures associated with managing stones once they have formed.

### 10. What is the single most important therapeutic intervention in *any* patient with a history of nephrolithiasis?

Increase the urine output to greater than 2 L/day by increasing the oral intake of water (reduce urinary supersaturation).

### 11. What is medullary sponge kidney?

Medullary sponge kidney is a disorder in which the collecting ducts of the kidney are patulous and dilated. As a result, urine flow is slowed as it moves from the tubule into the renal pelvis. The disorder is usually asymptomatic. However, crystals forming in a supersaturated urine are more likely to adhere to the urothelium in the presence of low urinary flow, leading to increased nucleation, aggregation, and stone formation.

### 12. True or false: One way to reduce stone formation is to decrease the dietary intake of calcium?

False. Unless the patient has marked or excessive calcium intake (milk-alkali syndrome), absorption of calcium reflects underlying pathophysiology more than intake. It is more important to reduce the dietary intake of oxalate.

Calcium in the diet may actually help to bind oxalate in the intestine and reduce its absorption. A recent 5-year randomized study showed that restriction of animal protein and salt combined with a normal calcium intake decreased the risk of stone recurrence more effectively than a traditional low-calcium diet. In support of this observation, post-menopausal women treated with calcium supplements do not have any increase in the risk of stone formation.

### 13. What is the treatment for cystinuria and cystine stone formation?

Alkalize the urine to increase cystine solubility. Chelating agents, d-penicillamine, and alpha-mercaptopropionyl glycine (Thiola) reduce cystine excretion but have some toxic side effects.

### 14. Describe the outpatient work-up of a patient with nephrolithiasis.

Review the history and physical exam. If the patient was hospitalized during an episode of renal colic, review diagnostic x-rays. For example, the chest x-ray may demonstrate granulomatous disease. The following studies will confirm the results of stone analysis and lead to appropriate therapy of the underlying cause of nephrolithiasis.

| TEST | RESULT | RESPONSE |
|---|---|---|
| Urinalysis | Specific gravity > 1.020 | Urine is too concentrated; encourage ↑ oral intake of fluids |
| | Urine pH > 6.0 with ↓ serum $HCO_3$ | Suggests RTA |
| | Pyuria | Send for urine culture and treat with appropriate antibiotic |
| | Cystine crystals | Send urine for quantitative urine cystine |
| Serum calcium | > 10.5 mg/dl | Consider primary hyperparathyroidism; send for PTH |
| | < 10.5 mg/dl | Normal |
| Serum phosphate | < 2.8 mg/dl | If patient is calcium stone former, add $KPO_4$, 250 mg q.i.d., to thiazide regimen |
| Serum uric acid | > 8.0 mg/dl | If hyperuricosuria or uric acid stones also present, decrease dietary intake of purines and consider Rx with allopurinol |
| Serum $HCO_3$ | < 22 mEq/L | Consider RTA or incomplete distal RTA. Document with acid loading test. Treat with potassium citrate (1 mEq/kg/day) |
| 24-hour urine | Volume < 1500 ml/24 hours | Increase oral fluid intake |
| Creatinine | > 1.0–1.5 gm/24 hours | Adequate 24-hour urine collection |
| | < 1.0 gm/24 hours | Collection may be inaccurate, affecting other values |
| Urinary calcium | > 300 mg/24 hours (males); > 250 mg/24 hours (females); *or* > 4 mg/kg/24 hours | If stone analysis is consistent, begin hydrochlorothiazide, 25–50 mg q.d., and potassium citrate (20–40 mEq/day) |
| | > 150 mg/24 hours | If calcium stones are present, benefit from thiazide and potassium citrate is still seen |
| Urinary uric acid | > 700 mg/day | Urinary alkalization (potassium citrate, 50 mEq/day); allopurinol, 300 mg/day |

*Table continued on next page*

| TEST | RESULT | RESPONSE |
|------|--------|----------|
| | < 700 mg/day | If uric acid stones are present, begin treatment as above |
| Urinary phosphate | Calculate tubular reabsorption of phosphate: $$TRP = \frac{U/P \text{ phosphate}}{U/P \text{ creatinine}} - 1.0$$ | |
| | < 0.8 | Renal wasting of phosphate may be secondary to renal tubular defect or hyperparathyroidism |
| Urinary citrate | Normal range: 140–940 mg/24 hours | Low urinary citrate suggests RTA |
| Urinary oxalate | > 25–50 mg/24 hours | Reduce dietary oxalate intake |
| | > 50 mg/24 hours | Suggests hyperoxaluria secondary to gastro-intestinal disease. Correct underlying cause and/or add cholestyramine to bind bile acids (8–10 gm/day PO) |
| | > 150 mg/24 hours | Primary hyperoxaluria. Treat with pyridoxin (150–400 mg/24 hours) |

## 15. What is the relationship between bacteria and the formation of struvite stones?

Infection stones are formed largely through the action of bacterial urease. This urea-splitting enzyme is most commonly produced by gram-negative organisms such as *Proteus, Pseudomonas*, and *Klebsiella* and by gram-positive organisms such as *Streptococcus faecalis*. Bacterial urease generates increased amounts of ammonium with consequent urinary alkalization. The characteristic lamellated structure of the struvite stone represents layers of bacterial products and mineral. The stone acts as a foreign body, difficult to penetrate with antibiotics. If possible, complete removal of the stone and appropriate antibiotic therapy are the most definitive therapy.

## 16. Are nanobacteria the cause of stones, or a lab artifact?

Nanobacteria, as small as the largest viruses, have been found to live in urine. Antigens from these bacteria have also been found in a variety of human kidney stones. By precipitating calcium and other minerals around themselves, they may be the source of nucleation in urine. However the existence of nanobacteria and their role in disease is considered controversial.

### BIBLIOGRAPHY

1. Asplin JR, Favus MJ, Coe FL: Nephrolithiasis. In Brenner BM (ed): Brenner and Rector's The Kidney, 6th ed. Philadelphia, W.B. Saunders, 2000, pp 1774–1819.
2. Borghi L, Schianchi T, Meschi T, et al: Comparison of two diets for the prevention of recurrent stones in idiopathic hypercalciuria. N Engl J Med 346:77–84, 2002.
3. Coe FL, Parks JH: New insights into the pathophysiology and treatment of nephrolithiasis. J Bone Min Res 12:522–533, 1997.
4. Kajander EO, Ciftcioglu N: Nanobacteria: An alternative mechanism for pathogenic intra- and extracellular calcification and stone formation. Proc Natl Acad Sci U S A 95:8274–8279, 1998.
5. Kupin WL: A practical approach to nephrolithiasis. Hosp Pract 30:57–60, 63–64, 1995.
6. Pak CYC: Southwestern Internal Medicine Conference: Medical management of nephrolithiasis: A new, simplified approach for general practice. Am J Med Sci 313:215–219, 1997.
7. Parks JH, Coe FL: The financial effects of kidney stone prevention. Kidney Int 50:1706–1712, 1996.
8. Pearle MS, Roehrborn CG, Pak CYC: Meta-analysis of randomized trials for medical prevention of calcium oxalate nephrolithiasis. J Endourol 13:679–685, 1999.
9. Wasserstein AG: Nephrolithiasis: Acute management and prevention. Dis Mon 44:196–213, 1998.

# 19. URINARY TRACT INFECTION

*Carolyn P. Cacho, M.D.*

### 1. What are urinary tract infections and how are they classified?

The term *urinary tract infection* (UTI) refers to an infection occurring anywhere along the urinary tract from the perinephric fascia to the urethral meatus. UTIs have been classified based on the etiologic agent (e.g., bacterial, fungal, or mycobacterial), on the location in the genitourinary tract, and by complexity. In categorizing UTIs by location, a distinction generally is made between lower tract disease (e.g., cystitis, urethritis, prostatitis, and epididymitis) and upper tract disease (e.g., acute or chronic pyelonephritis). **Uncomplicated UTI** is an infection that occurs in a nonpregnant adult woman without structural or nephrologic dysfunction. This is the most common type of urinary tract infection and is usually responsive to appropriate antibiotic therapy. **Complicated UTI** includes infections at sites other than the bladder and those that occur in children, men, or pregnant women. They are more difficult to treat and may be associated with structural abnormalities of the urinary tract or with renal dysfunction.

### 2. What is the pathogenesis of UTI?

A urinary tract infection develops when the balance between the virulence and number of the infecting bacteria on the one hand and host defense mechanisms on the other is disrupted. The urinary tract can become infected by two major routes. Most infections occur by the **ascending route**. Bacteria, which have colonized the anus, distal urethra, or vagina, can enter and invade the proximal urethra and bladder. The mere presence of bacteria is not sufficient to cause infection, however. Invasion also depends on the virulence of the organism. Infection of the renal parenchyma generally occurs when bacteria in the bladder multiply and ascend up the ureters to the renal pelvis and kidney parenchyma. Vesicoureteral reflux or obstruction anywhere in the urinary tract enhances this process. A much less common route of infection of the urinary tract is the **hematogenous route**. For example, the kidneys can become infected in the presence of *Staphylococcus aureus* bacteremia or *Candida fungemia*.

### 3. Who gets UTIs?

UTIs are common and account for more than 7 million outpatient visits per year. In the neonatal period, UTIs are more common in boys than in girls. In childhood and throughout adulthood, females are at higher risk than males. Indeed, reports indicate that 20–50% of women will have at least one UTI in their lifetime. UTI continues to be a problem in the later stages of life for both men and women. The incidence of complicated UTI increases with advanced age because of the prevalence of urinary tract abnormalities such as prostatic disease, neurogenic disease, and a higher likelihood of urethral catheterization. Additionally, in postmenopausal women, lower levels of circulating estrogen may lead to decreased colonization of the vagina by lactobacilli, which lower vaginal pH and decrease adherence of pathogenic organisms to the uroepithelium. Age, however, is not the only risk factor predisposing to infection of the urinary tract. Recent sexual intercourse, use of a diaphragm with spermicide, pregnancy, and diabetes mellitus are all associated with increased incidence of UTI.

### 4. Which organisms most commonly cause UTI?

Seventy percent to 95% of UTIs are caused by *Escherichia coli*. Five percent to 20% of cases are caused by *Staphylococcus saprophyticus*. In patients with complicated UTI or who have risk factors such as hospitalization or diabetes mellitus, other fecal flora such as *Proteus mirabilis, Klebsiella* species, or *Enterococcus* may be the etiologic agents.

### 5. Can UTIs be prevented?

Yes. Prophylaxis of UTI should be considered in a number of clinical scenarios. In the woman with uncomplicated, recurrent UTIs, nonpharmacologic measures such as voiding immediately after intercourse, increasing fluid intake, and avoiding the use of a diaphragm with spermicide for contraception are often recommended but have not been confirmed in prospective studies to significantly decrease the risk of infection. On the other hand, consumption of cranberry juice has been shown to decrease bacteriuria and pyuria, likely by inhibiting the adherence of prefimbriated *E. coli* to uroepithelial cell surfaces by tannin compounds (proanthocyanidins) present in cranberries and blueberries.

A number of prophylaxis protocols using low doses of antibiotics are effective in the treatment of recurrent uncomplicated UTIs. These protocols use one of three strategies: continuous antibiotic prophylaxis, postcoital prophylaxis, or patient-administered self-treatment. In addition to antibiotic prophylaxis, institution of estrogen replacement therapy in postmenopausal women may favorably alter the vaginal flora and reduce the incidence of UTIs. Because pregnant women with bacteriuria have a twofold increase in the risk of premature delivery compared to those without bacteriuria, prevention of UTI is important in improving peripartum outcomes. Indications for prophylaxis in pregnant women include treatment of all women with a prepartum history of recurrent UTI, a single UTI early in pregnancy, and asymptomatic bacteriuria in early pregnancy. Both continuous and postcoital regimens have been shown to be effective (see question 13).

### 6. What are the signs and symptoms of UTI?

Symptoms include frequency, urgency, dysuria, hematuria, suprapubic tenderness, and flank pain. These classic signs and symptoms may be absent in elderly patients who sometimes present with gastrointestinal complaints (e.g., nausea and vomiting) or even with mental status changes.

### 7. How is UTI diagnosed?

In the patient with acute dysuria, cystitis must be distinguished from urethritis and vaginitis. A patient with frequency, dysuria, pyuria, and hematuria is likely to have a UTI, but the definite diagnosis depends on the demonstrated presence of white cells and bacteria in the urine. A urine dipstick test can rapidly demonstrate the presence of inflammation by the detection of leukocyte esterase. The leukocyte esterase test is generally positive when more than 10–20 leukocytes per milliliter are detected; however, this test does not specifically indicate bacterial infection. The presence of nitrites is highly specific for bacteria but is relatively insensitive, leading to many false negatives. In addition, the nitrite test is not positive in the presence of bacteria that do not produce nitrate reductase (e.g., *Staphylococcus, Enterococcus,* and *Pseudomonas* species). Gram stain of uncentrifuged urine is a useful diagnostic tool with a sensitivity and specificity that approach 90%. The presence of bacteria on Gram stain of uncentrifuged urine corresponds to a urine culture colony count of $10^5$ organisms. The gold standard for establishing the diagnosis of a UTI is a urine culture detecting greater than $10^5$ organisms per milliliter of urine. More recent data have shown that colony counts as low as $10^2$ colony-forming units per milliliter in a female with acute symptoms is sufficient to establish this diagnosis. Similarly, in symptomatic men, the presence of $10^3$ or greater colony-forming units per milliliter is sufficient to establish the diagnosis of a UTI.

### 8. How is an uncomplicated UTI treated?

Although nonspecific therapies such as hydration, urine acidification, cranberry juice, and urinary tract analgesics play a limited role in the treatment of UTIs, the mainstay of treatment is antimicrobial therapy. Acute uncomplicated cystitis, such as commonly occurs in young women of childbearing age, has traditionally been treated with trimethoprim-sulfamethoxazole or amoxicillin for 7 days. Shorter 3-day and single-dose regimens have been developed in an effort to reduce cost, increase compliance, reduce the emergence of resistant organisms, and decrease the risk of adverse drug effects. The relative efficacy of single-dose therapy in comparison to 3-day therapy varies but appears to be related to the half-life of the antimicrobial agent. For example, a single dose of trimethoprim-sulfamethoxazole maintains adequate urine concentrations for approximately 48 hours when compared to 24 hours for the quinolones and 18 hours for the beta-lactams. The current recommendation is for a 3-day course of therapy with trimethoprim-sulfamethoxazole or a quinolone. Beta-lactam regimens are less desirable because of the high rate of resistance to these drugs.

### 9. What is the approach to treatment of UTI in the pregnant patient?

When UTI occurs in pregnancy, the chosen antimicrobial agent and duration of therapy should be effective in eradicating the infecting organism but also must be safe for the fetus. Trimethoprim-sulfamethoxazole should be avoided, especially in the third trimester, because of the potential for hyperbilirubinemia in the neonate. Quinolones have been studied inadequately and should probably also be avoided. The safest agents are the beta-lactams. However, as noted above, these agents have a short half-life, which makes short-course regimens less effective. Thus, most authorities currently recommend a 7-day course of amoxicillin, ampicillin, or a first-generation cephalosporin for treatment of cystitis in a pregnant woman.

### 10. How should adult males with UTI be treated?

Cystitis should always be considered a complicated UTI when it occurs in an adult male. Studies have shown that both single-dose and 3-day courses of therapy are unsuccessful in men and that cure rates are much higher when the antimicrobial (i.e., trimethoprim-sulfamethoxazole or a quinolone) is used for 7 or more days.

### 11. What is the approach to the geriatric patient with a positive urine culture?

Elderly patients frequently have asymptomatic bacteriuria. While initial studies shown a link between bacteriuria and mortality in this population, more recent studies have shown that the increase in mortality is related more to other comorbid factors than to bacteriuria per se. Accordingly, most experts currently recommend no treatment for elderly or institutionalized persons with asymptomatic bacteriuria. In the geriatric patient who is symptomatic with significant levels of bacteriuria, a 7-day course of therapy with trimethoprim-sulfamethoxazole, a quinolone, or a beta-lactam is suggested. Because renal function declines with age, the creatinine clearance should be estimated in order to adjust the dosage of these medications to the patient's level of renal function.

### 12. What is the approach to the patient with an upper tract UTI?

Like other forms of complicated UTI, treating acute pyelonephritis with a short course of therapy is inappropriate. Traditionally, these infections were treated for 4–6 weeks. However, recent studies show good recovery within 2 weeks of therapy. When the infection is mild and patients show no signs of dehydration or renal failure, admission to the hospital may not be required. A 14-day course of oral therapy with trimethoprim-sulfamethoxazole, a quinolone, or ampicillin-clavulanate is appropriate depending on culture results. Many patients with acute pyelonephritis, however, experience significant nausea, vomiting, or dehydration and may even exhibit overt signs of sepsis. In these cases, admission to hospital and initiation of therapy with intravenous antibiotics such as trimethoprim-sulfamethoxazole, a quinolone, or ampicillin plus an aminoglycoside is appropriate. A clinical response to therapy should be apparent in 24–48 hours. Once the patient is afebrile, the patient may be changed to oral therapy based on the results of urine culture. The 14-day course may be completed at home either with oral therapy or with intravenous antibiotics administered by a home care service.

### 13. What is the strategy for managing recurring UTIs?

Treatment of recurrent UTI poses a challenge. First, repeated urine cultures should be obtained to determine whether the patient is having a relapse or reinfection. A **relapse** occurs when the infecting agent has not been eradicated. This condition will yield a positive culture at the end of therapy. When the culture obtained after treatment is negative and the patient has another infection, this is considered a **reinfection**. Relapses and reinfections are treated differently. If the patient is having a relapse, the appropriate initial step would be to administer antibiotics for a longer duration. If this strategy is unsuccessful, the likelihood that structural problems are contributing to the pathogenesis of infection is increased, and further work-up should be initiated. In patients who have frequent reinfections, risk factors should be investigated. When the infections are related to sexual intercourse, postcoital voiding may be helpful. Additionally, women experiencing this problem who use diaphragms or spermicides may benefit from alternative methods of birth control. When these nonantibacterial measures fail, antibiotic prophylaxis should be considered. Trimethoprim-sulfamethoxazole may be taken as a single dose immediately before or after intercourse. Similarly, in women with frequent recurrences of UTI that are not related to sexual intercourse or birth control methods and in whom a work-up to rule out structural causes of the UTI has proven negative, self-initiated therapy is often successful. Both single-dose and short-course regimens as previously described for acute cystitis (see question 8) can be helpful in a compliant patient who is able to determine that she has a UTI. In those patients who cannot reliably self-diagnose UTI and who have recurrent infections, a continuous low dose of antibiotics for a 6-month period may prevent further recurrences.

### 14. How should fungal infections be treated?

Immunocompromised and catheterized patients are at increased risk for fungal infections of the urinary tract. These infections are often mild and asymptomatic; however, on occasion, they may be complicated by fungus balls in the bladder and renal parenchymal infection with dissemination. When a catheterized patient develops candiduria, removal of the catheter is sufficient to treat the condition if the patient is asymptomatic. When the catheter cannot be removed, or when the patient is symptomatic, amphotericin B bladder washes or fluconazole is appropriate. Patients with severe fungal urinary tract infection should be treated with intravenous amphotericin B.

BIBLIOGRAPHY

1. Barnett BJ, Stephens DS: Urinary tract infection: An overview. Am J Med Sci 314:245–249, 1997.
2. Hooton TM, Stamm WE: Diagnosis and treatment of uncomplicated urinary tract infection. Infect Dis Clin North Am 11:551–581, 1997.
3. Rushton HG: Urinary tract infections in children: Epidemiology, evaluation, and management. Pediatric Clin North Am 44:1133–1169, 1997.
4. Sobel JD: Pathogenesis of urinary tract infection. Role of host defenses. Infect Dis Clin North Am 11:531–549, 1997.
5. Stapleton A, Stamm WE: Prevention of urinary tract infection. Infect Dis Clin North Am 11:719–733, 1997.
6. Svanborg C, Godaly GD: Bacterial virulence in urinary tract infection. Infect Dis Clin North Am 11:513–529, 1997.
7. Warren JW: Catheter-associated urinary tract infections. Infect Dis Clin North Am 11:609–622, 1997.

# 20. DISORDERS OF TUBULAR FUNCTION

R. Tyler Miller, M.D.

**1. How are disorders of renal tubules different from interstitial diseases?**

Disorders of renal tubular function are characterized by abnormalities of transport with preserved renal architecture. In general, filtered substances including glucose, amino acids, phosphate, bicarbonate, potassium, sodium, calcium, magnesium, and uric acid are reabsorbed in bulk in the proximal tubule, and their excretion is regulated in the distal nephron. A reduction in the transport capacity for a substance in any segment can result in inadequate reabsorption and its appearance in the urine. If the blood levels of a substance such as glucose is high enough that the tubule cannot reabsorb it, it may also appear in the urine. Defects in the transport of a single substance or multiple substances with similar characteristics or that share transport mechanisms may be observed. These defects in transport may be genetic or acquired and usually represent loss of function of a protein or group of proteins. The dysfunctional proteins are commonly transporters or channels but also may be signaling proteins or proteins involved in metabolism. Interstitial diseases are characterized be inflammation or fibrosis between tubules that may result in transport abnormalities, but the transport abnormalities are secondary to the inflammatory or fibrotic processes.

**2. What is the Fanconi syndrome?**

The Fanconi syndrome is a generalized disorder of renal tubular transport that leads to phosphaturia, glucosuria, aminoaciduria, and, in some situations, urinary loss of bicarbonate, uric acid, and potassium. Although traditionally associated with transport abnormalities of the proximal tubule, these abnormalities also may be present in the distal nephron. Some patients may have a partial Fanconi syndrome, meaning that only some of these transport processes are affected. Interference with multiple transport processes indicates that common processes required for transport such as the Krebs cycle or Na,K$^+$-ATPase are defective. Ultrastructural abnormalities may be found in the endoplasmic reticulum and mitochondria, and these morphologic changes are compatible with this interpretation. Clinically, the Fanconi syndrome is characterized by rickets or osteomalacia, metabolic acidosis, reduced growth (children), and hypokalemia. In adults, hypophosphatemia may be symptomatic. In the pediatric population, cystinosis is associated with Fanconi syndrome, whereas in adults it is acquired and associated with multiple myeloma (Bence Jones proteinuria), Wilson's disease, and tubular toxins (e.g., heavy meals, outdated tetracycline, Lysol, and vitamin D intoxication). The Fanconi syndrome may be an early feature of multiple myeloma.

**3. Does the presence of glucose in the urine always mean that the patient has diabetes mellitus?**

No. Glucose is reabsorbed in the proximal tubule from the filtrate by a specific transport protein. The most common cause of glucose in the urine is hyperglycemia in diabetes mellitus where the serum glucose level becomes high enough (usually on the order of 250 mg/dl) that the transporters in the proximal tubule are saturated and cannot completely remove glucose from the filtrate. However, glucosuria can occur in the presence of normal serum glucose levels (or levels below 250 mg/dl) if an abnormality of the glucose transporter is present. Genetic abnormalities of the renal glucose transporter occur as an autosomal recessive syndrome with variable penetrance and are benign conditions.

#### 4. What conditions cause loss of amino acids in the urine?

Amino acids are transported by proteins that carry a unique amino acid or a family of related amino acids. The immunoglycinuria, characterized by loss of L-proline, hydroxy-L-proline, and glycine, and dicarboxylic aminoaciduria are benign conditions, and no therapy is required. However, Hartnup disease, caused by a defect in intestinal and renal absorption of neutral monoamino-monocarboxylic amino acids (e.g., L-tryptophan) results in pellagra due to the inability of the patient to synthesize nicotinamide. These patients should be treated with nicotinic acid. Cystinuria is caused by an autosomal recessive disorder that results in increased urinary concentrations of cysteine and dibasic amino acids. Because cysteine is insoluble at normal urine pH, cysteine stones form and cause pain and obstruction. Treatment is induction of high-volume dilute urine and alkalization of the urine. Patients are also treated with thiols such as penicillamine or captopril to increase the solubility of the cysteine.

#### 5. What defects in tubular transport lead to metabolic alkalosis and hypokalemia?

Metabolic alkalosis and hypokalemia are associated with two genetic syndromes, Bartter's syndrome and Gitelman's syndrome, each of which is associated with mutations in transport proteins in the distal nephron. Bartter's syndrome is characterized by hypokalemia, metabolic alkalosis, and secondary hyperreninemic hyperaldosteronism with normal blood pressure. Bartter's syndrome is caused by defects in one of the molecules primarily or secondarily involved in transepithelial NaCl transport across the TAL. These proteins include the genes encoding the luminal bumetanide-sensitive $Na^+$-$K^+$-$2Cl^-$ cotransporter (NKCC2), the luminal potassium channel, ROMK (KCJN1), and the *CLCNKB* gene, which codes for the basolateral renal chloride channel CLC-Kb (responsible for most of the cases of the classical variant, which is characterized by a milder phenotype beginning in infancy or childhood, hypomagnesemia in 40% of cases and normo- or hypercalciuria). Recently, a new gene (*BSND*) responsible for the antenatal variant of Bartter's syndrome with sensorineural deafness has been identified and encodes a new protein, barttin. This protein is an essential subunit for basolateral Cl channels. Gitelman's syndrome is characterized by urinary K wasting, hypokalemia, tetany if the hypokalemia is severe, hypocalciuria, and hypomagnesemia. It is caused by loss of function mutations in the thiazide-sensitive NaCl cotransporter in the collecting duct.

#### 6. Can tubular disorders lead to metabolic acidosis?

Some types of metabolic acidosis are caused by abnormalities of proton transporters in the proximal or distal nephron. This group of disorders is referred to as **renal tubular acidosis** and is described in detail in Chapter 65.

#### 7. Are mutations in transport proteins a common cause of hypertension?

No, although mutations in several proteins that are involved in Na transport can lead to hypertension; these are rare genetic conditions. The proteins identified in these conditions may also exist in polymorphic forms that contribute to hypertension or may be therapeutic targets. Liddle's syndrome, also know as pseudoaldosteronism, is characterized by hypokalemia, growth failure, Na retention, hypertension, and reduced levels of plasma renin and aldosterone. The syndrome is caused by gain of function mutations in the epithelial Na channel α subunit. The syndrome of apparent mineralocorticoid excess (AME) is characterized by hypertension and hypokalemia. It is caused by loss of function of 11-β-hydroxysteroid dehydrogenase, the principal cell enzyme that alters glucocorticoids so that they do not activate mineralocorticoid receptors.

#### 8. What causes nephrogenic diabetes insipidus?

Nephrogenic diabetes insipidus results from the inability of the collecting duct to respond to vasopressin. This failure of response can be a result of toxic or obstructive injury to the tubule (see Chapter 65) or genetic loss of function of proteins including the V2 vaso-pressin receptor and the water channel, aquaporin-2. The common toxic causes include amphotericin and Li therapy, hypercalcemia, severe hypokalemia, and distal nephron injury by a variety of mechanisms.

BIBLIOGRAPHY

1. Bonnardeaux A, Bichet DG: Inherited disorders of the renal tubule. In Brenner BM (ed): The Kidney, 6th ed. Philadelphia, W.B. Saunders, 2000, pp 1621–1678.
2. Chesney RW: Noncystic hereditary diseases of the kidney. In Brady HR, Wilcox CS (eds): Therapy in Nephrology and Hypertension. Philadelphia, W.B. Saunders, 1999, pp 375–381.
3. Lifton RP: Molecular genetics of blood pressure control. Science 272:676–680, 1996.
4. Palacin M, Estevez R, Zorzano A: Cystinuria calls for heteromultimeric amino acid transporters. Curr Opin Cell Biol 10:455–461, 1998.
5. Simon DB, Lifton RP: Mutations in Na(K)Cl transporters in Gitelman's and Bartter's syndromes. Curr Opin Cell Biol 10:450–454, 1998.

# 21. RENAL DISEASE AND HYPERTENSION IN PREGNANCY

*Donald E. Hricik, M.D.*

### 1. How does pregnancy normally influence renal function?

Renal plasma flow increases up to 70% by the second trimester and remains elevated throughout pregnancy. The glomerular filtration rate begins to increase by the fourth week of gestation, peaks at 150% of normal by 13 weeks, and remains elevated until term. Given these expected changes, a serum creatinine concentration greater than 0.9 mg/dl is generally indicative of renal impairment in the pregnant woman. The kidneys enlarge by 1–1.5 cm during pregnancy, and hormonal changes lead to dilatation of the ureters, giving the appearance of hydronephrosis on imaging studies. Pregnancy also affects renal tubular function, leading to hyperuricosuria (and hypouricemia) and occasionally to glycosuria in the absence of hyperglycemia.

### 2. How common is urinary tract infection during pregnancy?

Asymptomatic bacteriuria occurs in 5% of pregnant women and may be associated with low birth weight. If untreated, 30% of pregnant women with asymptomatic bacteriuria will develop pyelonephritis. Thus, monthly screening for urinary tract infection is warranted and even asymptomatic bacteriuria should be treated.

### 3. How does pregnancy affect women with underlying renal disease?

In women with impaired renal function, the ability to conceive decreases proportionally with the level of renal impairment. Women with underlying renal disease generally exhibit higher rates of urinary protein excretion during pregnancy, partly reflecting an increase filtered load of protein resulting from the increased glomerular filtration rate. When underlying renal disease is present, the most important determinant of whether renal function deteriorates during pregnancy is the level of renal function at the time of conception. Women with a serum creatinine concentration greater than 1.4 mg/dl at conception are at increased risk for a decline in renal function during pregnancy. Underlying renal disease increases the risk of preeclampsia (see question 11).

### 4. How does underlying renal disease influence fetal outcome?

Fetal outcome is worse than for the general population. Approximately 10% of pregnancies that continue beyond the second trimester end in stillbirth. Twenty percent of infants are born prematurely.

### 5. Can women on dialysis become pregnant?

Infertility is the rule in women with end-stage renal disease. However, 0.5% of women of childbearing age on chronic dialysis conceive each year. Approximately 30% of pregnancies in women who conceive while on dialysis result in surviving infants. However, the infants are almost always premature and usually small for gestational age. Increasing the dose of dialysis has become a common practice in managing pregnancy in the dialysis-dependent patient. However, the benefit of this practice has not been proven.

### 6. How does kidney transplantation influence fertility?

Fertility is often restored in women who achieve satisfactory allograft function. In general, women are advised to wait 1–2 years after transplantation and then to consider pregnancy only if the serum creatinine concentration is less than 2.0 mg/dl.

### 7. What is postpartum hemolytic uremic syndrome (HUS)?

This is an unusual form of acute renal failure that typically occurs several days to 2 months after a normal pregnancy. Clinical features are similar to those described in other forms of HUS (see Chapter 38) and include severe renal failure, thrombocytopenia, microangiopathic hemolytic anemia, and neurologic dysfunction. The prognosis is poor, and permanent renal failure is common in survivors.

### 8. How does pregnancy normally influence systemic blood pressure?

During normal pregnancy, systolic blood pressure changes little. However, diastolic pressure decreases by an average of 10 mmHg by the 20th week of gestation and rises back to baseline levels in the third trimester. The normal decrease in blood pressure early in gestation may mask the presence of antecedent chronic hypertension. Third-trimester hypertension is generally defined as a diastolic blood pressure of 85 mmHg or higher.

### 9. What is the clinical importance of hypertension associated with pregnancy?

Hypertensive disorders are the most common medical complications of pregnancy, occurring in up to 20% of all cases. They are an important cause of maternal and fetal morbidity and mortality.

### 10. Classify the hypertensive disorders associated with pregnancy.

Traditionally, four categories of gestational hypertension are recognized:
1. Preeclampsia/eclampsia
2. Chronic hypertension
3. Chronic hypertension with superimposed preeclampsia
4. Late or transient hypertension

As discussed below, it can be difficult to clinically differentiate these various forms of gestational hypertension.

### 11. What is preeclampsia/eclampsia?

Preeclampsia is a hypertensive disorder associated with proteinuria, edema, and sometimes coagulation and liver function abnormalities in pregnant women. The disorder occurs in 5–10% of all pregnancies and occurs most often in nulliparas, usually after the 20th week of gestation. Preeclampsia can progress rapidly to eclampsia, a state characterized by seizures and often preceded by severe hypertension, headache, and hyperreflexia. The convulsive, eclamptic phase can occur suddenly in seemingly stable women with mild blood pressure elevations. Thus, third-trimester hypertension should be regarded and treated as preeclampsia until proven otherwise.

### 12. Define chronic hypertension associated with pregnancy.

Most women with this category have essential hypertension, but secondary forms of hypertension always merit consideration. Patients with preexisting hypertension may exhibit elevated blood pressures during the first two trimesters. Women with pregestational hypertension are more prone to superimposed preeclampsia (category 3 in the classification scheme in question 10).

### 13. Define late or transient hypertension associated with pregnancy.

This term refers to the development of hypertension in the third trimester without associated proteinuria. Typically, maternal and fetal outcomes are normal, and blood pressure returns to normal within a week or two of delivery.

## 14. What is the pathophysiology of preeclampsia?

The pathophysiologic mechanisms underlying preeclampsia remain a subject of controversy. The vasculature of women with this disorder is intensely sensitive to endogenous pressor peptides and catecholamines as well as to exogenous infusions of pressors such as angiotensin, norepinephrine, and vasopressin. This vascular sensitivity may be related to decreased levels of eicosanoids such as prostaglandins E and I. The hemodynamic profile of the preeclamptic woman is characterized by volume depletion, salt retention, and edema. One theory regarding the pathogenesis is that a primary reduction in intravascular volume leads to placental hypoperfusion and release of pressor substances by the uterus. Other theories suggest that primary vasoconstriction leads secondarily to the observed reduction in plasma volume.

## 15. Besides proteinuria, what are the other renal manifestations of preeclampsia?

Glomerular filtration rate decreases in preeclampsia in association with a renal lesion called *glomerular endotheliosis* and is characterized by swelling of glomerular endothelial cells. Varying degrees of renal sodium retention contribute to the pathogenesis of edema in this disorder.

## 16. In a pregnant woman, how does one distinguish preeclampsia from underlying renal disease associated with hypertension?

Unless the woman's past medical history is well known, it can be difficult to distinguish these two entities. Furthermore, many nephrologists are reluctant to perform a kidney biopsy in a pregnant woman to help make this differentiation. When doubt exists, it is probably prudent to manage the patient as though she has preeclampsia, particularly since underlying renal disease increases the risk of superimposed preeclampsia. Because the clinical manifestations of preeclampsia resolve following delivery, persistence of proteinuria and hypertension several weeks following delivery strongly suggest underlying parenchymal renal disease.

## 17. How does eclampsia differ from hypertensive encephalopathy?

The seizures that occur in eclampsia have been attribute to intense cerebral vasoconstriction or to platelet thrombi that obstruct the cerebral microcirculation. The ophthalmologic hallmarks of hypertensive encephalopathy (i.e., retinal hemorrhages, exudates, and papillary edema) are uncommon in eclampsia.

## 18. How is preeclampsia managed?

Delivery is the ultimate cure but may not be feasible when preeclampsia occurs relatively early in pregnancy. There is disagreement about the need for bed rest, prolonged hospitalization, antihypertensive drug therapy, and anticonvulsant prophylaxis in women with *mild* preeclampsia; however, bed rest at home or in the hospital is still recommended commonly. Results of randomized trials designed to test the efficacy of antihypertensive drug therapy in preventing the progression of preeclampsia have yielded conflicting results.

In women with *severe* preeclampsia remote from term, the objective of treatment is to prevent cerebral complications. The aim of therapy is to keep the diastolic blood pressure below 105 mmHg (but not below 90 mmHg). Intravenous hydralazine (administered as a 5-mg bolus every 20 minutes up to a cumulative dose of 20 mg) is probably the drug of choice. Nifedipine and labetalol have also been found to be safe and effective. Although routine anticonvulsant prophylaxis remains controversial, intravenous magnesium sulfate is the treatment of choice for eclamptic seizures and is still used by some obstetricians in a prophylactic manner in women with severe preeclampsia.

### 19. Are there other preventive modalities for preeclampsia?

Early single-center studies suggested that aspirin reduced the incidence and severity of preeclampsia. However, subsequent large, randomized trials demonstrated no benefit compared with placebo. Aspirin may still be useful in women with hypercoagulable states such as the antiphospholipid antibody syndrome. Epidemiologic studies have suggested an inverse relationship between dietary calcium intake and the incidence of preeclampsia. The results of randomized trials comparing calcium supplementation with placebo suggest that calcium supplements may reduce the risk of gestational hypertension, but they have little impact on the incidence or severity of preeclampsia.

### 20. What drugs are favored for the treatment of chronic hypertension associated with pregnancy?

Methyldopa is the drug most often used to treat chronic hypertension in pregnant women. Hydralazine and labetalol have also been shown to be effective and safe. Atenolol and diuretics may be effective, but some studies suggest that these agents adversely affect fetal growth. Angiotensin-converting enzyme (ACE) inhibitors are contraindicated in pregnancy because these drugs are associated with fetal growth retardation, congenital malformations, and neonatal renal failure.

BIBLIOGRAPHY

1. Caroli G, Duley L, Belizan JM, Villar J: Calcium supplementation during pregnancy. A systemic review of randomized controlled trials. Br J Obstet Gynaecol 101:753–758, 1994.
2. Davison JM: Pregnancy in renal allograft recipients: Prognosis and management. Clin Obstet Gynaecol 8:501–525, 1994.
3. Hou SH: Peritoneal and haemodialysis in pregnancy. Clin Obstet Gynaecol 8:481–500, 1994.
4. Jones DC, Hayslett JP: Outcome of pregnancy in women with moderate or severe renal insufficiency. N Engl J Med 335:226–232, 1996.
5. Lindheimer MD: Preeclampsia–eclampsia 1996: Preventable? Have disputes on its treatment been resolved? Curr Opin Nephrol Hypertens 5:452–458, 1996.
6. Lindheimer MD, Katz AI: Hypertension in pregnancy. N Engl J Med 313:675–680, 1985.
7. Schobel HP, Fischer T, Heuszer K, et al: Preeclampsia: A state of sympathetic overactivity. N Engl J Med 335:1480–1485, 1996.
8. Sibai BM: Treatment of hypertension in pregnant women. N Engl J Med 335:257–265, 1996.

# III. Primary Glomerular Disease

## 22. MINIMAL CHANGE DISEASE

*Katherine MacRae Dell, M.D.*

**1. What is the nephrotic syndrome?**

Nephrotic syndrome is a disorder defined by four features: edema, proteinuria (> 3.5 gm/24 hr in adults, > 40 mg/m$^2$/hr in children), hypoalbuminemia, and hyperlipidemia. Primary renal diseases that present as nephrotic syndrome include minimal change nephrotic syndrome, focal segmental glomerulosclerosis and membranous nephropathy.

**2. What is minimal change nephrotic syndrome?**

Minimal change nephrotic syndrome (MCNS), also called "nil disease" or lipoid nephrosis, is a disease that occurs primarily in young children. It is characterized histologically by normal light microscopy and immunofluorescence. Effacement and widening of epithelial cell foot processes with loss of slit diaphragms are seen on electron microscopy.

**3. What causes MCNS?**

Although the pathogenesis remains unclear, it is thought to be an immune-mediated disease. Initial episodes and relapses of nephrotic syndrome are often triggered by viral or bacterial infections, suggesting a role for activation of the immune system. Furthermore, effective therapies for MCNS, such as corticosteroids, act as immunosuppressants.

**4. How common is MCNS?**

Nephrotic syndrome in children occurs at an incidence of 2/100,000. Approximately 77% of children with nephrotic syndrome have MCNS. In adults, MCNS is less common, accounting for 20–30% of patients with nephrotic syndrome.

**5. What are the typical clinical features of MCNS?**

Patients are usually between the ages of 2 and 6 years, and boys are affected more often than girls (3:2 ratio). Children typically present with the insidious onset of edema progressing to frank anasarca. Decreased urine output is often noted. Patients also may have diarrhea or abdominal pain, poor appetite, and irritability.

**6. How is MCNS diagnosed?**

Diagnosis in children is usually based on the presence of the typical clinical features outlined above, as well as response to therapy (see below). For these "typical" patients who respond to therapy, a renal biopsy is not performed. However, certain clinical features may suggest a diagnosis other than MCNS. These include age older than 10 years, hypertension, abnormal serum creatinine, and microscopic or macroscopic hematuria. A renal biopsy may be performed in patients with one or more of these features prior to initiating therapy.

**7. What is the standard therapy for treatment of the initial episode of nephrotic syndrome when MCNS is suspected?**

High-dose prednisone at a dose of 60 mg/m$^2$/day (maximum 80 mg/day) in 2–3 divided doses initially for 4–6 weeks is the accepted standard therapy for this disease. However,

recent data suggest that a longer initial treatment period of 6 weeks may decrease the incidence of subsequent relapses. The prednisone is then decreased to a single dosage of 40
mg/m$^2$ on alternate days for 1 month, before discontinuing the prednisone using a slow taper
over a 1–2-month period. In addition, a low-sodium diet is recommended to control edema.

### 8. What therapies are used to treat symptomatic edema?

Judicious use of oral diuretics may be helpful in patients with moderate edema. With
more severe edema (such as severe scrotal swelling, tense ascites, or impaired ambulation),
intravenous infusions of 25% albumin (0.5 gm/kg) and loop diuretics given slowly over 2–4
hours once or twice daily will provide improvement in symptoms. However, the effects of
albumin and diuretics are generally short-lived. Complications of therapy include volume
depletion, hypertension, and pulmonary edema. Sodium restriction is also an essential part
of edema management in MCNS.

### 9. What are the complications of nephrotic syndrome?

Patients with MCNS have an increased risk of infection with encapsulated organisms,
such as *Streptococcus pneumoniae, Escherichia coli,* and *Haemophilus influenzae.* This
increased risk may be due to loss of opsinizing antibodies and complement proteins as well
as defective cell-mediated immunity. Spontaneous bacterial peritonitis, pneumonia, bacteremia, and cellulitis may occur. Prophylactic antibiotics, such as amoxicillin, are advocated by some practitioners, but this remains controversial. Patients with MCNS are also
hypercoagulable, possibly due to an imbalance in the loss of anticoagulant versus procoagulant factors in the urine. Venous thrombosis may occur, including renal vein and sagittal
sinus thromboses. Arterial thrombosis also may occur, and arterial puncture should be
avoided in these patients unless absolutely necessary. Overly aggressive diuresis may
increase the risk of thrombotic events.

### 10. How long does it take for a child with MCNS to go into remission when treated with prednisone?

Among patients with MCNS who are steroid responsive, 75–80% go into remission
within 2 weeks of therapy, and 94% achieve a remission by 4 weeks of therapy.

### 11. Does MCNS recur or relapse?

Yes. Approximately 60–75% of children with MCNS will have at least one relapse of
their nephrotic syndrome. In adults, about 60% of patients with MCNS will have a relapse.
Younger adults generally have a greater risk of relapse and experience relapses earlier than
older adults.

Furthermore, 50% of children with MCNS will have a **frequently relapsing course**,
defined as at least two relapses in a 6-month period. Frequent relapses during the initial 6
months after diagnosis of MCNS appear to predict which patients will have a frequently
relapsing course during subsequent years. An additional subgroup of patients, called
**steroid-dependent**, will enter remission but will relapse while still on a steroid taper or
within 4 weeks of discontinuing a steroid therapy.

### 12. How are relapses treated?

Relapses typically are treated with repeat courses of prednisone, 60 mg/m$^2$/day (maximum 80 mg/day) in 2–3 divided doses, until the patient is in remission for 3 days. Once a
remission is achieved, prednisone is tapered to a single dose of 40 mg/m$^2$ on alternate days
for 1 month followed by either a rapid (over 2 months) or a slow (over 6–12 months) taper.
Steroid-dependent patients or those with a frequent relapsing course and signs of steroid
toxicity (e.g., growth retardation, obesity, cataracts, hypertension, hyperglycemia) may ben-

efit from treatment with other immunosuppressive agents such as cyclophosphamide, cyclosporine, levamisole, or mycophenolate mofetil.

**13. What if the patient fails to respond to the initial trial of prednisone therapy?**

Patients who do not achieve a remission after 4 weeks of prednisone, 60 mg/m$^2$/day in divided doses, and 4 weeks of a once-daily dose of prednisone, 60 mg/m$^2$/day, are considered **steroid resistant**. Approximately 50% of children younger than 6 years of age with steroid-resistant nephrotic syndrome will have MCNS on renal biopsy. Less than 5% of steroid-resistant patients older than 6 years of age have MCNS. Pathologic lesions such as mesangial proliferative glomerulonephritis, focal segmental glomerulosclerosis, and membranous nephropathy are more common in these patients.

**14. What is the long-term prognosis for children with MCNS?**

Patients with steroid-responsive MCNS have excellent survival and normal renal function. The frequency of relapses diminishes with advancing age. Patients with steroid-resistant nephrotic syndrome secondary to MCNS have a poorer long-term prognosis. Even when the initial renal biopsy shows MCNS, these patients often have mesangial proliferative glomerulonephritis or focal segmental glomerulosclerosis on follow-up biopsies. The latter lesions are associated with a 30–50% chance of progressing to end-stage renal disease within 5 years.

BIBLIOGRAPHY

1. Clark AG, Barratt TM: Steroid-responsive nephrotic syndrome. In Barratt TM, Avner ED, Harmon WE (eds): Pediatric Nephrology, 4th ed. Baltimore, Lippincott Williams & Wilkins, 1999, pp 731–748.
2. Hogg R, Portman RJ, Milliner D, et al: Evaluation and management of proteinuria and nephrotic syndrome in children: Recommendations from a pediatric nephrology panel established at the National Kidney Foundation Conference on Proteinuria, Albuminuria, Risk Assessment, Detection, and Elimination (PARADE). Pediatrics 105:1242–1249, 2000.
3. International Study of Kidney Disease in Children: Early identification of frequent relapses among children with minimal change nephrotic syndrome. J Pediatr 101:514–518, 1982.
4. International Study of Kidney Disease in Children: The primary nephrotic syndrome in children: Identification of patients with minimal change nephrotic syndrome from initial response to prednisone. J Pediatr 98:561–564, 1981.
5. International Study of Kidney Disease in Children: Nephrotic syndrome in children: Prediction of histopathology from clinical and laboratory characteristics at time of diagnosis. Kidney Int 113:159–165, 1978.
6. Nakayama M, Katafuchi R, Yanase T, et al: Steroid responsiveness and frequency of relapse in adult-onset minimal change nephrotic syndrome. Am J Kidney Dis 39:503–512, 2002.
7. Niadet P: Steroid-resistant nephrotic syndrome. In Barratt TM, Avner ED, Harmon WE (eds): Pediatric Nephrology, 4th ed. Baltimore, Lippincott Williams & Wilkins, 1999, pp 749–764.
8. Trompeter RS, Lloyd B, Hicks J, et al: Long-term outcome for children with minimal-change nephrotic syndrome. Lancet 1:368–370, 1985.
9. Tune BM, Mendoza SA: Treatment of the idiopathic nephrotic syndrome: Regimens and outcomes in children and adults. J Am Soc Nephrol 8:824–832, 1997.

# 23. FOCAL SEGMENTAL GLOMERULOSCLEROSIS

*John R. Sedor, M.D.*

**1. What is focal segmental glomerulosclerosis (FSGS) and what is the typical clinical presentation of a patient with FSGS?**

FSGS is a glomerular disease defined by a characteristic histologic pattern that occurs either as a primary kidney disease (primary FSGS) or as a result of a systemic illness (secondary FSGS). Sclerosis, or scarring, is present in parts (segmental) of some (focal) glomeruli. Proteinuria, often in the nephrotic range, is the hallmark of FSGS. Hypertension is a presenting feature in approximately one third of patients, and some degree of renal insufficiency is present in one third of patients at the time of diagnosis. Over half the patients with FSGS have hematuria. Proteinuria without hypertension is more common in children than in adults with FSGS.

**2. What is the characteristic pathology of FSGS?**

When examined with light microscopy, the typical FSGS lesion demonstrates mesangial collapse, scarring in parts of glomerular capillary tufts, and adhesions to Bowman's capsule. However, the light microscopic changes are nonspecific and can be seen in other renal diseases associated with glomerular inflammation. Immunoglobulin and complement deposition is generally not detected, although IgM and, less frequently, C3 staining can be detected in nonsclerotic glomeruli of some patients with FSGS. Demonstration of abundant immunoglobulin deposits by immunofluorescence should suggest a primary or secondary glomerulonephritis. Similar to light microscopy, ultrastructural analysis by electron microscopy shows nonspecific changes, predominantly foot process effacement in FSGS patients with heavy proteinuria, but electron microscopy can demonstrate other causes of glomerular disease that were not apparent by light microscopy. Sometimes, the focal, segmental glomerular scar is identified only by electron microscopy.

**3. Are there variants of FSGS histology? Do the histopathologic variants predict the clinical course of the disease?**

In addition to the typical lesion described in question 2, there are two additional structural variants of FSGS. The **glomerular tip lesion** is characterized by swelling, vacuolation, and proliferation of visceral epithelial cells (podocytes) and by sclerosis in the glomerular segments closest to the proximal tubule. Limited evidence suggests that patients with this histology tend to exhibit a more benign course and to be more responsive to steroid therapy compared to patients with classic FSGS. A second variant is characterized by **focal** or **global glomerular capillary collapse** and sclerosis with visceral epithelial cell swelling. This lesion is associated with a less favorable prognosis and is identified more commonly in African-American patients and in patients with human immunodeficiency virus (HIV) nephropathy (see Chapter 31, HIV-associated Renal Disorders). Severe tubulointerstitial disease associated with any of the three structural FSGS lesions correlates with poor long-term renal survival.

**4. Is there a racial predilection for the development of FSGS?**

Yes. FSGS is the most common cause of idiopathic nephrotic syndrome among African Americans. However, patients with FSGS constitute an increasingly larger fraction of adult patients with idiopathic nephrotic syndrome. For example, one survey of renal biopsies in adult patients with idiopathic nephrotic syndrome from 1995 to 1997 showed that FSGS is the most common lesion, accounting for 35% of all patients and 50% of cases in African-American patients.

## 5. What are the causes of FSGS?

FSGS may be idiopathic or secondary (see table). By definition, the term *idiopathic FSGS* is used only if evidence is lacking for other causes of focal glomerulonephritis that could result in focal scarring after healing.

| CLASSIFICATION OF FSGS | CAUSE |
|---|---|
| Primary | Idiopathic FSGS |
| |     Classic |
| |     Glomerular tip variant |
| | Collapsing or "malignant" variant |
| | Superimposed on minimal change nephropathy |
| | Familial (caused by mutations in podocyte genes |
| |     encoding slit diaphragm proteins) |
| Secondary | Sickle-cell disease |
| | Unilateral renal agenesis |
| | HIV infection |
| | Intravenous drug abuse |
| | Vesicoureteral reflux |
| | Diabetes mellitus (rare) |
| | Postinflammatory scarring |
| | Morbid obesity |

## 6. Describe the clinical course of FSGS.

The prognosis and clinical course of patients with idiopathic FSGS are determined primarily by the severity of proteinuria. Persistent non–nephrotic-range proteinuria is associated with good long-term renal survival. In contrast, declining glomerular filtration rates characterize patients with persistent nephrotic-range proteinuria. In this latter group of FSGS patients, the prevalence of end-stage renal disease 10 years after initial diagnosis is greater than 50%. Patients with HIV-induced FSGS or the collapsing variant of FSGS may progress rapidly to end-stage renal disease, often requiring dialysis from several months to 2–3 years after diagnosis. The course of secondary forms of FSGS varies according to the severity and activity of the underlying disease.

## 7. Does FSGS recur after kidney transplantation?

Yes. The reported recurrence rates among patients with idiopathic FSGS range between 20% and 40%. Secondary FSGS may not recur if the underlying disease is inactive after transplantation. FSGS patients with high-grade proteinuria and a rapid course to renal failure are at highest risk for recurrence. Interestingly, FSGS recurs less often in African-American patients, despite the higher prevalence of progressive FSGS in this population.

## 8. What are the general principles of management for patients with FSGS?

1. Blood pressure should be normalized, if possible, in all hypertensive patients with FSGS.

2. All patients with nephrotic-range proteinuria and FSGS should be treated with angiotensin-converting enzyme (ACE) inhibitors or angiotensin-1 (AT1) receptor antagonists, unless otherwise contraindicated. Nephrotic-range proteinuria of any cause is an independent risk factor for progression of chronic renal failure, and ACE inhibitors and AT1-receptor blockers are the most potent antiproteinuric agents available. Angiotensin stimulates aldosterone synthesis, and small case series suggest that spironolactone, an aldosterone antagonist, also may slow progression in patients with parenchymal renal disease.

3. Hyperlipidemia should be controlled with appropriate medications to lower elevated cholesterol and triglycerides, if dietary modifications fail to achieve target serum levels.

4. Salt restriction and diuretics should be used to control edema in nephrotic FSGS patients.

## 9. Should FSGS patients be treated with corticosteroids?

The therapy of FSGS remains controversial, and data for evidence-based decisions are lacking. Most studies of therapy for FSGS patients have employed regimens used for treatment of minimal change nephropathy and have reported poor response to therapy. However, recent case series, in which FSGS patients were treated with high-dose corticosteroids (1 mg/kg/day) for prolonged courses (at least 16 weeks and for as long as 6 months), report response rates of up to 60–70% and improved long-term renal survival.

## 10. What factors influence the decision to treat a patient who has FSGS?

The potential efficacy and side effects of therapy must be considered for each patient. The amount of proteinuria, the presence and degree of renal insufficiency, and the extent of scarring on biopsy are appropriate variables to evaluate before administering anti-inflammatory drugs. Nonspecific therapy (see question 8) is probably an appropriate first approach in patients with mild proteinuria and normal renal function. In contrast, patients with persistent nephrotic proteinuria and renal insufficiency should be considered for more aggressive therapy with corticosteroids or other immunosuppressants.

## 11. Outline specific treatment options for patients with idiopathic FSGS.

Prednisone, 1 mg/kg/day for at least 4 months, is now the recommended treatment regimen for patients with FSGS and is usually continued for 1–2 weeks after induction of remission and then tapered slowly. A prolonged prednisone therapy of 5–8 months has been advocated by some experts. Some patients who initially respond to prednisone therapy may exhibit frequent relapses or become steroid-dependent. High-quality evidence for the use of other immunosuppressive agents in patients with FSGS who do not respond to corticosteroids alone, who are steroid-dependent, or who frequently relapse is not available. However, the North American Nephrotic Syndrome Study Group recently demonstrated in a randomized controlled trial that steroid-resistant FSGS patients treated with cyclosporine and prednisone had better outcomes compared to patients who were not treated with cyclosporine. Relapse is common when cyclosporine is discontinued, but cyclosporine-treated FSGS patients have a long term decrease in proteinuria and better preservation of glomerular filtration rate. Cyclosporine itself can be nephrotoxic and should be used judiciously. Cyclophosphamide or other cytotoxic drugs can be added to the therapeutic regimen, and small case series suggest that these drugs may induce complete or partial remission in up to 75% of these individuals.

## 12. What factors are associated with steroid resistance?

Significant tubulointerstitial disease on renal biopsy, an elevated creatinine, and massive proteinuria of more than 10 gm daily suggest that the clinical response to steroid therapy may be poor. Patients with these risk factors may be candidates for early withdrawal from treatment if the steroids are tolerated poorly or cause significant side effects.

## 13. Is there a genetic basis for FSGS?

The molecular etiology of the sporadic forms of FSGS has not been determined, but several landmark studies have identified genetic mechanisms of FSGS and nephrotic syndromes, which cluster in families and are often steroid-resistant. Mutations in several genes have be linked to familial FSGS, demonstrating the genetic heterogeneity of this disorder. The protein products of the human FSGS and nephrotic syndrome genes, identified to date, appear necessary for the maintenance of the filtration barrier (specifically the slit diaphragm) by the podocyte. These genes include *NPHS1* (encoding the slit diaphragm protein nephrin), *NPHS2* (encoding the slit diaphragm protein podocin), and *ACTN4* (encoding the cytoskeletal protein α-actinin-4). By defining pathways that prevent pathologic proteinuria, we may be able to define the mechanisms that are responsible for the idiopathic variants of FSGS.

### BIBLIOGRAPHY

1. Appel GB: Focal segmental glomerulosclerosis. In Greenberg A (ed): Primer on Kidney Diseases, 2nd ed. San Diego, Academic Press, 1998, pp 160–164.
2. Burgess E: Management of focal segmental glomerulosclerosis: Evidence-based recommendations. Kidney Int 55:S26–S32, 1999.
3. Cattran DC, Appel GB, Hebert LA, et al: A randomized trial of cyclosporine in patients with steroid-resistant focal segmental glomerulosclerosis. Kidney Int 56:2220–2226, 1999.
4. Haas M, Meehan SM, Karrison TG, Spargo BH: Changing etiologies of unexplained adult nephrotic syndrome: A comparison of renal biopsy findings from 1976–1979 and 1995–1997. Am J Kidney Dis 30:621–631, 1997.
5. Kaplan J, Pollak MR: Familial focal segmental glomerulosclerosis. Curr Opin Nephrol Hypertens 10:183–187, 2001.
6. Korbet SM: Primary focal segmental glomerulosclerosis. J Am Soc Nephrol 79:1333–1342, 1998.
7. Lewis EJ: Recurrent focal sclerosis after renal transplantation. Kidney Int 22:315–323, 1982.
8. Ponticelli C, Rizzoni G, Edefonti A, et al: A randomized trial of cyclosporine in steroid-resistant idiopathic nephrotic syndrome. Kidney Int 43:1377–1384, 1993.
9. Rydel JJ, Korbet SM, Borok RZ, Schwartz MM: Focal segmental glomerular sclerosis in adults: Presentation, course, and response to treatment. Am J Kidney Dis 25:534–542, 1995.
10. Schwartz MM, Korbet SM, Rydell J, et al: Primary focal segmental glomerulosclerosis in adults: Prognostic value of histologic variants. Am J Kidney Dis 25:845–852, 1995.
11. Seney FD Jr, Burns DK, Silva FG: Acquired immunodeficiency syndrome and the kidney. Am J Kidney Dis 16:1–13, 1990.
12. Tune BM, Mendoza SA: Treatment of idiopathic nephrotic syndrome: Regimens and outcomes in children and adults. J Am Soc Nephrol 8:824–832, 1997.
13. Winn MP, Conlon PJ, Lynn KL, et al: Clinical and genetic heterogeneity in familial focal segmental glomerulosclerosis. International Collaborative Group for the Study of Familial Focal Segmental Glomerulosclerosis. Kidney Int 55:1241–1246, 1999.

# 24. MEMBRANOUS GLOMERULOPATHY

Patrick S. T. Hayden, M.D.

### 1. What is membranous glomerulopathy?

Membranous glomerulopathy is a morphologic entity defined by biopsy. Pathologic examination reveals subepithelial immune complex deposition within the glomerular basement membrane (see figure) without associated mesangial hypercellularity or matrix expansion.

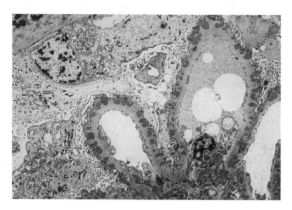

Electron micrograph from a patient with membranous glomerulopathy showing irregularly distributed electron-dense immune deposits in the subepithelial portion of the glomerular basement membrane.

### 2. What are some synonyms for membranous glomerulopathy?

*Epimembranous*, *perimembranous*, and *extramembranous glomerulonephritis* have been used interchangeably in the literature to refer to membranous glomerulopathy. Sometimes, it is called *membranous nephropathy* or *membranous glomerulonephritis*. The latter term is probably inappropriate because this entity is generally not associated with the cellular proliferation or evidence of inflammation commonly associated with the term *nephritis*.

### 3. What are the major constituents of the immune complexes implicated in membranous glomerulopathy?

Immunoglobulin G (IgG) and complement factor 3 (C3), although other complement components can rarely be seen.

### 4. What percentage of adult patients with nephrotic syndrome have membranous glomerulopathy?

Idiopathic membranous nephropathy accounts for about 20% of all adult cases of nephrotic syndrome, although focal and segmental glomerulosclerosis (FSGS) has now emerged as the leading cause of nephrotic syndrome in African-Americans. For those older than 50 years of age, idiopathic membranous glomerulopathy is the etiology in nearly 40% of cases; in children, by contrast, it accounts for less than 5% of cases. The peak occurrence of membranous glomerulopathy is in the fifth decade; 80–95% of patients are diagnosed after the age of 30.

**5. Does gender confer susceptibility to membranous glomerulopathy?**

Although equal numbers of men and women present with membranous glomerulopathy, nearly three times as many men as women progress to end-stage renal disease (ESRD). Of note, no racial predominance has been identified.

**6. What disease entities need to be excluded to make a diagnosis of primary idiopathic membranous glomerulopathy?**

A secondary cause for membranous glomerulopathy can be found in 15–30% of adults and up to 80% of children (see table). Of these, up to 75% of secondary cases are associated with systemic lupus erythematosus, hepatitis B, medications (e.g., gold, penicillamine), or malignancies.

*Secondary Causes of Membranous Glomerulopathy*

| CAUSES | EXAMPLES | |
| --- | --- | --- |
| Infections | Hepatitis B | Schistosomiasis |
| | Hepatitis C | Filariasis |
| | Malaria | Scabies |
| | Syphilis | Hydatid disease |
| | Leprosy | Castleman's disease |
| | *Helicobacter pylori* | |
| Autoimmune | Systemic lupus erythematosus | Hashimoto's thyroiditis |
| | Rheumatoid arthriti | Dermatitis herpetiformiss |
| | Sjögren's syndrome | Myasthenia gravis |
| | Dermatomyositis | Guillain-Barré syndrome |
| | Sarcoidosis | Weber-Christian panniculitis |
| | Mixed connective tissue disease | Bullous pemphigoid/pemphigus |
| | Crohn's disease | Ankylosing spondylitis |
| | Anticardiolipin antibody syndrome | Graves' disease |
| | Urticarial vasculitis | Graft-versus-host disease |
| Malignancies | Carcinoma (lung, colon, breast, stomach, esophagus, carotid body) | |
| | Melanoma | |
| | Leukemia/lymphoma (non-Hodgkin's type) | |
| Medications | Organic gold | |
| | D-Penicillamine | |
| | Mercury-containing compounds | |
| | Captopril | |
| | Probenecid | |
| | Trimethadione | |
| | NSAIDs (ketoprofen, fenoprofen) | |
| Genetic | Sickle cell disease | |
| | Fanconi's syndrome | |
| | Sclerosing cholangitis | |
| | (?) Diabetes—increased incidence of membranous glomerulonephritis | |
| Others | Kimura's disease | |
| | Gardner-Diamond syndrome | |
| | Hydrocarbon exposure | |
| | Systemic mastocytosis | |
| | De novo in renal allografts | |

## 7. What is the most common clinical presentation of membranous glomerulopathy?

Membranous glomerulopathy presents with the nephrotic syndrome in more than 80% of patients. Some patients, though, present with asymptomatic proteinuria. Up to 50% will have accompanying microhematuria. The onset of membranous glomerulopathy is typically insidious and generally not associated with antecedent or concomitant infection.

## 8. Does membranous glomerulopathy present with renal failure?

Only 5–10% of patients present with renal insufficiency. Patients will more often complain of edema and sometimes anasarca. Nonspecific symptoms such as nausea, anorexia, and malaise may be present. Hypertension and azotemia are usually absent on initial presentation but may develop in the course of membranous glomerulopathy.

## 9. How is the diagnosis of membranous glomerulopathy made?

Biopsy, as in most forms of primary glomerular disease, is necessary for definitive diagnosis. Although the clinical picture may suggest the possibility of membranous glomerulopathy, confirmation by biopsy is required. Again, one must carefully exclude secondary causes of membranous glomerulopathy by clinical evaluation for systemic disease.

## 10. Describe the biopsy findings in membranous glomerulopathy.

| EXAMINATION | FINDINGS |
| --- | --- |
| Light microscopy | Initially, the glomeruli and mesangial areas appear normal; later, capillary wall thickening appears as the disease progresses. Methenamine silver staining may reveal characteristic epithelial projections ("spikes") along the capillary walls, which represent new basement membrane material that surrounds the subepithelial deposits. |
| Immunofluorescence | Granular staining for IgG with some C3 (occasionally weak IgA and IgM) |
| Electron microscopy | May be classified under four stages (I–IV) with common features of variable subepithelial immune complex depositions and no obvious mesangial changes. The development, size, and frequency of the immune deposits determine the stage. Early and irregularly placed deposits are classified under stage I, whereas stage IV represents late, lightly staining, "burned out" deposits. |

## 11. What causes primary membranous glomerulopathy?

The most commonly accepted mechanism in the pathogenesis of membranous glomerulopathy is in situ immune complex formation against antigens that have become implanted within the glomerular basement membrane. The antibody is thought to find its way to the subepithelial antigen, form immune complexes, and deposit there. Another theory proposes that preformed circulating immune complexes deposit in the subepithelial space. In some secondary forms of membranous glomerulopathy, the antigen is known and can be demonstrated in the glomerulus by immunofluorescence (e.g., hepatitis B surface and core antigens). A rat model of membranous glomerulopathy known as Heymann's nephritis produces lesions similar to human membranous glomerulopathy. Immune complex deposition mediates proteinuria in part by activating the complement cascade. The activated terminal complex C5b-C9 is cytotoxic for glomerular epithelial cells in vitro and results in proteinuria in vivo.

## 12. What laboratory tests are useful in patients with membranous glomerulopathy?

Laboratory studies should include a chemistry profile to measure renal function and electrolyte status, a urinalysis to document proteinuria and hematuria, a 24-hour urine collection to quantitate the proteinuria and glomerular filtration rate, a serum albumin, and a lipid profile. Proteinuria can also be estimated reliably using the protein-to-creatinine ratio obtained from a random or "spot" urine sample. Ancillary tests may be used to rule out other etiologies as noted in question 6, depending on the clinical manifestations. Serum complement levels should be normal; therefore, low complements should prompt a search for other causes of glomerular disease.

## 13. What is the incidence of ESRD in patients with membranous glomerulopathy?

The natural history of membranous glomerulopathy varies depending on several factors. The overall prognosis in children is excellent, with less than 5% progressing to renal failure. The 10-year renal survival in children is over 80–90%. In adults, 20–40% undergo complete remission, and 20–35% undergo partial remission. Thus, depending on the series, 5-year renal survival is approximately 80–85%, 10-year renal survival is over 65–75%, and in one study, 15-year renal survival was 59% in adults. Membranous glomerulopathy appears to have an indolent course among most patients. However, 10–30% of patients do progress to ESRD over 10–20 years. In summary, the "rule of thirds" applies quite well: one-third spontaneously remit, one-third remain proteinuric with stable renal function, and one-third progress to ESRD, although 10% will die from nonrenal causes.

## 14. What factors indicate a poor prognosis in patients with membranous glomerulopathy?

The degree and duration of proteinuria appear to be the best indicators validated in the literature so far. Patients with nephrotic-range proteinuria in excess of 8 gm/day for at least 6 months appear to have a 66% chance of developing renal insufficiency. Other indicators of poor prognosis include the presence of hypertension, older age, male sex, and decreased renal function at presentation. Morphologically, superimposed crescentic glomerulonephritis and chronic tubulointerstitial disease further portend a worse outcome.

## 15. If an individual has idiopathic membranous glomerulopathy but normal renal function, is there any pressing need to treat?

This is a difficult question, and treatment decisions should be made on an individual basis. When making treatment decisions about idiopathic membranous glomerulopathy, the biopsy (as discussed previously) provides valuable prognostic information, as do the clinical presentation (age, gender, creatinine, blood pressure) and accumulated follow-up information (e.g., sustained proteinuria and elevated creatinine). Because over a quarter of patients experience a complete spontaneous remission in the absence of any treatment within 5 years of initial diagnosis, empirically treating *all* patients—thus subjecting some patients to toxic therapies who likely would have remitted without any intervention—remains a controversial issue. However, in a review of treatment modalities, Ponticelli et al. found that nearly 50% of *untreated* patients with membranous nephropathy die or enter ESRD within 10 years of diagnosis, suggesting that watchful waiting may prove detrimental for many patients.

## 16. What therapeutic regimens have been employed to treat membranous nephropathy? Which work the best?

Steroids, azathioprine, intravenous immunoglobulin, cyclosporine A, probucol, angiotensin-converting enzyme (ACE) inhibitors, chlorambucil, and cyclophosphamide have all been used to treat membranous glomerulopathy. The data on steroid efficacy have been mixed at best, with some prospective randomized trials finding efficacy and others showing lack of effect. Data are clearer and more promising with chlorambucil and cyclophosphamide. In a 1995 randomized trial, Ponticelli and colleagues showed that methylprednisolone and chlorambucil achieved a 10-year renal survival in 92% of treated patients compared with just 60% of untreated controls. A subsequent controlled trial demonstrated that steroids and chlorambucil achieved remission more effectively (64%) and more quickly than did supportive treatment or steroid therapy (34%) alone. A third trial demonstrated that cyclophosphamide and methylprednisolone worked as well as chlorambucil and methylprednisolone.

**17. How about supportive care for patients with membranous glomerulopathy?**
    Symptomatic therapy with diuretics and control of hypertension remain standard in the care of the patient with membranous glomerulopathy. Some authors have advocated low-protein diets, control of cholesterol intake, and use of lipid-lowering agents. ACE inhibitors have been used to decrease proteinuria. Some have tried nonsteroidal anti-inflammatory drugs (NSAIDs) as well. Prophylactic anticoagulation with warfarin, aspirin, or dipyridamole have been advocated, especially in patients with persistent nephrotic syndrome. However, the data supporting the use of aspirin and prophylactic anticoagulation are weak.

**18. Does transplantation play a role in membranous glomerulopathy?**
    Yes. Transplantation has an excellent prognosis for patients with membranous glomerulopathy who have reached ESRD. Membranous glomerulopathy remains, nevertheless, one of the most common types of immune complex–mediated glomerulopathy in renal allografts, occurring both as a recurrent disease, particularly in individuals whose original biopsy demonstrated crescent formation, and as a de novo one. The prevalence of membranous glomerulopathy in renal allografts is 1.3–2.1%, with the vast majority of cases (about 90%) due to de novo disease. Multiple series have shown variable recurrence rates, ranging from 7% to 50%; one review found a 72% risk of graft loss at 5 years due to recurrent membranous glomerulopathy.

BIBLIOGRAPHY

1. Austin HA, Falk RJ: Idiopathic membranous nephropathy. In Brady HR, Wilcox CS (eds): Therapy in Nephrology and Hypertension. Philadelphia, W.B. Saunders, 1999, pp 189–198.
2. Cattran DC: Membranous nephropathy: Quo vadis? Kidney Int 61:349–350, 2002.
3. Cattran DC: Idiopathic membranous glomerulonephritis. Kidney Int 59:1983–1994, 2001.
4. Geddes CC, Cattran DC: The treatment of idiopathic membranous nephropathy. Semin Nephrol 20:299–308, 2000.
5. Horl WH: Membranous glomerulonephritis (MGN). J Nephrol 13:291–316, 2000.
6. Ponticelli C, Altieri P, Scolari F, et al: A randomized study comparing methylprednisolone plus chlorambucil versus methylprednisolone plus cyclophosphamide in idiopathic membranous nephropathy. J Am Soc Nephrol 9:444–450, 1998.
7. Ponticelli C, Passerini P: Treatment of membranous nephropathy. Nephrol Dial Transplant 16(suppl 5):8–10, 2001.
8. Torres A, Dominguez-Gil B, Carreno A, et al: Conservative versus immunosuppressive treatment of patients with idiopathic membranous nephropathy. Kidney Int 61:219–227, 2002.

# 25. IgA NEPHROPATHY

*Donald E. Hricik, M.D.*

### 1. What is IgA nephropathy?

IgA (immunoglobulin A) nephropathy is a common form of mesangioproliferative glomerulonephritis characterized pathologically by mesangial deposition of IgA (detected by immunofluorescence microscopy) and varying degrees of mesangial cell proliferation and expansion of mesangial matrix. Codeposits of IgG, IgM, or terminal components of the complement system are present in the majority of cases.

### 2. What is the cause of IgA nephropathy?

This disorder probably results from altered regulation of the production or structure of IgA. Circulating IgA immune complexes are detectable in many cases and roughly parallel the severity of the disease. Glomerular deposits in IgA nephropathy consist primarily of abnormally glycosylated polymeric forms of the isotype subclass IgA1. The underlying cause of the abnormalities are unknown. However, the common association of gross hematuria with infections of the respiratory or gastrointestinal tract suggests that abnormal production of IgA may be triggered by mucosal exposure to environmental antigens. Recent genetic linkage analyses have identified the chromosomal locus (at 6q22-23) of a disease gene highly associated with the development of IgA nephropathy.

### 3. How common is IgA nephropathy?

The exact prevalence is difficult to determine because it is likely that the vast majority of cases are subclinical. Nevertheless, IgA nephropathy is now recognized as the most common form of glomerulonephritis worldwide. The prevalence varies considerably between and within countries, with high rates in the western Pacific rim and relatively low rates in the United States and northern Europe. The disorder occurs in all age groups with a peak incidence in the second and third decades. There is a male predominance of at least 2:1. IgA nephropathy is uncommon in African Americans.

### 4. What explains the geographic variation in the prevalence of IgA nephropathy?

Variations in the prevalence of the disease may reflect differences in genetic tendencies to develop the disorder. Because many patients with IgA nephropathy present with otherwise symptomless hematuria, it is also possible that geographic variations in prevalence rates reflect local health screening practices or locally accepted indications for renal biopsy.

### 5. How is IgA nephropathy related to Henoch-Schönlein purpura?

Henoch-Schönlein purpura is a systemic disease characterized by cutaneous purpura, arthritis, colitis, and glomerulonephritis. The glomerular findings in Henoch-Schönlein purpura are morphologically indistinguishable from those observed in primary IgA nephropathy so that these disorders often are considered to be related components of a pathophysiologic spectrum.

### 6. Are IgA levels elevated in patients with IgA nephropathy?

Plasma concentrations of IgA are elevated in up to 50% of cases. However, measurement of IgA levels is neither sensitive nor specific enough to be of use in the diagnosis of IgA nephropathy.

**7. How do patients with IgA nephropathy present?**

The most common clinical presentation (50–60% of cases) consists of episodic gross hematuria frequently associated with simultaneous respiratory or gastrointestinal infection. Persistent microscopic hematuria, typically discovered during screening examinations, occurs in 30% of cases. Finally, 10% of patients present either with acute glomerulonephritis or with nephrotic syndrome.

**8. What treatments are available?**

Curative therapy is lacking. However, a variety of therapies have been attempted in an effort to retard the progression of the disease. Angiotensin inhibitors are probably more effective than other antihypertensive agents in slowing the progression of IgA nephropathy. Steroids and cytotoxic drugs may have some benefit in reducing rates of urinary protein excretion. It remains unclear whether these agents beneficially influence long-term renal function. However, a recent randomized trial suggests that a 6-month course of steroid treatment was more effective than supportive therapy alone in preventing deterioration of renal function. Based on the premise that $\omega$-3 fatty acids may limit the actions of cytokines and eicosanoids induced by glomerular depositions of IgA, fish oil has proved to be of benefit in some trials. Several other treatment regimens, including high-dose immunoglobulin therapy, phenytoin, antiplatelet agents, urokinase, dapsone, plasma exchange, and tonsillectomy, have been attempted without conclusive results.

**9. What is the prognosis of patients with IgA nephropathy?**

Although IgA nephropathy commonly presents with asymptomatic or "benign" hematuria, end-stage renal disease ultimately develops in 20–40% of patients 5–25 years after diagnosis. Risk factors for progression to end-stage renal disease include older age, male gender, hypertension, persistent heavy proteinuria, impaired renal function at the time of diagnosis, the absence of gross hematuria, the presence of glomerulosclerosis or interstitial fibrosis on renal biopsy, and presence of the DD genotype for the deletion polymorphism in the angiotensin-converting enzyme gene.

BIBLIOGRAPHY

1. Donadio JV, Bergstralh ES, Offord KP, et al: A controlled trial of fish oil in IgA nephropathy. N Engl J Med 331:1194–1199, 1994.
2. Emancipator SN: IgA nephropathy: Morphologic expression and pathogenesis. Am J Kidney Dis 23:451–462, 1994.
3. Galla JH: IgA nephropathy. Kidney Int 47:377–387, 1995.
4. Gharavi AG, Yan Y, Scolari F, et al: IgA nephropathy, the most common cause of glomerulonephritis, is linked to 6q22-23. Nature Genet 26: 354-357, 2000.
5. Hricik DH, Chung-Park M, Sedor JR: Glomerulonephritis. N Engl J Med 339:888–899, 1998.
6. Ibels LS, Ayory AZ: IgA nephropathy: Analysis of the natural history, important factors in the progression of renal disease, and a review of the literature. Medicine 73:79–102, 1994.
7. Mestecky J, Tomana M, Crowley-Nowick PA, et al: Defective galactosylation and clearance of IgA1 molecules as a possible etiopathogenic factor in IgA nephropathy. Contrib Nephrol 104:172–182, 1993.
8. Pozzi C, Bolasco P, Fogazzi G, et al: Corticosteroids in IgA nephropathy: A randomised, controlled trial. Lancet 353:883–887, 1999.
9. Rostoker G, Desvaux-Belghiti D, Pilatte Y, et al: High-dose immunoglobulin therapy for severe IgA nephropathy and Henoch-Schönlein purpura. Ann Intern Med 120:476–484, 1994.
10. Schena FP, Montenegro M, Scivittaro P: Meta-analysis of randomized controlled trials in patients with IgA nephropathy (Berger's disease). Nephrol Dial Transplant 5:47–52, 1990.

# 26. MEMBRANOPROLIFERATIVE GLOMERULONEPHRITIS

*Ira D. Davis, M.D., M.S.*

### 1. What is membranoproliferative glomerulonephritis (MPGN)?

MPGN is a morphologic entity defined by mesangial proliferation and thickening of the glomerular capillary walls as seen on light microscopy. The capillary wall thickening is due to immune deposits and interposition of mesangial matrix that results in double contours ("tram tracks") of the glomerular basement membrane, best appreciated on silver-stained specimens. Both primary and secondary forms of MPGN occur. Idiopathic MPGN is one of the least common types of glomerulonephritis.

### 2. What are some synonyms for MPGN?

- Mesangiocapillary glomerulonephritis
- Lobular glomerulonephritis
- Hypocomplementemic persistent glomerulonephritis

### 3. Describe the three types of primary MPGN.

The three types are shown in the table below and differ with reference to pathology and prevalence. The pathologic differentiation is based definitively on electron microscopic findings.

*Pathology of MPGN*

| TYPE | MICROSCOPY LIGHT | IMMUNO-FLUORESCENCE | ELECTRON MICROSCOPY |
|------|------------------|---------------------|---------------------|
| Type I (most common) | Focal mesangial deposits with a nodular quality and double contours best seen with the Jones methenamine silver stain | IgG and C3 predominate in a granular mesangial and subendothelial pattern | Mesangial proliferation with immune deposition. Mesangial cell "interposition" noted between the GBM and endothelium. Subendothelial electron-dense deposits surrounded by new basement membrane producing double contours |
| Type II or dense deposit disease (least common) | Less uniform hyper cellularity with band-like thickening of the lamina densa containing intramembranous PAS-positive, silver-positive deposits | C3 only in a linear or double-contoured distribution along the GBM with occasional nodular mesangial deposition | Highly electron-dense deposits replacing the lamina densa to create smooth and ribbon-like depositions. Nodular mesangial deposits present |

*Table continued on next page*

99

*Pathology of MPGN (continued)*

| TYPE | MICROSCOPY LIGHT | IMMUNO-FLUORESCENCE | ELECTRON MICROSCOPY |
|---|---|---|---|
| Type III (uncommon) | Combined double contour and "spikes" denoting presence of subendothelial and subepithelial deposits seen best with silver stain | Mostly C3 with variable IgG deposition in the subendothelial, subepithelial, and mesangial areas | Electron-dense deposits in mixed subendothelial and subepithelial lesions producing "tram tracks" on the inner aspect and "spikes" on the outer aspect |

PAS = periodic acid–Schiff stain, GBM = glomerular basement membrane.

**4. What secondary causes of MPGN must be excluded in order to call it a primary glomerular disease?**

*Secondary Causes of MPGN*

| CAUSES | EXAMPLES |
|---|---|
| Infections | Hepatitis B |
| | Hepatitis C + cryoglobulinemia |
| | Infective endocarditis |
| | Visceral abscesses |
| | Infected ventriculoatrial shunts |
| | Angiofollicular lymph node syndrome (Castleman's disease) |
| | Malaria |
| | Schistosomiasis |
| | Epstein-Barr virus |
| | HIV |
| | Mycoplasma |
| Autoimmune | Systemic lupus erythematosus |
| | Rheumatoid arthritis |
| | Sjögren's syndrome |
| | Scleroderma |
| | Sarcoidosis |
| | Celiac disease |
| Chronic liver disease | Cirrhosis of any etiology |
| Thrombotic microangiopathies | Hemolytic uremic syndrome–thrombotic thrombocytopenic purpura |
| | Antiphospholipid antibody syndrome |
| | Sickle cell nephropathy |
| | Chronic allograft failure |
| | Radiation nephritis |
| Malignancies | B-cell lymphomas |
| | Chronic lymphocytic leukemia |
| | Other carcinoma (rarely) |

*Table continued on next page*

*Secondary Causes of MPGN (continued)*

| CAUSES | EXAMPLES |
|---|---|
| Genetic disorders | Alpha$_1$-antitrypsin disease |
| | Complement deficiency (C2 or C3) with or without partial lipodystrophy |
| | Kartagener's syndrome |
| | Renal artery dysplasia |
| | Buckley's syndrome |
| Dysproteinemias | Cryoglobulinemia |
| | Light chain deposition disease |
| | Waldenström's macroglobulinemia |

### 5. What causes primary MPGN?

The pathogenesis is largely speculative. However, intermittently low complement levels (70% of cases) and circulating immune complexes (found in 50%) do support the role of immune complex deposition in the etiology of MPGN type I. The pathophysiology of types II and III remains unknown.

### 6. What is the most common clinical presentation of MPGN?

Fifty percent of patients present with nephrotic syndrome, 30% present with asymptomatic proteinuria (with or without recurrent gross or microscopic hematuria), and 20% present with acute glomerulonephritis. Type I MPGN especially tends to present with nephrotic syndrome. Some patients report a respiratory illness preceding the overt signs and symptoms of renal disease.

### 7. What age groups are most commonly affected by MPGN?

MPGN occurs most commonly between the ages of 7 and 30 years. Seventy percent of cases present in the second decade.

### 8. Is there any gender or racial predominance in MPGN?

There is near equal incidence between males and females, although, in some series, there is a slight female predominance in type I disease. Although it is seen in most races, MPGN appears to predominate among caucasians.

### 9. How is the diagnosis of MPGN made?

Biopsy, biopsy, biopsy! As stated in question 1, this is a morphologic diagnosis, and definitive diagnosis can be made only with renal tissue and confirmation by electron microscopy.

### 10. What laboratory tests are useful in patients suspected of having MPGN?

Helpful tests include a chemistry profile to assess renal function and electrolyte status, a urinalysis to document proteinuria and hematuria, a renal ultrasound to exclude obstruction, serum complements to support the diagnosis (usually a low C3), and a 24-hour urine specimen to quantitate proteinuria and glomerular filtration rate. Other ancillary tests to rule out secondary causes of MPGN will be needed depending on the clinical presentation.

### 11. Does complement pattern have a bearing in diagnosis?

Type I MPGN is most often associated with panhypocomplementemia including decreased levels of C3, C4, and C5. Patients with type II MPGN tend to have only low C3, suggesting activation of the alternative complement pathway. Type III has low C3 or C5 but usually normal C4. This is only a rough guide, and there is a moderate degree of overlap in the complement patterns associated with the three entities.

## 12. What is the C3 nephritic factor?

This term refers to an antibody that is responsible for binding C3 convertase. As a result, the C3 convertase becomes stable and resistant to degradation by C3b inactivator, thus increasing its half-life tenfold. Consequently, it acts on the C3b amplification loop, markedly lowering C3 levels. C3 nephritic factor is found mostly in type II MPGN (40–50%) but also is present in up to 20% of MPGN type I and some cases of MPGN type III.

## 13. What are poor prognostic signs for patients with MPGN?

Rapidly progressing renal failure, severe hypertension, and persistent nephrotic syndrome are poor prognostic signs. Renal biopsy findings of glomerular crescents and interstitial fibrosis are also associated with a poor prognosis leading to chronic renal failure.

## 14. What is the treatment for MPGN?

No consensus has been reached regarding the ideal treatment for MPGN. For all age groups, for idiopathic MPGN with normal renal function and asymptomatic non–nephrotic-range proteinuria, no specific therapy is necessary. Close follow-up every 3–4 months, with specific attention to renal function, proteinuria, and blood pressure control, is recommended. In children with MPGN and nephrotic syndrome or azotemia, a trial of alternate-day steroids (40 mg/m$^2$) for 6–12 months is recommended. A randomized, controlled trial by the International Study of Kidney Disease in Children showed a significant beneficial effect of steroids but with some steroid toxicity, including hypertension. If no benefit is seen, steroids are discontinued, and patients are managed with diuretics and angiotensin-converting enzyme (ACE) inhibitors. Less well-designed trials also support the efficacy of steroid therapy in children, but good evidence for the benefit of steroids in adults with MPGN is lacking. Only small, uncontrolled case series support the use of steroids in adults with MPGN. Some studies have suggested benefit using antiplatelet agents such as aspirin and dipyridamole. A low-protein diet has been advocated by some authors. In addition, control of blood pressure is advocated to help retard progression of renal disease. The empiric use of ACE inhibitors or angiotensin II receptor antagonists to decrease proteinuria is also practiced by many physicians.

## 15. What are renal survival rates in primary MPGN?

Although older studies reported a 50% 10-year survival, recent studies quote survival rates of 60–85% in 10 years. The Cincinnati group reports a 20-year renal survival rate of 59% for patients on alternate-day steroid therapy.

## 16. Does transplantation play a role in MPGN patients who reach end-stage renal disease?

Yes. Transplantation is an option for patients with this disease. However, recurrence rates in post-transplant patients with MPGN type I and type II are 30% and 80%, respectively. Furthermore, the recurrent disease causes graft failure in 40% of type I and 10–20% of type II MPGN patients. Risk of recurrence in type III disease is not known.

## 17. Are there any new treatments on the horizon for MPGN?

Plasmapheresis, angiotensin II receptor antagonists, cyclosporine, and mycophenolate mofetil have been used for MPGN, but reports of their use are largely anecdotal. Newer therapies will undoubtedly arise as we gain more understanding of the biomolecular basis and pathogenesis of this disease.

## BIBLIOGRAPHY

1. D'Agati V: Membranoproliferative glomerulonephritis. In Greenberg A (ed): Primer on Kidney Diseases, 2nd ed. San Diego, Academic Press, 1998, pp 153–160.
2. Donadio JV, Offord KP: Reassessment of treatment results in membranoproliferative glomerulonephritis, with emphasis on life-table analysis. Am J Kidney Dis 14:445–451, 1989.
3. Glassock RJ, Cohen AH, Adler SG: Mesangiocapillary glomerulonephritis. In Brenner BM (ed): The Kidney, 5th ed. Philadelphia, W.B. Saunders, 1996, pp 1458–1466.
4. Levin A: Management of membranoproliferative glomerulonephritis: Evidence-based recommendations. Kidney Int 55:S41–S46, 1999.
5. McEnery PT: Membranoproliferative glomerulonephritis: The Cincinnati experience: Cumulative renal survival from 1957 to 1989. J Pediatr 116:S109–S114, 1990.
6. McEnery PT, McAdams AJ, West CD: The effect of prednisone in a high-dose, alternate-day regimen on the natural history of idiopathic membranoproliferative glomerulonephritis. Medicine 64:401–424, 1986.
7. Milford DV, Mathieson PW: Membranoproliferative glomerulonephritis. In Barratt TM, Avner ED, Harmon WE (eds): Pediatric Nephrology, 4th ed. Baltimore, Lippincott Williams & Wilkins, 1999, pp 707–718.
8. Tarshish P, Bernstein J, Tobin JN, Edelmann CM Jr: Treatment of mesangiocapillary glomerulonephritis with alternate-day prednisone: A report of the International Study of Kidney Disease in Children. Pediatr Nephrol 6:123–130, 1992.
9. West CD: Idiopathic membranoproliferative glomerulonephritis in childhood. Pediatr Nephrol 6:96–103, 1992.

# IV. Secondary Glomerular Disease

## 27. DIABETIC NEPHROPATHY

*Thomas Zipp, M.D., and Jeffrey R. Schelling, M.D.*

**1. What renal pathologic lesions are characteristic in diabetic nephropathy?**

Nodular glomerulosclerosis, which is characterized by the presence of eosinophilic Kimmelstiel-Wilson nodules at the glomerular periphery, is the most pathognomonic finding of diabetic nephropathy but is present in only about 10–20% of patients with diabetic renal disease. Other characteristic pathologic features of diabetic nephropathy include a thickened glomerular basement membrane, glomerular epithelial cell foot-process fusion, and glomerular enlargement due to extracellular mesangial matrix expansion. With advanced disease, tubular atrophy and interstitial fibrosis can be observed.

**2. What are the risk factors for progression of diabetic nephropathy?**

In general, about 1 out of 3 patients with type 1 or type 2 diabetes will proceed to develop significant diabetic nephropathy, but identification of susceptible patients has been problematic. Over the past decade, several longitudinal studies have suggested that microalbuminuria, defined as urine albumin excretion ranging between 30 and 300 mg/24 hours, predicts progression to overt proteinuria and then renal insufficiency. By definition, microalbuminuria is urine protein concentration below the detection limits of standard urine dipsticks. However, use of a more sensitive laboratory assay to detect microalbuminuria has become standard. In patients who do develop it, microalbuminuria is generally observed 5–10 years after the onset of diabetes, with nephrotic-range proteinuria occurring at 10–15 years and severe renal insufficiency with progression to end-stage renal disease occurring within 15–20 years. Once clinical albuminuria (> 300 mg/24 hours) develops, progression of renal disease is virtually certain.

Multiple intervention trials also have demonstrated that blood pressure and glycemic control delay the progression of renal disease (see question 5), indicating that hypertension and hyperglycemia, in the context of diabetes, also may pose risks for progressive diabetic nephropathy. There is fairly tight concordance of retinopathy and neuropathy with nephropathy in patients with type 1 diabetes. Discordance in expression of these manifestations of diabetic end-organ damage is more common in type 2 diabetics. Finally, there is increased concordance for diabetic nephropathy within families and in certain racial groups (African Americans, Native Americans), suggesting a genetic component to diabetic renal disease. The specific genes that regulate the expression of diabetic nephropathy have yet to be discovered, however.

**3. Is renal biopsy necessary in the diagnosis of patients with suspected diabetic nephropathy?**

Although the histologic features of diabetic nephropathy are well described, the diagnosis usually is made using clinical criteria, and patients require biopsy only if the clinical presentation is unusual. A biopsy diagnosis is commonly considered if the duration of diabetes is less than 10 years (as it often is in type 2 diabetes), in the absence of accompanying retinopathy, or for clinical suspicion of an alternative diagnosis. An estimated 25% of patients with type 2 diabetic nephropathy also may have another concomitant renal lesion. Additional renal pathology is much rarer in patients with type 1 diabetic nephropathy.

### 4. What are the typical urinalysis findings in patients with diabetic nephropathy?

The hallmark of the urinalysis in diabetic nephropathy is proteinuria. The predominant protein in the urine is albumin. A minority of patients with diabetic nephropathy will demonstrate microscopic hematuria. The presence of cellular casts should prompt careful consideration of other diagnoses, but cellular casts have been described in patients with diabetic renal disease.

### 5. What treatments should be considered to slow the progression of diabetes mellitus nephropathy?

1. **Blood pressure control**. Blood pressure control is one of the mainstays in the treatment of diabetic nephropathy. In particular, antihypertensive treatment with angiotensin-converting enzyme (ACE) inhibitors or angiotensin-receptor blockers (ARBs) may be preferred over other antihypertensive regimens. Lowering blood pressure with an ARB or ACE inhibitor–containing regimen has been associated with enhanced slowing of diabetic nephropathy progression when compared with equivalent blood pressure control with regimens that do not contain an ACE inhibitor. The mechanism by which ARBs and ACE inhibitors achieve this "renoprotective" effect is debated. ACE inhibitors and ARBs reduce both systemic and intraglomerular pressures. An alternative or additional renoprotective mechanism may be through inhibition of glomerular sclerosis and interstitial fibrosis, because in vitro studies have shown that angiotensin II promotes extracellular matrix deposition and fibrosis. Most studies that have demonstrated benefit from ARB or ACE inhibitor therapy in diabetic nephropathy have enrolled patients with mild to moderate renal disease (e.g., serum creatinine < 2.0 mg/dl). It remains to be determined if conclusions from these studies can be extrapolated to patients with more advanced renal disease. Lowering blood pressure to less than 130/80 mmHg is desirable in all diabetics, even in those without albuminuria. Multiple antihypertensive agents may be required to achieve this goal.

2. **Glycemic control**. Well-designed studies definitively demonstrate that glycemic control results in slowing of diabetic renal disease progression. In the Diabetes Control and Complications Trial, tight glycemic control, which was achieved with multiple daily insulin injections, was associated with a 40–50% decrease in the incidence of proteinuria.

3. **Dietary protein restriction**. Use of dietary protein restrictions as a therapeutic maneuver was initially identified using animal models of diabetic renal disease. The purported mechanism of action was reduction in glomerular capillary pressures. Initial human studies confirmed these results, although these data have been difficult to corroborate. In the Modification of Diet in Renal Disease study, which was designed to answer this question, there was no clear benefit to patients with established renal disease after 3 years of dietary protein restriction. However, type 1 diabetics were excluded from this study, and the type 2 diabetic cohort comprised only 3% of the study population.

### 6. Should calcium channel blockers be recommended for the treatment of hypertension in diabetic nephropathy?

Fairly good evidence exists to support the use of the nondihydropyridine classes of calcium channel blockers (verapamil and diltiazem family) for the treatment of hypertension in diabetic nephropathy. In animal models of diabetic renal disease, as well as human studies, benefit has been shown with respect both to preservation of glomerular filtration rate and to diminution of proteinuria. The data are much less compelling with dihydropyridine calcium channel blocker, particularly the older generation short-acting agents (e.g., nifedipine). Some studies have shown no effect on, or even increases in, proteinuria with these agents.

However, the Appropriate Blood Pressure Control in Diabetes study found that a dihydropyridine agent was as efficacious as an ACE inhibitor, suggesting that it is the target blood pressure and not the agent used that is the key goal.

## 7. How does the development of diabetic nephropathy alter the management of blood glucose?

Because the kidney both metabolizes and excretes glucose, the half-life of endogenously and exogenously administered insulin is prolonged in the setting of decreased glomerular filtration rate (GFR). Therefore, to avoid hypoglycemia, the dose of oral hypoglycemic agents or insulin often needs to be decreased in patients with diabetic nephropathy.

## 8. What are the renal replacement therapy options in patients with end-stage renal disease caused by diabetic nephropathy?

Diabetic nephropathy is now the most common cause of end-stage renal disease (ESRD), accounting for 1 in 3 patients entering renal replacement therapy programs. Similar to other causes of chronic renal disease, the optimum treatment is kidney transplantation. The 10-year survival rate in some series is as high as 40%, which is superior to mortality figures for diabetics on dialysis (see question 9). The data should be viewed with some caution, however, because there is a selection bias toward transplantation of diabetics with fewer comorbid medical problems. As with other types of glomerular disease, diabetic nephropathy may recur in the transplant allograft. A combined kidney and pancreas transplantation may be the preferred treatment for diabetic nephropathy, but this is an option at only a few medical centers. Because of the relatively small supply of donor organs and the high incidence of comorbid conditions in diabetics, which may preclude a transplant, the majority of patients with diabetic ESRD are treated with either hemodialysis or peritoneal dialysis (see figure). Outcome studies comparing hemodialysis versus peritoneal dialysis have yielded mixed results. Therefore, either modality is generally considered acceptable. The rates of peritoneal dialysis catheter infection and malfunction are higher in diabetics versus nondiabetics. Finally, mortality with all forms of renal replacement therapy is higher in diabetics compared to nondiabetics.

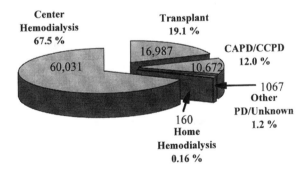

Distribution of patients with end-stage renal disease caused by diabetes mellitus to various renal replacement modalities. (From Friedlander MA, Hricik DE: Optimizing end-stage renal disease therapy for the patient with diabetes mellitus. Sem Nephrol 17:331–345, 1997, with permission.)

## 9. What is the mean life expectancy of diabetics on dialysis, and what are the major causes of death?

The life expectancy of diabetics with ESRD depends on age and comorbid conditions. In general, however, the mean life expectancy on hemodialysis is approximately 2–3 years.

The leading cause of death is cardiovascular disease, which reflects the increased incidence of macrovascular and microvascular disease in the setting of diabetes. Infection or sepsis is the second most common cause of death. Mortality is similar in diabetics on peritoneal dialysis, although cardiovascular disease and infection are roughly equal as the most common cause of death.

### BIBLIOGRAPHY

 1. American Diabetes Association: Position statement: Diabetic nephropathy. Diabetes Care 25:S85–S89, 2002.
 2. Bakris GL, Williams M, Dworkin L, et al: Preserving renal function in adults with hypertension and diabetes: A consensus approach. Am J Kidney Dis 36:646–661, 2000.
 3. Bloembergen WE, Port FP, Mauger EA, Wolfe RA: A comparison of mortality between patients treated with hemodialysis and peritoneal dialysis. J Am Soc Nephrol 6:177–183, 1995.
 4. Diabetes Control and Complications Trial Research Group: The effect of intensive treatment of diabetes on the development and progression of long-term complications in insulin-dependent diabetes mellitus. N Engl J Med 329:977–986, 1993.
 5. Fenton SSA, Schaubel DE, Desmeules M, et al: Hemodialysis versus peritoneal dialysis: A comparison of adjusted mortality rates. Am J Kidney Dis 30:334–344, 1997.
 6. Friedlander MA, Hricik DE: Optimizing end-stage renal disease therapy for the patient with diabetes mellitus. Semin Nephrol 17:331–345, 1997.
 7. Klahr S, Levey AS, Beck GJ, et al: The effects of dietary protein restriction and blood-pressure control on the progression of chronic renal disease. Modification of Diet in Renal Disease Study Group. N Engl J Med 330:877–884, 1994.
 8. Kloke HJ, Branten AJ, Huysmans FT, Wetzels JF: Antihypertensive treatment of patients with proteinuric renal diseases: Risks or benefits of calcium channel blockers? Kidney Int 53:1559–1573, 1998.
 9. Lewis EJ, Hunsicker LG, Bain RP, Rohde RD: The effect of angiotensin-converting enzyme inhibition on diabetic nephropathy. N Engl J Med 329:1456–1462, 1993.
10. Lewis EJ, Hunsicker LG, Clarke WR, et al: Renoprotective effect of the angiotensin-receptor antagonist irbesartan I patients with nephropathy due to type 2 diabetes. N Engl J Med 345:851–860, 2001.
11. Maki DD, Ma JZ, Louis TA, Kasiske BL: Long-term effects of antihypertensive agents on proteinuria and renal function. Arch Intern Med 155:1073–1080, 1995.
12. Mogensen CE, Christensen CK: Predicting diabetic nephropathy in insulin-dependent patients. N Engl J Med 311:89–93, 1984.
13. Ravid M, Brosh D, Levi Z, et al: Use of enalapril to attenuate decline in renal function in normotensive, normoalbuminuric patients with type 2 diabetes mellitus. A randomized, controlled trial. Ann Intern Med 128:982–988, 1998.
14. Reichard P, Nilsson BY, Rosenqvist U: The effect of long-term intensified insulin treatment on the development of microvascular complications of diabetes mellitus. N Engl J Med 329:204–309, 1993.
15. Schrier RW, Estacio RO, Esler A, Mehler P: Effects of aggressive blood pressure control in normotensive type 2 diabetic patients on albuminuria, retinopathy, and strokes. Kidney Int 61:1086–1097, 2002.

# 28. LUPUS NEPHRITIS

*Marcia R. Silver, M.D.*

**1. What proportion of patients with systemic lupus erythematosus (SLE) develop lupus nephritis?**

The kidney is the most common site of major organ system involvement in SLE. About 40% of patients with SLE develop lupus nephritis. Nearly 100% of those with major organ system involvement, such as lupus cerebritis, pneumonitis, or vasculitis, will have lupus renal disease as well.

**2. How are the lesions of lupus nephritis classified?**

Based on pathologic findings, the World Health Organization (WHO) developed the following classification:

*World Health Organization Classification of Lupus Nephritis Lesions*

| CLASS | DESCRIPTION |
|---|---|
| I | Normal glomeruli |
| II | Pure mesangial alterations (mesangial widening with or without hypercellularity) |
| III | Focal segmental glomerulonephritis (associated with mild or moderate mesangial alterations) |
| IV | Diffuse glomerulonephritis (severe mesangial, endocapillary, or mesangiocapillary proliferation and/or extensive subendothelial deposits with mesangial deposits present invariably and subepithelial deposits present often) |
| V | Diffuse membranous glomerulonephritis (but if associated with proliferative lesions, go to class IV) |
| VI | Advanced sclerosing glomerulonephritis |

**3. Do nonglomerular renal diseases occur in patients with SLE?**

The frequent use of nonsteroidal anti-inflammatory drugs (NSAIDs) for the management of arthritis may result in renal impairment. Pure interstitial nephritis may occur. A renal thrombotic microangiopathy has been described in the presence of antiphospholipid antibodies and in the absence of other findings of renal vasculitis or antibody-mediated glomerulonephritis. This antiphospholipid syndrome nephropathy has been described in up to a third of renal biopsies from patients with SLE.

**4. What are the usual presenting signs and symptoms of lupus nephritis?**

Many patients are asymptomatic. Early detection (highly desirable!) may be accomplished through regular monitoring of the urinalysis in patients with SLE for onset of hematuria or proteinuria or the presence of casts. Hypertension also may be a clue to the presence of renal disease. Edema may occur in patients with nephrotic-range proteinuria. Uremic signs and symptoms are very late findings—the renal disease is rarely reversible at this stage.

**5. What is the prognosis of patients with lupus nephritis?**

Overall survival for patients with SLE is about 70% at 10 years. Infection and renal failure are the most common causes of death. Outcomes are worse in African Americans, Hispanics, Asians, poor people, and patients with evidence of disease affecting major organs such as the brain, kidneys, lungs, or heart.

Outcomes for patients with lupus nephritis appear to have improved substantially over the past 4 decades. In the 1950s and 1960s, the 5-year survival rate was 45% for all patients with lupus and 20% for patients with class IV lupus nephritis. Since the early 1990s, 5-year survival for all patients with lupus nephritis has increased to approximately 80%. Some of these dramatic improvements, based on historical controls, may be the result of more aggressive and judicious use of immunosuppressive agents to treat lupus but also probably reflect increased sensitivity and availability of serologic tests for the disease, leading to earlier diagnosis and diagnosis of patients with milder disease. Also, patients who develop end-stage renal disease (ESRD) can now be managed successfully with dialysis and transplantation. Extrarenal manifestations of lupus tend to become quiescent when lupus patients develop ESRD, an improvement usually sustained in patients who receive a kidney transplant. Immunosuppressive effects of ESRD may have a salutary impact on extrarenal manifestations. After transplantation, the immunosuppressive agents required to prevent rejection of the transplanted organ may act similarly.

**6. How is the diagnosis of lupus nephritis made? When should a renal biopsy be performed?**

The presence of an abnormal urinalysis, hypertension, elevated serum creatinine concentration, edema, or other elements of the nephrotic syndrome (see Chapter 17, Nephrotic Syndrome) should trigger a thorough evaluation for the presence of lupus nephritis or other forms of kidney disease. The indications for renal biopsy in patients with SLE are controversial. Some experts think that patients with an established diagnosis of SLE who develop typical findings consistent with lupus nephritis can be treated empirically, avoiding the risks and expense of renal biopsy. Renal biopsy would still be indicated for those who fail to respond to initial treatment or for those with an atypical clinical presentation. Other authors propose that every patient suspected of having lupus nephritis requires a biopsy to determine the nature of the renal pathology. The benefits of this approach include (1) ensuring that one is not dealing with allergic interstitial nephritis or pure antiphospholipid syndrome, disorders that are associated with different diagnostic and management implications; (2) promptly determining the pathologic classification of the lupus nephritis, so that the best therapy can be selected and instituted early in the course of the disease (see question 7); and (3) allowing assessment of the degree of chronicity (scarring and other irreversible changes) on the biopsy, findings that may serve to temper the aggressive use of immunosuppressive agents. Also, up to 40% of patients with lupus nephritis may show changes in renal pathology on repeat biopsy, especially in the setting of changing clinical findings (e.g., new red cell casts, new hypertension, or new nephrotic syndrome).

**7. Does the classification scheme help the nephrologist make management decisions?**

Yes. Patients with class II (pure mesangial) and class V (pure membranous) lesions appear to have a better prognosis than those with proliferative lesions (classes III and IV). Treatment with potentially toxic immunosuppressive regimens is usually reserved for patients with more aggressive lesions.

**8. How should lupus nephritis be managed?**

Vigorous management of hypertension delays the progression of all forms of renal disease. The goal should be a blood pressure of $\leq$ 120/80 mmHg in most patients. Measures to decrease proteinuria (e.g., use of angiotensin-converting enzyme [ACE] inhibitors) probably are also beneficial in delaying the progression of any proteinuric renal disease, including aggressive forms of lupus nephritis. Although clinical data are somewhat limited, many nephrologists also believe that vigorous management of persistent hyperlipidemia may have a beneficial effect on renal and cardiovascular outcomes.

The data supporting the widely accepted notion that steroids are of significant benefit in lupus would not likely meet today's standards for evidence-based medicine. Nevertheless, the limited randomized trials of management of lupus nephritis include only a few hundred patients worldwide and generally compare some form of aggressive management using steroids with steroid-sparing alternative immunosuppressive agents such as cyclophosphamide or azathioprine. Evidence from a number of such trials suggests that the prognosis of patients with proliferative lupus nephritis (class III or IV) is substantially improved by treatment with cyclophosphamide and reduced doses of prednisone compared with prednisone alone. Pulse intravenous cyclophosphamide is about as effective as daily oral cyclophosphamide, but IV administration has become popular because of reduced gonadal and bladder toxicities. The data on azathioprine are mixed, with some evidence suggesting that it may be as effective as cyclophosphamide, perhaps with less long-term toxicity. In particular, it seems not to interfere with fertility or pregnancy, often an important issue for the many young women suffering with this disease. Mycophenolate mofetil is a newer agent that may be of benefit in patients who are unresponsive to cyclophosphamide. The combination of mycophenolate mofetil and prednisolone was as effective as a regimen of cyclophosphamide and prednisolone followed by azathioprine and prednisolone but was less toxic in a small, randomized trial, which studied 42 Chinese patients with WHO class IV lupus nephritis. Pulse methylprednisolone may be less toxic and equally efficacious compared to prolonged therapy with high doses of oral steroids in managing acute exacerbations of lupus renal disease. A randomized, controlled trial of plasmapheresis in severe lupus nephritis showed no benefit.

## BIBLIOGRAPHY

1. Austin HA 3d, Klippel JH, Balow JE, et al: Therapy of lupus nephritis: Controlled trial of prednisone and cytotoxic drugs. N Engl J Med 314:614–619, 1986.
2. Balow JE, Boumpas DT, Fessler BJ, Austin HA 3d: Management of lupus nephritis. Kidney Int 49:S88–S92, 1996.
3. Berden JHM: Lupus nephritis. Kidney Int 52:538–558, 1997.
4. Cameron JS: The long-term outcome of glomerular diseases. In Schrier RW, Gottschalk CW (eds): Diseases of the Kidney, 6th ed. Boston, Little, Brown, 1997, pp 1919–1982.
5. Chan TM, Li FK, Tang CS, et al: Efficacy of mycophenolate mofetil in patients with diffuse proliferative lupus nephritis. Hong Kong-Guangzhou Nephrology Study Group. N Engl J Med 343:1156–1162, 2000.
6. Donadio JV Jr, Glassock RJ: Immunosuppressive drug therapy in lupus nephritis. Am J Kidney Dis 21:239–250, 1993.
7. Daugas E, Nochy D, Huong du LT, et al: Antiphospholipid syndrome nephropathy in systemic lupus erythematosus. J Am Soc Nephrol 12:42–52, 2002.
8. Falk RJ: Treatment of lupus nephritis: A work in progress. N Engl J Med 343:1182–1183, 2000.
9. Glicklich D, Acharya A: Mycophenolate mofetil therapy for lupus nephritis refractory to intravenous cyclophosphamide. Am J Kidney Dis 32:318–322, 1998.
10. Levey AS, Lan SMPH, Corwin HL, et al: Progression and remission of renal disease in the lupus nephritis collaborative study. Results of treatment with prednisone and short-term oral cyclophosphamide. Ann Intern Med 116:114–123, 1992.
11. Lewis EJ, Hunsicker LG, Lan SP, et al: A controlled trial of plasmapheresis therapy in severe lupus nephritis. N Engl J Med 326:1373–1379, 1992.
12. Sloan RP, Schwartz MM, Korbet SM, et al: Long-term outcome in systemic lupus erythematosus membranous glomerulonephritis. Lupus Nephritis Collaborative Study Group. J Am Soc Nephrol 7:299–305, 1996.
13. Zimmerman R, Radhakrishnan J, Valeri A, Appel G: Advances in the treatment of lupus nephritis. Annu Rev Med 52:63–78, 2001.

# 29. POSTINFECTIOUS GLOMERULONEPHRITIS

Ira D. Davis, M.D.

**1. What common infections are associated with postinfectious glomerulonephritis?**

Acute pharyngitis, upper respiratory infections, and skin infections are the most frequent infections associated with postinfectious glomerulonephritis. This entity also may be seen following infection of ventriculoatrial or ventriculoperitoneal shunts or in association with acute and subacute bacterial endocarditis.

**2. What is the most common cause of acute postinfectious glomerulonephritis?**

Specific nephritogenic strains of group A beta-hemolytic streptococci are the most common organisms associated with acute glomerulonephritis. These strains differ from the strains associated with rheumatic fever.

**3. What other infectious agents are associated with acute postinfectious glomerulonephritis?**

Other infectious organisms that cause acute postinfectious glomerulonephritis include a variety of bacteria and viruses. *Staphylococcus aureus* is often seen in cases of shunt infections, whereas *Staphylococcus epidermidis* and various streptococcal species are frequently seen in glomerulonephritis associated with subacute bacterial endocarditis. Viruses associated with acute postinfectious glomerulonephritis include enteric cytopathic human orphan (ECHO) viruses, human immunodeficiency virus (HIV), adenovirus, and influenza A. Acute glomerulonephritis also has been reported following Rocky Mountain spotted fever, cat-scratch fever, trichinosis, and toxoplasmosis.

**4. What is the pathogenesis of acute poststreptococcal glomerulonephritis?**

Acute poststreptococcal glomerulonephritis is an immune-complex–mediated glomerular disease, although the precise nature of the antigen-antibody complex remains undefined. Unique streptococcal antigens associated with nephritogenic strains of streptococci have been found in immune complexes in the glomerulus. Glomerular immune deposits result from deposition of circulating immune complexes or binding of immunoglobulin to streptococcal antigens "planted" in glomerular structures, leading to in situ development of immune complexes.

**5. What are the typical pathologic changes of the glomerulus in acute postinfectious glomerulonephritis?**

The glomeruli are often enlarged, swollen, and bloodless with an intense diffuse cellular infiltrate of polymorphonuclear leukocytes, eosinophils, and monocytes. Capillary lumina are occluded by proliferating mesangial and endothelial cells and infiltrating leukocytes, resulting in a diffuse proliferative glomerulonephritis on light microscopy. The typical immunofluorescence finding is fine granular deposition of IgG and C3 in capillary walls, sometimes referred to as a "starry sky" pattern. Predominant immunoglobulin or C3 deposition in the axial or stalk region of the glomerulus is another immunofluorescent pattern. Characteristic findings on electron microscopy include "hump" electron-dense deposits on the epithelial side of the basement membrane (see figure, top of next page) and less discrete deposits in the mesangium and endothelial side of the basement membrane.

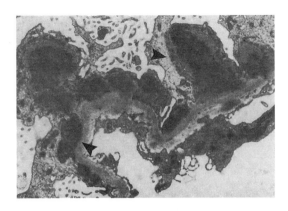

Large, nodular, subepithelial immune deposits (arrows), referred to as "humps," in an electron micrograph taken from a patient with poststreptococcal glomerulonephritis. (From Hricik DE, Chung-Park M, Sedor JR: Glomerulonephritis. N Engl J Med 339:888–889, 1998, with permission.)

**6. When do symptoms of renal disease occur in relation to the timing of the infection in acute postinfectious glomerulonephritis?**

A latency period of a few days to 3 weeks is typically seen in cases of acute glomerulonephritis following a streptococcal infection. The latency periods following pharyngitis and impetigo infections are typically 10 days and 21 days, respectively.

**7. What are the most common presenting complaints of patients with acute postinfectious glomerulonephritis?**

These patients commonly present with the abrupt onset of edema and cola-colored (or tea-colored) urine. Other symptoms may include malaise, lethargy, anorexia, fever, abdominal pain, weakness, and headache.

**8. How common is hypertension in acute postinfectious glomerulonephritis?**

Hypertension occurs in over 75% of children requiring hospitalization for acute glomerulonephritis. Approximately 5% of hospitalized patients develop severe hypertension that may be associated with encephalopathy (see Chapter 63, Hypertensive Emergencies). Hypertension usually resolves within 3–4 weeks of disease onset.

**9. What is the etiology of hypertension in acute postinfectious glomerulonephritis?**

The primary cause is expansion of the extracellular fluid compartment due to an increased avidity of the kidney for sodium and water. Interestingly, the renin-angiotensin-aldosterone axis appears to be suppressed. Because some patients are resistant to diuretics, other unknown factors also contribute to the development of hypertension in this disorder.

**10. How often is the complement component C3 depressed in patients with acute postinfectious glomerulonephritis?**

C3 levels and total hemolytic complement activity ($CH_{50}$) are depressed in 90% of patients and usually return to normal within 8 weeks. By contrast, patients with membranoproliferative glomerulonephritis or lupus nephritis exhibit depressed levels of C3 (often associated with a low C4) that persist for more than 8 weeks following the initial presentation with acute glomerulonephritis.

**11. How often are the streptozyme test and antistreptolysin O (ASO) titers elevated in patients with acute poststreptococcal glomerulonephritis?**

Streptozyme test positivity and elevated ASO titers occur in 90% and 70% of patients, respectively. However, early treatment of the infection may limit the ability of the patient to mount a serologic response to the streptococcal infection.

**12. Does treatment of the infection clear the glomerulonephritis?**

No. Once the immunologic response to the offending organism occurs, treatment with antibiotics does not limit pathologic injury to the kidney.

**13. Does acute postinfectious glomerulonephritis recur?**

Long-term studies suggest that recurrent active disease, manifested primarily by gross hematuria, occurs in approximately 10% of patients. This usually occurs within 1 year of the initial episode of acute glomerulonephritis.

**14. What other renal diseases must be considered in the differential diagnosis of acute postinfectious glomerulonephritis?**

Acute exacerbation of a chronic glomerulonephritis
Henoch-Schönlein purpura
IgA nephropathy
Thin basement membrane disease
Hereditary nephritis (Alport's syndrome)

**15. What is the long-term prognosis of patients with acute postinfectious glomerulonephritis?**

The long-term prognosis in children is very good, with complete recovery in most cases. However, chronic renal disease may occur in as many as 1–2% of patients. This favorable prognosis contrasts with reports of postinfectious glomerulonephritis in the adult population, in which over 50% of patients may have evidence of persisting renal disease.

BIBLIOGRAPHY

1. Baldwin DS, Melvin C, Gluck MC, et al: The long-term course of poststreptococcal glomerulonephritis. Ann Intern Med 80:342–358, 1974.
2. Brouhard BH, Travis LB: Acute postinfectious glomerulonephritis. In Edelmann CM, Bernstein J, Meadow SR, et al (eds): Pediatric Kidney Disease. Boston, Little, Brown, 1992, pp 1199–1221.
3. Cole BR, Salinas-Madrigal L: Acute proliferative glomerulonephritis and crescentic glomerulonephritis. In Barratt TM, Avner ED, Harmon WE (eds): Pediatric Nephrology, 4th ed. Baltimore, Williams & Wilkins, 1994, pp 669–690.
4. Dodge WF, Spargo BH, Travis LB, et al: Poststreptococcal glomerulonephritis. A prospective study in children. N Engl J Med 286:273–278, 1972.
5. Hricik DE, Chung-Park M, Sedor JR: Glomerulonephritis. N Engl J Med 339:888–899, 1998.
6. Perlman LV, Herdman RC, Kleinman H, et al: Poststreptococcal glomerulonephritis: A ten-year follow-up of an epidemic. JAMA 194:175–182, 1965.
7. Potter EV, Lipschultz SA, Abidh S, et al: Twelve to seventeen-year follow-up of patients with poststreptococcal acute glomerulonephritis in Trinidad. N Engl J Med 307:725–729, 1982.

# 30. HEPATITIS-ASSOCIATED GLOMERULONEPHRITIS

*Ashwini R. Sehgal, M.D.*

### 1. What types of hepatitis are associated with glomerulonephritis?

Chronic infection with hepatitis B or C is associated with glomerulonephritis. Hepatitis A does not result in chronic infection and is not associated with glomerulonephritis. The newly discovered hepatitis G virus recently was reported to cause membranoproliferative glomerulonephritis, but data are limited on the role of this virus as a cause of kidney disease.

### 2. How does hepatitis viral infection cause glomerulonephritis?

Immune complexes containing hepatitis B or C antigens, either deposited from the circulation or formed in situ, are frequently found in affected glomeruli. These may elicit an inflammatory response involving complement activation and infiltration by monocytes and neutrophils. These leukocytes can release oxidants and proteases that damage both endogenous glomerular cells and the glomerular basement membrane, resulting in altered permeability.

### 3. Name the types of glomerular disease associated with hepatitis B and C.

*Glomerular Diseases Associated with Hepatitis B and C*

|  | COMMON TYPES | LESS COMMON TYPES |
| --- | --- | --- |
| Hepatitis B | Membranous nephropathy | Polyarteritis nodosa Membranoproliferative glomerulonephritis |
| Hepatitis C | Essential mixed cryoglobulinemia | Membranoproliferative glomerulonephritis Membranous nephropathy |

### 4. How common is hepatitis-associated glomerulonephritis?

In the United States, the prevalence of renal disease associated with hepatitis B is relatively low. By contrast, hepatitis C infection is found in 80–90% of patients with essential mixed cryoglobulinemia, in 10–20% of patients with membranoproliferative glomerulonephritis, and in < 10% of patients with membranous nephropathy.

### 5. How are hepatitis B and C acquired?

In developed countries, hepatitis B is acquired from sexual activity, intravenous drug use, or occupational exposure (e.g., needle sticks). Hepatitis C usually is acquired from intravenous drug use or blood transfusions. In about 25% of cases, the mode of transmission of hepatitis B or C is unclear.

### 6. What is the natural history of hepatitis B and C infection?

Whereas acute hepatitis B infection tends to be symptomatic, less than 5% of patients go on to develop chronic hepatitis. By contrast, acute hepatitis C infection is generally mild and asymptomatic. However, persistent viremia is typical, and chronic hepatitis C infection eventually develops in two-thirds of patients.

**7. How long does it take for hepatitis-associated glomerulonephritis to develop?**

Hepatitis B–associated glomerulonephritis develops several months to several years after acute hepatitis B infection. Hepatitis C–associated glomerulonephritis generally develops more than 10 years after acute hepatitis C infection.

**8. What is the liver function of patients with hepatitis-associated glomerulonephritis?**

Most patients with hepatitis B–associated glomerulonephritis have elevated transaminase levels. However, transaminase levels may be normal, and a history of acute hepatitis may be absent in these patients.

**9. How is hepatitis-associated glomerulonephritis diagnosed?**

• Hepatitis C RNA levels in serum
• Serologic evidence of hepatitis antigens or antibodies
• Kidney biopsy findings of an immune complex glomerulonephritis with glomerular deposits containing hepatitis antigens

**10. Describe the pathologic findings in hepatitis-associated glomerulonephritis.**

The glomerular lesions in hepatitis C–associated cryoglobulinemia are diverse, but membranoproliferative glomerulonephritis accounts for 80% of cases. Hepatitis-associated membranoproliferative glomerulonephritis, with or without cryoglobulinemia, is histologically similar to idiopathic type I membranoproliferative glomerulonephritis (see Chapter 26, Membranoproliferative Glomerulonephritis). Light microscopy shows increased mesangial matrix and cellularity and basement membrane thickening; immunofluorescence shows immunoglobulin M (IgM), IgG, and C3 deposits in the mesangium and in capillary walls. Electron microscopy shows mesangial and subendothelial immune deposits. Hepatitis C–associated membranoproliferative glomerulonephritis differs from idiopathic membranoproliferative glomerulonephritis in that additional deposits with ultrastructural features characteristic of cryoglobulins sometimes fill the capillary lumen.

Hepatitis-associated membranous nephropathy is histologically similar to idiopathic membranous nephropathy (see Chapter 24, Membranous Glomerulopathy). Light microscopy shows normal cellularity with basement membrane thickening, immunofluorescence shows IgG and C3 deposits in capillary walls, and electron microscopy shows subepithelial immune deposits and effacement of podocyte foot processes. Hepatitis B–associated membranous nephropathy differs from idiopathic membranous nephropathy in that additional subendothelial or mesangial deposits are frequently present as well. Hepatitis B–associated polyarteritis nodosa results in necrotizing inflammation of medium-sized arteries and is similar to polyarteritis nodosa not associated with hepatitis (see Chapter 37, Renal Vasculitis).

**11. What is the prognosis of hepatitis-associated glomerulonephritis?**

Hepatitis B–associated membranous nephropathy generally resolves spontaneously in children but tends to be progressive in adults. Hepatitis C–associated glomerulonephritis is generally slowly progressive.

**12. How is hepatitis-associated glomerulonephritis treated?**

Optimal therapy for these disorders has yet to be defined. Antiviral therapy with interferon may be helpful, but relapses often occur once treatment is stopped. Immunosuppressive treatment should be avoided because steroid and cyclophosphamide use may result in increased viral replication that can accelerate progression of liver disease.

**13. Can patients with hepatitis B or C receive a renal transplant?**

Renal transplantation may be performed in patients with asymptomatic hepatitis B or hepatitis C infection. However, the presence of hepatitis B infection may adversely affect allograft survival. Furthermore, there is a risk of accelerated liver disease when patients with hepatitis B are treated with immunosuppressive drugs. Most transplant centers are willing to offer a kidney transplant to patients who are hepatitis B surface antigen–positive, as long as they have normal liver function tests and no serologic evidence of active viral replication (i.e., a positive hepatitis E antigen or high DNA titers). Experience with renal transplantation in patients with hepatitis C is limited. Unequivocal evidence demonstrates that hepatitis C–negative recipients can acquire hepatitis C from the kidney of an infected donor. Although kidneys from hepatitis C–positive donors are transplanted into hepatitis C–positive recipients, hepatitis C–associated liver disease may be more aggressive in renal transplant recipients, who are immunosuppressed, compared with immunocompetent patients with chronic hepatitis C infection. Various factors can affect the progression of hepatitis C in the renal transplant population, including coinfection with hepatitis B virus, type of immunosuppressive treatment, and alcohol abuse. The natural history of hepatitis C infection after renal transplantation is under evaluation; however, recent surveys with long follow-ups have documented adverse effects of hepatitis C infection on patient and graft survival in renal transplant recipients.

## BIBLIOGRAPHY

1. Carithers RL Jr: Hepatitis C and renal failure. Am J Med 107:S90–S94, 1999.
2. Daghestani L, Pomeroy C: Renal manifestations of hepatitis C infection. Am J Med 106:347–354, 1999.
3. D'Amico G: Renal involvement in hepatitis C infection: Cryoglobulinemic glomerulonephritis. Kidney Int 54:650–671, 1998.
4. Fabrizi F, Martin P, Ponticelli C: Hepatitis C virus infection and renal transplantation. Am J Kidney Dis 38:919–934, 2001.
5. Giannico G, Manno C, Schena FP: Treatment of glomerulonephritides associated with hepatitis C virus infection. Nephrol Dial Transplant 15:S34–S38, 2000.
6. Jefferson JA, Johnson RJ: Treatment of hepatitis C–associated glomerular disease. Semin Nephrol 20:286–292, 2000.
7. Morales JM, Campistol JM: Transplantation in the patient with hepatitis C. J Am Soc Nephrol 11:1343–1353, 2000.
8. Stehman-Breen C, Johnson RJ: Hepatitis C virus–associated glomerulonephritis. Adv Intern Med 43:79–97, 1998.
9. Willson RA: Extrahepatic manifestations of chronic viral hepatitis. Am J Gastroenterol 92:4–17, 1997.

# 31. HIV-ASSOCIATED RENAL DISORDERS

*Patrick S. T. Hayden,* M.D.

**1. What is the first issue to be addressed when confronted with an abnormal creatinine in a patient infected with human immunodeficiency virus (HIV)?**
The clinician needs to determine whether the renal failure is acute or chronic. As in any other situation, one must start with a careful history and physical exam.

**2. What are the usual causes of acute renal failure (ARF) in an HIV-infected patient?**
The typical causes of ARF in this population are similar to those seen in non–HIV-infected patients: volume depletion, obstructive uropathy, acute tubular necrosis (ATN) associated with hypoperfusion, sepsis, nephrotoxic medications, and contrast. An acute interstitial nephritis resulting from sulfa-based medicines, antibiotics, or nonsteroidal anti-inflammatory drugs (NSAIDs) is also not uncommon.

**3. Which antiviral treatments for HIV have an association with crystalluria and obstructive uropathy?**
Indinavir, a protease inhibitor, has this association. A 1999 study from the urologic literature found a 12.4% incidence rate of nephrolithiasis in HIV patients treated with indinavir. Both sulfadiazine and acyclovir have also caused obstructive uropathy in HIV-infected patients due to crystal formation.

**4. List three broad categories of acute and chronic renal failure associated with HIV infection. Which is most common?**
- Thrombotic microangiopathies (thrombotic thrombocytopenic purpura–hemolytic uremic syndrome [TTP-HUS])
- Immune-complex renal disease (IgA nephropathy)
- HIV-associated nephropathy (HIVAN)—this is, by far, the most commonly encountered

**5. True or false: TTP-HUS is frequently associated with nephrotic-range proteinuria.**
False. Nephrotic-range proteinuria is uncommon with this entity; hematuria, however, is often present. The nephrotic syndrome is very common, however, with HIVAN.

**6. What glomerulonephritides have been diagnosed in patients with HIV?**
- Cryoglobulinemia (associated with hepatitis C infection)
- Membranoproliferative glomerulonephritis (associated with hepatitis C infection)
- Membranous nephropathy (associated with hepatitis B infection)
- IgA nephropathy
- Postinfectious glomerulonephritis

**7. What is the most common cause of chronic renal disease in HIV-infected patients, and how is it usually manifested?**
HIVAN is the most common cause of chronic renal disease in seropositive HIV patients, usually evidenced by an elevated creatinine and significant proteinuria.

## 8. What does a biopsy typically show in a patient with HIVAN?

The biopsy shows focal segmental glomerulosclerosis of the collapsing type coupled with an interstitium marked by edema, fibrosis, and a mononuclear cell infiltrate (see figure; see Chapter 23, Focal Segmental Glomerulosclerosis). Whereas tubule atrophy and microcysts are common although variable, mesangial expansion and basement membrane thickening are usually absent. A pseudocrescent, a hypertrophied visceral epithelial cell, is formed in Bowman's space, and recent data demonstrate that this glomerular epithelial cell is an HIV reservoir. Although tubuloreticular inclusions, demonstrated by electron microscopy, previously have been the rule, they are now present in only a quarter of biopsies, coincident with the widespread use of highly active antiretroviral therapy (HAART). As in other forms of focal sclerosis, immunofluorescence microscopy typically reveals IgM and C3 in sclerotic segments of glomeruli.

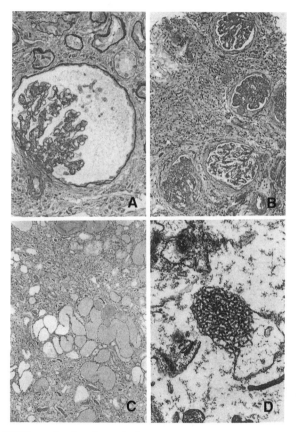

Histopathology of HIV-associated nephropathy from renal biopsies of patients with HIVAN. *A,* Collapse of the glomerular tuft. *B,* Focal segmental glomerulosclerosis. *C,* Microcysts containing proteinacious casts. *D,* Tubuloreticular inclusion in a glomerular endothelial cell. (All photomicrographs courtesy of Leslie A. Bruggeman, Ph.D.; the electron-micrograph is courtesy of Moonja Chung-Park, M.D.)

## 9. Does HIVAN appear disproportionately in certain racial groups?

Yes. Over 90% of patients are African American. There is a male sex preponderance as well. Interestingly, the IgA variant of HIV-associated glomerular disease is more common in white patients than in African Americans.

**10. Where does HIVAN place among the major causes of end-stage renal disease (ESRD) in African-American patients between the ages of 20 and 64 years?**
It now places third, behind diabetes mellitus and hypertension.

**11. What is currently known about the pathogenesis of HIVAN?**
This is an area of intense research. Initially, HIV-infected infiltrating mononuclear cells were thought to initiate kidney injury, exposing healthy, "bystander" renal cells to damaging viral products and cytokines. Others have speculated that dysregulated cytokine production from leukocytes may play the pivotal role in HIVAN pathogenesis. More recently, however, the renal epithelial cell has been studied since the tubule epithelial cell and glomerular visceral epithelium (podocyte) function and architecture are most dramatically altered in HIVAN, suggesting that this cell is a major target of HIV infection. New evidence from Bruggeman and Klotman demonstrates that the renal epithelial cell *is* directly infected by HIV. The authors not only have detected HIV DNA and mRNA in renal epithelial cells, which is highly indicative of localized viral replication, but also have shown evidence of kidney-specific viral evolution, leading many to speculate that the podocyte is an HIV reservoir.

**12. Describe the gross appearance of the kidneys in a person with HIVAN.**
As viewed with ultrasound, the patient's kidneys remain normal in size or may even enlarge as renal disease progresses, testifying to the dramatic epithelial cell proliferation that ensues. The kidneys are usually echogenic, correlating with the degree of microcystic tubular dilatation that is present.

**13. What is the natural history of HIVAN?**
In the absence of treatment, rapid progression to ESRD in weeks to months is the rule; heavy proteinuria is a clinical hallmark. Although an asymptomatic seropositive person can develop HIVAN, the typical patient already has an AIDS-defining illness when HIVAN is detected, with CD4 counts usually $< 200/m^3$.

**14. Is hypertension a common finding in the individual with HIVAN?**
Despite the preponderance of black patients, hypertension is not common in the patient with HIVAN and, indeed, normotension is more the rule than the exception.

**15. What acid-base abnormality is not infrequently associated with HIVAN?**
Renal tubular acidosis type IV.

**16. How is the diagnosis of HIVAN established?**
A kidney biopsy is necessary to make the diagnosis of HIVAN. Some experts recommend obtaining a biopsy once daily protein excretion reaches 1 gm in HIV-infected patients whose serum creatinine is > 2 mg/dl.

**17. What are effective treatments in HIVAN?**
Decreasing viral replication is the first-line therapy. The use of highly active antiretroviral therapy (HAART) in the mid-1990s was associated with the first decrease in HIVAN nephropathy incidence rates, a decline in all opportunistic infections, and a decline in HIV-associated mortality overall. In fact, a 1998 *Lancet* case report describes not only improved glomerular filtration rate (GFR) but also normalizing renal architecture by biopsy in a patient with HIVAN treated with HAART.

Angiotensin-converting enzyme inhibition (ACE-I) also has been shown to reduce the progression of renal disease in HIVAN. As in other proteinuric diseases, ACE-I favorably alters hemodynamics across the glomerulus, decreasing transglomerular passage of proteins.

A 1997 cohort study by Burns et al. demonstrated that ACE-I stabilized serum creatinine and 24-hour protein excretion in patients with both nephrotic and non-nephrotic proteinuria, whereas all untreated controls progressed to ESRD. Further, angiotensin II is a growth factor, and blocking it likely constitutes an antiproliferative effect, another therapeutic adjunct in curbing viral replication in dysregulated renal cells.

Steroids offer short-term improvement, removing from the interstitium the infiltrating leukocytes.

**18. Is there any evidence that HIVAN has a genetic predisposition?**

Yes. As discussed previously, HIVAN demonstrates a racial predilection for African-Americans, who already at increased risk for a variety of kidney diseases versus whites. A case-control study of incident HIVAN patients with ESRD (from the period 1991 to 1995, using Medicare data) found that approximately 88% were black and only 9% were white. Moreover, kidney disease clusters in families of African-American patients with HIVAN. Nearly 25% of the African-American HIVAN patients reported relatives with ESRD compared with 6% of the HIV-infected patients with normal renal function.

**19. Do the majority of HIV-infected black patients develop HIVAN?**

No. Only a minority of African-American HIV-positive patients develop HIVAN. Depending on the geographic locale, prevalence rates vary from 1% to 10% among the HIV-infected population.

**20. Is there good evidence supporting the use of corticosteroid therapy in treating HIVAN?**

Although randomized, controlled trials are lacking, several prospective and retrospective cohort studies have demonstrated improved GFR and decreased protein excretion in HIVAN patients treated with steroids, although benefits in terms of renal survival were usually not long-lasting. Importantly, nevertheless, steroid therapy was not associated with an increased incidence of infectious complications.

**21. Describe the mechanism by which steroids induce a stabilization or improvement in renal function, albeit short-term.**

Corticosteroid therapy is associated with a clearing of the parenchymal renal infiltrate, which likely limits interstitial inflammation and the production of damaging cytokines (such as IL-6).

**22. What is the experience with renal replacement therapy in patients with HIV nephropathy who progress to ESRD?**

Both hemodialysis and peritoneal dialysis have been used to treat HIV patients with ESRD. Not surprisingly, the average time between onset of ESRD and death is far shorter in the HIV population than in other dialysis patients. Most transplant centers currently do not offer renal transplantation to patients infected with HIV, regardless of the underlying cause of renal failure. However, the risks, benefits, and cost-effectiveness of transplanting such patients have not been fully explored.

**23. What electrolyte abnormalities occur in patients infected with HIV?**

A number of acid-base and electrolyte abnormalities have been reported in this patient population. In many cases, the abnormalities can be attributed to comorbid conditions (e.g., specific infections) or drug therapy. These abnormalities include:

- Hyponatremia—including syndrome of inappropriate secretion of antidiuretic hormone (SIADH) associated with pulmonary or intracranial disease

- Hypernatremia—e.g., from drug-induced diabetes insipidus (foscarnet, amphotericin)
- Hypokalemia—e.g., from chronic diarrheal disorders or infections
- Hyperkalemia—including drug effects (trimethoprim-sulfamethoxazole, pentamidine)
- Hypocalcemia—including drug effects (foscarnet, pentamidine)
- Hypercalcemia—e.g., related to granulomatous infections or lymphoma
- Hyperphosphatemia—e.g., in renal failure or secondary to foscarnet
- Hyperuricemia—including drug effects (pyrazinamide, rifampin, didanosine [DDI])

## BIBLIOGRAPHY

1. Burns GC, Paul SK, Toth IR, Sivak SL: Effect of angiotensin-converting enzyme inhibition in HIV-associated nephropathy. J Am Soc Nephrol 8:1140–1146, 1997.
2. D'Agati V, Appel GB: HIV infection and the kidney. J Am Soc Nephrol 8:138–152, 1997.
3. Eustace JA, Nuermberger E, Choi M, et al: Cohort study of the treatment of severe HIV-associated nephropathy with corticosteroids. Kidney Int 58:1253–1260, 2000.
4. Freedman BI, Soucie JM, Stone SM, Pegram S: Familial clustering of end-stage renal disease in blacks with HIV-associated nephropathy. Am J Kidney Dis 34:254–258, 1999.
5. Kimmel PL: The nephropathies of HIV infection: Pathogenesis and treatment. Curr Opin Nephrol Hypertens 9:117–122, 2000.
6. Marras D, Bruggeman LA, Gao F, et al: Replication and compartmentalization of HIV-1 in kidney epithelium of patients with HIV-associated nephropathy. Nature Med 8:522–526, 2002.
7. Monahan M, Tanji N, Klotman PE: HIV-associated nephropathy: An urban epidemic. Semin Nephrol 21:394–402, 2001.
8. Reiter WJ, Schon-Pernerstorfer H, Dorfinger K, et al: Frequency of urolithiasis in individuals seropositive for human immunodeficiency virus treated with indinavir is higher than previously assumed. J Urol 161:1082–1084, 1999.
9. Rodriguez RA, Humphreys MH: Therapy of HIV-related renal diseases. In Brady HR, Wilcox CS (eds): Therapy in Nephrology and Hypertension. Philadelphia, W.B. Saunders, 1999, pp 209–216.
10. Wali RK, Drachenberg CI, Papadimitriou JC, et al: HIV1-associated nephropathy and response to highly-active antiretroviral therapy. Lancet 352:783–784, 1998.
11. Winston JA, Bruggeman LA, Ross MD, et al: Nephropathy and establishment of a renal reservoir of HIV type 1 during primary infection. N Engl J Med 344:1979–1984, 2001.
12. Winston JA, Burns GC, Klotman PE: Treatment of HIV-associated nephropathy. Semin Nephrol 20:293–298, 2000.

# V. Other Parenchymal Renal Diseases

## 32. RENAL DYSPLASIA

*Beth A. Vogt, M.D.*

### 1. What is renal dysplasia?
Renal dysplasia defines a spectrum of a congenital renal anomalies in which one or both kidneys develop abnormally in utero. A dysplastic kidney is composed of primitive ducts surrounded by sheaths of fibromuscular and undifferentiated cells, often with islands of cartilage and renal cysts.

### 2. How common is renal dysplasia?
The exact incidence of renal dysplasia is unknown. However, renal dysplasia accounts for 15–20% of children with chronic renal insufficiency and end-stage renal disease.

### 3. What causes renal dysplasia?
The exact cause of renal dysplasia is unknown. Current theories include:
- Mutations in renal developmental genes
- Altered interaction of the ureteric bud with extracellular matrix
- Abnormalities of renal growth factors
- Antenatal urinary tract obstruction

### 4. What other types of urinary tract developmental anomalies are associated with renal dysplasia?
Posterior urethral valves, prune-belly (Eagle-Barrett) syndrome, ureteropelvic junction obstruction, and ureterovesicular junction obstruction are all associated with renal dysplasia. The timing and severity of the obstruction in utero are believed to correlate with the severity of renal dysplasia.

### 5. What other conditions are associated with renal dysplasia?
Although most cases of renal dysplasia are sporadic, a minority is associated with other anomalies or congenital syndromes. Some examples include VACTERL (*v*ertebral, *a*nal, *c*ardiac, *t*racheal, *e*sophageal, *r*enal, and *l*imb) syndrome; branchio-oto-renal syndrome; CHARGE (*c*oloboma of the eye, *h*eart anomaly, choanal *a*tresia, *r*etardation, and *g*enital and *e*ar anomalies) syndrome; trisomies 13, 18, and 21; and Jeune's syndrome.

### 6. What is the clinical course of patients with renal dysplasia?
Although the function of dysplastic kidneys is quite variable, children with bilateral involvement generally develop progressive renal insufficiency during early childhood. Nephrogenic diabetes insipidus, salt wasting, and distal renal tubular acidosis are commonly seen in children with renal dysplasia. Hematuria, heavy proteinuria, and hypertension can occur but are unusual clinical features.

### 7. What is a multicystic dysplastic kidney (MCDK)?
An MCDK is the most severe form of renal dysplasia. Just as in a dysplastic kidney, the normal renal parenchyma is replaced by cartilage and disorganized epithelial structures in

the form of primitive ducts. In addition, the MCDK is characterized by the presence of multiple cysts of varying size and atresia of the renal pelvis and ureter (see figure).

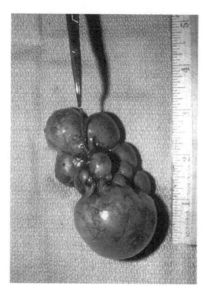

Multicystic dysplastic kidney.

### 8. Is an MCDK functional?

In general, an MCDK has no appreciable function. In fact, on a radionuclide renal scan, no tracer appears in the area of an MCDK.

### 9. How common is MCDK?

The incidence of unilateral MCDK has been estimated to be 1 in 4300 live births. MCDK is the most common cause of a unilateral abdominal mass in the neonatal period.

### 10. What causes MCDK?

MCDK is believed to result from an abnormal induction of the metanephric blastema by the ureteric bud. Although some families appear to have a genetic predisposition to MCDK and other urologic abnormalities, MCDK usually occurs as a sporadic event.

### 11. What other conditions are associated with MCDK?

VACTERL syndrome
Branchio-oto-renal syndrome
Williams syndrome
Beckwith-Wiedemann syndrome
Trisomy 18

### 12. What other urinary tract malformations are associated with MCDK?

Other urinary tract abnormalities are present in about 50% of patients with MCDK. Contralateral vesicoureteral reflux is present in 10–30% of individuals with MCDK. Other associated abnormalities include ureteropelvic junction obstruction, renal agenesis, renal hypoplasia, renal dysplasia, horseshoe kidney, ureterocele, bladder wall diverticulum, ectopic kidney, crossed fused renal ectopia, patent urachus, and posterior urethral valves.

**13. How are MCDKs discovered?**
Prior to the advent of fetal ultrasonography, the most common presentation of MCDK was discovery of an abdominal mass in a healthy newborn infant. Currently, most MCDKs are detected by antenatal ultrasonography and may be detected as early as the second trimester.

**14. What other conditions mimic MCDK?**
A severe ureteropelvic junction obstruction may be difficult to distinguish from MCDK.

**15. What is the natural history of bilateral MCDK?**
Bilateral MCDK usually results in stillbirth or death shortly after birth due to the consequences of pulmonary hypoplasia and renal failure.

**16. What is the natural history of a unilateral MCDK?**
The majority of unilateral MCDKs undergo spontaneous involution, a process that may begin even before birth. The contralateral kidney, if unaffected by other urologic malformations, grows larger than expected due to compensatory hypertrophy.

**17. Are there any complications related to unilateral MCDK?**
Hypertension has been reported in less than 2% of patients with MCDK and, in several cases, has been cured by surgical removal of the MCDK. In the past 20 years, there have been fewer than 10 reports of renal malignancy, including Wilms' tumor, embryonal cell tumor, and renal cell carcinoma, in patients with MCDK.

**18. How should an MCDK be managed?**
When an MCDK is suspected, an ultrasound should be obtained to rule out contralateral renal dysplasia and other urinary tract anomalies. Antibiotic prophylaxis should be given until a voiding cystourethrogram rules out vesicoureteral reflux or bladder abnormality. A radionuclide renal scan may be considered to confirm the diagnosis of MCDK, although this test is not mandatory.

Optimal long-term management of MCDK remains controversial. Some clinicians advocate conservative management with surveillance renal ultrasounds and ongoing monitoring of blood pressure. In view of the small but real risk of hypertension and malignancy, others advocate surgical removal in infancy.

BIBLIOGRAPHY

1. Atiyeh B, Husmann D, Baum M: Contralateral renal abnormalities in multicystic-dysplastic kidney disease. J Pediatr 121:65–67, 1992.
2. Becker N, Avner ED: Congenital nephropathies and uropathies. Pediatr Clin North Am 42:1319–1341, 1995.
3. Barratt TM, Avner ED, Harmon WE: Pediatric Nephrology, 4th ed. Baltimore, Williams & Wilkins, 1999.
4. Feldenberg LR, Siegel NJ: Clinical course and outcome for children with multicystic dysplastic kidneys. Pediatr Nephrol 14:1098–1101, 2000.
5. John U, Rudnik-Schoeneborn S, Zerres K, Misselwitz J: Kidney growth and renal function in unilateral multicystic dysplastic kidney disease. Pediatr Nephrol 12:567–571, 1998.
6. Robson WLM, Leung AKC, Thomason MA: Multicystic dysplasia of the kidney. Clin Pediatr 34:32–40, 1995.
7. Seeman T, John U, Glahova K, et al: Ambulatory blood pressure monitoring in children with unilateral multicystic dysplastic kidney. Eur J Pediatr 160:78–83, 2001.
8. Woolf AS: A molecular and genetic view of human renal and urinary tract malformations. Kidney Int 58:500–512, 2000.

# 33. CYSTIC DISEASES OF THE KIDNEYS

*Thomas Zipp, M.D., and John R. Sedor, M.D.*

### 1. What are the major types of renal cystic diseases?

Renal cystic disease can result from congenital diseases (e.g., renal cystic dysplasia and medullary sponge kidney), hereditary diseases with onset during fetal life (e.g., autosomal recessive medullary multicystic kidney disease), or hereditary diseases with onset during late childhood or early adulthood (e.g., autosomal dominant polycystic renal disease). Renal cysts also can be acquired later in life. Renal cysts are common and often are discovered as an incidental finding on a radiologic exam obtained for another purpose. Sometimes, renal cysts cause significant disease (see table).

*Renal Cystic Disease*

| CATEGORY | EXAMPLES |
|---|---|
| Congenital (results from abnormal development and not necessarily heritable) | Multiple anomaly syndromes (usually from toxic insult in vitro)<br>Cystic renal dysplasia<br>Multilocular cysts<br>Pyelocalyceal cysts |
| Hereditary | Fetal, infantile, or juvenile onset diseases<br>    Autosomal recessive polycystic kidney disease<br>    Autosomal dominant polycystic kidney disease<br>    Medullary sponge kidney<br>    Autosomal recessive medullary cystic disease (juvenile nephronophthisis)<br>    Hereditary and familial dysplasia<br>    Tuberous sclerosis<br>Adult onset<br>    Autosomal dominant medullary cystic disease (medullary cystic disease complex)<br>    von Hippel-Lindau disease |
| Acquired cystic disease | Simple cysts: single or multiple<br>Acquired cystic disease in patients with end-stage renal disease<br>Renal lymphangiomatosis<br>Hilar and perinephric pseudocysts |

Adapted from Welling LW, Grantham JJ: Cystic renal diseases. In Brenner BM (ed): The Kidney, 5th ed. Philadelphia, W.B. Saunders, 1996, pp 1828–1863.

### 2. Which renal cystic diseases are the most common?

Simple cysts are the most common renal cystic abnormality and can be single or multiple. Simple cysts are rare in children but increase in incidence with age and are found in approximately 20% of 40-year-old individuals. Autosomal dominant polycystic kidney disease (ADPKD) is the most common heritable cystic kidney disease, occurring in about 1 in 400 to 1 in 1000 individuals.

### 3. What is the genetic basis of ADPKD?

Two different genes for this disease have been identified. *ADPKD1* is located on the short arm of chromosome 16 and is responsible for 85–90% of the disease in the white population. *ADPKD2* is located on chromosome 4. A third gene, which has not been cloned, may also cause a small number of cases.

### 4. Does ADPKD have extrarenal manifestations?

Yes. ADPKD is a systemic disease that has multiple chemical manifestations, including renal cysts of varying sizes, hepatic cysts, pancreatic cysts, colonic diverticula, intracranial aneurysms, and thoracic and abdominal aortic aneurysms. In addition, hypertension prior to the development of end-stage renal disease (ESRD) is common. Certain manifestations of ADPKD tend to cluster in families. For example, some families of ADPKD patients have a high incidence of intracranial aneurysms, whereas other families do not. Most patients express manifestations of the disease after the age of 30, with highest incidence of onset occurring between ages 45 and 65.

### 5. What are the clinical features of autosomal recessive polycystic renal disease (ARPKD)?

ARPKD is a rare disease with incidence ranging from 1 in 6000 to 1 in 40,000. A gene for this disease is located on chromosome 6. The disorder is often diagnosed by ultrasonography in utero, when large echogenic kidneys and oligohydramnios are demonstrated. Renal cysts in ARPKD patients result from tubular ectasia of the collecting ducts. Liver abnormalities are universally identified in ARPKD patients. Severe liver fibrosis is the most common associated hepatic disease, but cholangitis and portal hypertension with variceal bleeding also can occur. In 75% of cases, ARPKD results in death in the perinatal period. The remainder of ARPKD patients present with milder disease later in infancy or childhood or even in early adulthood and may have a much better prognosis.

### 6. Which imaging studies are used to diagnose cystic diseases of kidneys?

Renal ultrasound is a commonly used, noninvasive screening tool. Computed tomography (CT) with contrast is another highly sensitive study that provides more accurate information about involvement of the pancreas, liver, and spleen. A CT scan can detect cysts as small as 1.5 cm.

### 7. What are the most reliable diagnostic criteria to differentiate ADPKD from ARPKD?

Differentiating ARPKD and ADPKD in children may be difficult. The best distinguishing criterion is a history of PKD in families with definitive inheritance patterns. Despite the identification of several ADPKD genes, genetic testing is not common in clinical practice as yet. Another reliable method to differentiate between these two inherited renal cystic diseases is to perform renal ultrasonography on parents. A negative renal ultrasound in both parents strongly supports a diagnosis of ARPKD in the proband but cannot rule out a de novo ADPKD mutation. Hepatic fibrosis with biliary dysgenesis occurs in virtually 100% of ARPKD patients but is rare in ADPKD patients. Hepatic biopsy may be necessary to differentiate ARPKD and ADPKD in children and young adults with PKD and no family history. The ultrasonographic appearance of the kidney in the index patient may also be a useful tool to distinguish ARPKD and ADPKD. Discrete fluid-filled cysts scattered in renal cortex and medulla favor a diagnosis of ADPKD (see figure, top of next page). In contrast, the typical sonogram in the ARPKD patient shows enlarged kidneys with increased cortical and medullary echogenicity. Discrete cysts are generally identified only in ARPKD patients with late onset of disease.

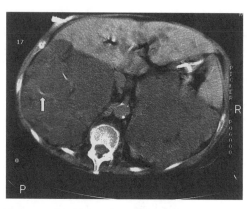

A CT scan of 70-year-old woman with ADPKD. The kidneys are massively enlaraged and compress other intra-abdominal viscera. Cyst walls are indistinct because the cysts have accumulated fluid and increased in size; the arrow indicates a portion of a remaining cyst wall.

### 8. Is it possible to have a normal renal ultrasound and still have ADPKD?

Yes. Up to 24% of adult ADPKD patients younger than 30 years and up to 40% of children younger than 5 years with ADPKD may have a normal renal ultrasound.

### 9. What are the most common clinical complications of ADPKD?

1. **Pain:** Abdominal or flank pain commonly occurs and usually results from rupture of cysts, hemorrhage into cysts, passage of kidney stones, or infection of cysts.

2. **ESRD:** About 50% of patients have progressed to ESRD by the age of 60 years. Male gender, African ethnicity, the presence of hypertension, early age of onset, and recurrent infections are predictors of a poor prognosis.

3. **Hematuria:** Either microscopic or macroscopic hematuria results from bleeding into a cyst or passage of a kidney stone.

4. **Hypertension:** Elevated blood pressure occurs in 30% of children and in 60% of adults prior to development of ESRD. Over 80% of adult ADPKD patients with ESRD are hypertensive.

5. **Nephrolithiasis:** Kidney stones occur in up to 34% of ADPKD patients and most likely result from urinary stasis and decreased excretion of citrate, an inhibitor of stone formation. Stones in ADPKD patients are most commonly composed of uric acid or calcium oxalate. Renal parenchymal calcifications or nephrocalcinosis also may occur. Therapy for stones in these patients is similar to treatment of kidney stones in patients without PKD.

6. **Recurrent urinary tract infections:** Recurrent urinary tract infections are a major problem for ADPKD patients, especially women. Cysts can become infected, essentially resulting in abscesses that are difficult to treat because these cysts no longer freely communicate with tubular lumens. A prolonged course of parenteral antibiotics may be required to treat these infections (see question 11).

7. **Stroke:** Five percent to 10% of ADPKD patients have intracranial aneurysms, which tend to cluster in families. Rupture of aneurysms usually occurs after the age of 30 years and in aneurysms larger than 10 mm in diameter. Individuals from ADPKD families with a history of aneurysm rupture may be candidates for screening using cerebral magnetic resonance imaging (MRI) or magnetic resonance angiography (MRA).

### 10. What are the indications for nephrectomy in ADPKD?

Nephrectomy is performed as a last resort and may be indicated in ADPKD patients with the following complications: (1) severe recurrent urinary tract infections that have not been eradicated after an appropriate course of antibiotic therapy; (2) intractable pain; (3) renal neoplasm; (4) compression of inferior vena cava or other intra-abdominal organs; (5) persistent gross hematuria; and (6) nephrolithiasis that is not successfully treated by lithotripsy or percutaneous nephrostolithotomy.

## 11. Which antibiotics should be used for treatment of urinary tract infection in ADPKD patients?

Most cysts are no longer connected to the tubule from which they originated. In contrast to patients with simple renal parenchymal infection (pyelonephritis), ADPKD patients with cyst infections usually present as treatment failures after an appropriate course of antibiotic therapy. Antibiotics chosen to treat urinary tract infections in PKD patients should penetrate well into the cysts. Quinolones (e.g., ciprofloxacin and norfloxacin), trimethoprim, chloramphenicol, and clindamycin are lipid-soluble antibiotics with good penetration into cysts. Ampicillin and aminoglycosides penetrate less well but can be used if the bacterial susceptibilities necessitate use of these drugs.

## 12. Which ADPKD patients should be screened for intracranial aneurysms?

Most authorities agree that ADPKD patients who have a family history of aneurysmal bleeding or who present with appropriate symptoms (such as new headache, change in headache pattern, nerve paresis, paralysis, meningeal irritation, or strokes) should undergo evaluation for intracranial aneurysm. ADPKD patients engaging in activities such as contact sports, working as pilots, or undergoing major surgery, which could result in hemodynamic instability and severe hypertension, should also be considered for radiographic screening with MRI or MRA.

## 13. What are the clinical characteristics of tuberous sclerosis?

Tuberous sclerosis is a disease complex characterized by epilepsy, mental retardation, skin abnormalities including adenoma sebaceum and "ash leaf" spots, and hamartomas of multiple organs. Patients with tuberous sclerosis may or may not have renal cysts. Renal hamartomas (angiomyolipomas) can be identified in as many as 50% of patients and should be distinguished from renal cysts. Renal cysts and hamartomas commonly are found in the same patients. The presence of renal cysts in the absence of renal hamartomas is relatively uncommon, occurring in only 18% of patients. Two defective genes on chromosomes 9 and 16 have been identified. Tuberous sclerosis frequency is approximately 1 in 10,000.

## 14. What are the major characteristics of von Hippel-Lindau disease?

Up to 75% of patients have numerous, irregularly distributed renal cysts. Other clinical features of this disorder include retinal angiomas, cerebellar and spinal hemangioblastomas, pancreatic cysts, renal cell carcinomas, and pheochromocytomas. The disease is inherited by autosomal dominant transmission, and the defective gene responsible for von Hippel-Lindau disease is on the short arm of chromosome 3. Its onset usually is in the third or fourth decade of life.

## 15. What are distinguishing radiographic characteristics of simple cysts?

Most simple cysts are found on radiographic exams of the urinary tract and abdomen that are obtained for other indications. They appear on ultrasound as smooth-walled, fluid-filled structures without internal debris. Simple cysts are acquired and increase in incidence with age. Although usually single and unilateral, simple cysts can be multiple and bilateral. Suggested CT criteria to differentiate a simple cyst from a more serious lesion include a homogenous attenuation value near water density, lack of enhancement after injection with radiocontrast, no measurable wall thickness, and a smooth interface with normal kidney parenchyma. In the absence of fever, leukocytosis, hematuria, or pain, no further evaluation of simple cysts is indicated.

### 16. What is nephronophthisis-medullary cystic kidney disease complex?

This hereditary disease has several variants that invariably progress to ESRD. The most common variants are familial juvenile nephronophthisis, an autosomal recessive disease that causes ESRD in affected individuals by age 20 years, and medullary cystic kidney disease, an autosomal dominant disease that affects young adults between the ages of 20 and 50 years. Both variants are characterized by multiple renal cysts arising from distal and collecting tubules located primarily at the corticomedullary junction and in the medulla. The cysts are characteristically small (approximately 2 cm) and contain fluid. However, almost 25% of patients will have no grossly identifiable cysts due to the small size of these cysts. Renal biopsy demonstrates tubular atrophy, cysts lined by a single epithelial layer, and nonspecific glomerular hyalinosis. The clinical manifestations of the disease reflect dysfunction of affected nephron segments, predominantly reduced concentrating ability, polyuria, polydipsia, hypovolemia, and hyponatremia early in the course of the disease. Subsequently, glomerular filtration declines as the glomerular hyalinosis develops and progresses. The best imaging modality for diagnosis is thin-section CT scan of kidneys.

### 17. How does medullary sponge kidney differ from other cystic diseases?

Medullary sponge kidney is a benign disease that results from a congenital anomaly. It is characterized by small and large cysts, which are limited to medulla and do not involve the cortex. Many patients are asymptomatic, but some individuals present with kidney stones, recurrent urinary tract infections, and hematuria. The diagnosis can be made only by intravenous pyelography. It has an excellent prognosis in most patients.

### 18. What is acquired cystic kidney disease (ACKD)?

ACKD is an acquired disorder, characterized by the development of multiple renal cysts in patients with progressive, noncystic renal disease. A minimum of five cysts is required for diagnosis. CT scan is more sensitive than ultrasound in establishing this diagnosis. ACKD occurs in up to 40% of patients who have been on hemodialysis for 3 years and in 80–90% of patients on dialysis for 5–10 years. Patients with significant renal failure, who have not yet started on dialysis, may also have ACKD.

### 19. Are renal tumors more common in patients with ESRD than in patients with ACKD?

Yes. The development of renal cell neoplasms, ranging from adenomas to renal cell carcinomas, is the most serious complication of ACKD. Patients with ACKD have a fiftyfold increased risk of renal carcinoma compared to the general population. ACKD-associated renal cell carcinoma predominates in males, is frequently bilateral (9%) and multicentric (50%), and often occurs in ESRD patients at an age younger than that of patients with renal cell carcinoma but without renal failure.

### 20. How are tumors in ACKD patients managed?

Tumors larger than 3 cm are treated by nephrectomy. Management of tumors smaller than 3 cm in patients with back pain or hematuria is controversial, but many authorities recommend nephrectomy because these tumors often are renal cell carcinomas. Asymptomatic patients with tumors smaller than 3 cm also can be followed with serial CT examinations.

## BIBLIOGRAPHY

1. Arnaout MA: Molecular genetics and pathogenesis of autosomal dominant polycystic kidney disease. Annu Rev Med 52:93–123, 2001.
2. Chapman AB, Rubinstein D, Hughes R, et al: Intracranial aneurysms in autosomal dominant polycystic kidney disease. N Engl J Med 327:916–920, 1992.
3. Elzouki AY, al-Suhaibani H, Mirza K, al-Sowailem AM: Thin-section computed tomography scans detect medullary cysts in patients believed to have juvenile nephronophthisis. Am J Kidney Dis 27:216–219, 1996.
4. Fick GM, Duley IT, Johnson AM, et al: The spectrum of autosomal dominant polycystic kidney disease in children. J Am Soc Nephrol 4:1654–1660, 1994.
5. Fick GM, Gabow PA: Hereditary and acquired cystic disease of the kidney. Kidney Int 46:951–964, 1994.
6. Gabow PA: Polycystic and acquired cystic disease. In Greenberg A (ed): Primer on Kidney Diseases, 2nd ed. San Diego, Academic Press, 1998, pp 313–318.
7. Griffin M, Torres VE, Kumar R: Cystic kidney diseases. Curr Opin Nephrol Hypertension 6:276–283, 1997.
8. Hildebrandt F, Jungers P, Grunfeld J-P: Medullary cystic and medullary sponge renal disorders. In Schrier RW, Gottschalk CW (eds): Diseases of the Kidney, 6th ed. Boston, Little, Brown, 1996, pp 499–520.
9. Truong LD, Krishnan B, Cao JT, et al: Renal neoplasm in acquired cystic kidney disease. Am J Kidney Dis 26:1–12, 1995.
10. Welling LW, Grantham JJ: Cystic renal diseases. In Brenner BM (ed): The Kidney, 5th ed. Philadelphia, W.B. Saunders, 1996, pp 1828–1863.
11. Wolf JS Jr: Evaluation and management of solid and cystic renal masses. J Urol 159:1120–1133, 1998.

# 34. OTHER HEREDITARY RENAL DISEASES

*Beth A. Vogt, M.D.*

### 1. What is Alport syndrome?

Alport syndrome is an inherited disorder characterized by persistent microscopic hematuria, progressive nephritis with proteinuria and declining renal function, sensorineural deafness, and ocular abnormalities. It is a generalized disorder of basement membranes resulting from mutations in basement membrane collagen.

### 2. How is Alport syndrome inherited?

Classic Alport syndrome (80% of cases) is inherited as an X-linked dominant trait. Other reported modes of inheritance include autosomal recessive (15% of cases) and autosomal dominant (5% of cases).

### 3. What is the genetic abnormality in Alport syndrome?

The classic or X-linked dominant form of Alport syndrome usually results from one of a variety of mutations in the gene for the alpha-5 chain of type IV collagen (*COL4A5*) on the X chromosome. The most common type of mutation involves the substitution of another amino acid for a glycine residue, which alters the structure of the A5 collagen chain, preventing normal incorporation of A3 and A4 collagen chains into basement membranes. Mutations in the *COL4A3* and *COL4A4* genes on chromosome 2 have been reported in autosomal recessive Alport syndrome. Mutations in *COL4A3* and *COL4A4* also have been identified in a family with autosomal dominant Alport syndrome.

### 4. How many children with asymptomatic microscopic hematuria will have Alport syndrome?

An estimated 20% of children with persistent microscopic hematuria evaluated by a nephrologist have Alport syndrome.

### 5. What are the clinical findings in males with Alport syndrome?

Persistent microscopic hematuria is usually present by the age of 10 years in all affected males. Episodes of macroscopic hematuria may be seen in children with Alport syndrome but become less common after adolescence. Proteinuria and chronic renal insufficiency may develop as early as the second decade of life but may not be present until well into adulthood. End-stage renal disease (ESRD) ultimately develops in virtually all affected males, but the rate of renal disease progression is variable between families. Overall, about 60% of males reach ESRD by age 30 years, and 80% by age 40 years. Bilateral, high-frequency, sensorineural hearing loss is seen in 80–90% of males with Alport syndrome by age 40 years.

### 6. What are the clinical findings in females with Alport syndrome?

Females with X-linked Alport syndrome have a much milder course than males. Microscopic hematuria is present in 90% of females with Alport syndrome but may be intermittent in nature. Significant proteinuria and renal insufficiency occur in only 15% of females. Approximately 20% of females with Alport syndrome have sensorineural hearing loss. Females with autosomal recessive Alport syndrome have a clinical course more similar to that of males, with persistent hematuria, proteinuria, and progressive renal dysfunction.

**7. What other abnormalities may be associated with Alport syndrome?**

Ocular abnormalities such as anterior lenticonus and perimacular flecks are identified in 30–40% of patients with Alport syndrome and are associated with early progression to ESRD. Leiomyomatosis and platelet abnormalities are occasionally seen.

**8. What are the characteristic renal biopsy findings in Alport syndrome?**

Light microscopy shows segmental or global glomerulosclerosis, interstitial fibrosis, and tubular atrophy. Immunofluorescence shows nonspecific deposition of immunoglobulin G (IgG), IgM, and C3. The pathognomonic renal biopsy finding in Alport syndrome, however, is diffuse thickening of the glomerular basement membrane with splitting of the lamina densa on electron microscopy. In young patients, both thickening and thinning of the glomerular basement membrane may be present, causing difficulty in distinguishing Alport syndrome from thin basement membrane nephropathy.

**9. What treatment is available for Alport syndrome?**

Currently, there is no definitive therapy for Alport syndrome. Treatment remains supportive in nature and should focus on control of hypertension, management of the consequences of progressive renal insufficiency, and early identification of all affected family members. Renal transplantation is successful in most patients.

**10. What is post-transplant antiglomerular basement membrane nephritis?**

Post-transplant antiglomerular basement membrane nephritis is a condition that occurs in 3–4% of transplanted males with Alport syndrome. The cause of this condition is not well understood but may represent an immunologic response by the recipient to the presentation of a previously unrecognized glomerular basement membrane antigen in the donor kidney. The subset of patients at highest risk for this complication is males with significant deafness who develop ESRD before 30 years of age. Allograft failure occurs in more than 75% of patients with this phenomenon.

**11. What is thin glomerular basement membrane disease?**

Thin glomerular basement membrane disease, also known as benign familial hematuria, is an inherited condition characterized by persistent microscopic hematuria and episodic gross hematuria. Unlike Alport syndrome, thin glomerular basement membrane disease is rarely associated with proteinuria, loss of renal function, or extrarenal abnormalities.

**12. What is the inheritance pattern of thin glomerular basement membrane disease?**

Thin glomerular basement membrane disease appears to follow an autosomal dominant pattern of inheritance. Recent studies have identified mutations in the type IV collagen gene (*COL4A3* and *COL4A4*) in some families, suggesting that thin glomerular basement membrane disease and Alport syndrome may be related disorders.

**13. What are the renal biopsy findings in thin glomerular basement membrane disease?**

The pathognomonic renal biopsy finding in thin glomerular basement membrane disease is irregular thinning of the glomerular basement membrane on electron microscopy, with attenuation of the lamina densa. Light and immunofluorescence microscopic analyses are usually normal.

**14. How many children with asymptomatic microscopic hematuria have thin glomerular basement membrane disease?**

An estimated 30% of children with persistent asymptomatic microscopic hematuria have thin glomerular basement membrane disease.

## 15. What is the natural history of thin glomerular basement membrane disease?

In the majority of patients, thin glomerular basement membrane disease is a benign condition in which progressive renal insufficiency does not occur. Rare patients, however, have been reported to develop significant proteinuria and chronic renal insufficiency.

## 16. What is the nephronophthisis–medullary cystic kidney disease complex?

The nephronophthisis–medullary cystic kidney disease complex (NPH-MCKD) is a group of renal cystic diseases characterized by inherited progressive tubulointerstitial nephropathy with eventual progression to end-stage kidney disease. In general, individuals with nephronophthisis present in childhood or adolescence, whereas those with medullary cystic kidney disease present in adulthood.

## 17. What is the genetic basis of NPH-MCKD?

Nephronophthisis is inherited in an autosomal recessive fashion. A gene for nephronophthisis (*NPHP1*) was recently mapped to the short arm of chromosome 2. The gene product, nephrocystin, is theorized to be involved in focal adhesion or adherens junction signaling. Medullary cystic kidney disease is inherited in an autosomal-dominant fashion, and at least two gene loci, on chromosome 1 and 16, have been identified, although the gene products and their functions remain unknown.

## 18. What are the clinical findings in NPH-MCKD?

The symptoms of the NPH-MCKD complex include polyuria, polydipsia, weakness, pallor, short stature, failure to thrive, and insidious onset of chronic renal insufficiency. Hematuria, proteinuria, urinary tract infection, and hypertension are very uncommon.

## 19. What extrarenal findings have been associated with NPH-MCKD?

Twenty-five percent to 33% of patients with nephronophthisis have retinal degeneration, which is detectable by 10 years of age. This condition can be confirmed by electroretinogram and is associated with progressive loss of vision. In this subset of patients with nephronophthisis, other abnormalities including mental retardation, cerebellar ataxia, skeletal abnormalities, and congenital hepatic fibrosis may be seen. Extrarenal findings have not been reported in medullary cystic kidney disease.

## 20. What are the ultrasound findings in NPH-MCKD complex?

The renal ultrasound of patients with NPH-MCKD complex shows small, hyperechoic kidneys with small medullary cysts, 1–2 mm in diameter, at the corticomedullary junction. These cysts correspond to the distal convoluted and medullary collecting tubules. Absence of medullary cysts does not rule out the diagnosis of NPH-MCKD complex.

## 21. What are the renal biopsy findings in NPH-MCKD complex?

Renal biopsy findings in advanced nephronophthisis or medullary cystic kidney disease show tubulointerstitial atrophy, interstitial fibrosis, and thickening of the tubular basement membrane. Electron microscopy reveals thickening and loss of definition of the tubular basement membrane.

## 22. What is the treatment for NPH-MCKD complex?

There is currently no definitive treatment for nephronophthisis or medullary cystic kidney disease. Treatment is focused on supportive therapy for progressive renal insufficiency, control of hypertension, and early identification of affected family members. Renal transplantation is successful, and recurrent disease in the renal allograft has not been reported.

## BIBLIOGRAPHY

1. Barratt TM, Avner ED, Harmon WE: Pediatric Nephrology, 4th ed. Baltimore, Williams & Wilkins, 1999.
2. Hildebrandt F, Otto E: Molecular genetics of nephronophthisis and medullary cystic kidney disease. J Am Soc Nephrol 11:1753–1761, 2000.
3. Hildebrandt F, Omram H: New insights: Nephronophthisis-medullary cystic kidney disease. Pediatr Nephrol 16:168–176, 2001.
4. Kashtan CE: Alport syndrome and thin glomerular basement disease. J Am Soc Nephrol 9:1736-1750, 1998.
5. Lemmink HH, Nillesen WN, Mochizuki T, et al: Benign familial hematuria due to mutation of the type IV collagen a4 gene. J Clin Invest 98:114–118, 1996.
6. Nieuwhof CMG, De Heer F, De Leeuw P, et al: Thin GBM nephropathy: Premature glomerular obsolescence is associated with hypertension and late onset renal failure. Kidney Int 51:1596–1601, 1997.

# 35. INTERSTITIAL RENAL DISEASES

*Bruce E. Berger, M.D.*

**1. What are the interstitial renal diseases?**

They are a heterogeneous group of disorders that histologically feature inflammation of the nonvascular regions of the kidneys, such as the tubules and interstitium.

**2. What are the histologic characteristics of tubulointerstitial diseases?**

The histologic presentation is nonspecific, making it difficult to establish a definitive diagnosis on the basis of biopsy findings alone. The histologic presentation may reflect **acute** injury, with a predominance of polymorphonuclear cells, eosinophils, and plasma cells. **Chronic** injury is suggested by a predominance of monocytes and lymphocytes, together with tubular atrophy and interstitial fibrosis. These tubulointerstitial findings sometimes accompany glomerular or vascular diseases. Thus, a histologic diagnosis of primary tubulointerstitial disease should be entertained only when the above findings are observed in the absence of glomerular or vascular pathology.

**3. How are the interstitial renal diseases classified?**

They can be classified either according to acuity or chronicity or based on the site of tubular injury or dysfunction as shown in the tables below.

| | ACUTE INTERSTITIAL NEPHRITIS | CHRONIC INTERSTITIAL NEPHRITIS |
|---|---|---|
| Drugs/toxins | Antibiotics: penicillins, cephalo-sporins, acyclovir, rifampin<br>NSAIDs<br>Diuretics<br>Other: captopril, phenytoin, allopurinol, interferon | Analgesics<br>Cadmium<br>Lead (plumbism)<br>Lithium<br>Cisplatin<br>Cyclosporine |
| Infections | Bacterial: *Legionella, Strepto-coccus, Staphylococcus*<br>Viral: EBV, CMV, HIV<br>Other: *Rickettsia, Leptospira,* toxoplasmosis | Bacterial: bacteremic/ascending, malacoplakia |
| Hereditary | | ADPKD<br>Medullary cystic disease |
| Metabolic | | Hypercalcemia/nephrocalcinosis<br>Hypokalemia<br>Hyperuricemia<br>Hyperoxaluria |
| Immunologic | | Allograft rejection<br>Vasculitides: Wegener's, Sjögren's, SLE, sarcoid |

*Table continued on next page*

| | ACUTE<br>INTERSTITIAL NEPHRITIS | CHRONIC<br>INTERSTITIAL NEPHRITIS |
|---|---|---|
| Hematologic | | Multiple myeloma/light chain<br>  deposition disease<br>Sickle cell disease<br>Lymphoma |
| Obstructive | | Stones, tumors, clots, reflux |
| Other | Antitubule basement membrane<br>  disease, tubulointerstitial<br>  nephritis and uveitis syndrome,<br>  sarcoidosis | Balkan nephropathy<br>Radiation<br>Hypertension<br>Ischemia<br>Response to primary glomerular disease |

NSAIDs = nonsteroidal anti-inflammatory drugs; EBV = Epstein-Barr virus; CMV = cytomegalovirus; ADPKD = autosomal dominant polycystic kidney disease; SLE = systemic lupus erythematosus.

*Interstitial Renal Disease Classified by Tubular Site of Dysfunction*

| CORTEX | MEDULLA | PAPILLA |
|---|---|---|
| Proximal tubule | Analgesics | Analgesics |
|   Heavy metals | Sickle cell disease | Diabetes mellitus |
|   Multiple myeloma | Hypercalcemia | Infection |
|   Immunologic | Hypokalemia | Sickle cell disease |
|   Hereditary | Hereditary | Obstruction |
| Distal tubule | Infections | |
|   Immunologic | Uric acid | |
|   Granulomatous | | |
|   Hereditary | | |
|   Hypercalcemia | | |
|   Obstruction | | |
|   Sickle cell disease | | |

**4. What are the common clinical presentations for interstitial renal diseases?**

Proteinuria is typically less than 2 gm per day and a urine protein electrophoresis reveals nonglomerular proteinuria (i.e., minimal albuminuria). Sterile pyuria is more common than microscopic hematuria. Anemia may be observed with less severe azotemia than is seen in patients with a primary glomerular diseases. Often, the tubular segment(s) involved can be identified based on the accompanying dysfunctions. **Proximal tubule** involvement can manifest with reabsorption defects for sodium, bicarbonate, glucose, uric acid, phosphorous and amino acids (e.g., type II renal tubular acidosis [RTA] or Fanconi syndrome). Proximal tubule defects are often associated with decreased production of erythropoietin and 1,25 vitamin $D_3$. **Distal tubule** involvement can manifest with decreased secretion of hydrogen ion (type I RTA), decreased potassium secretion (type IV RTA), or decreased sodium reabsorption (salt losing nephropathy). **Medullary and papillary segment** involvement can result in concentrating defects (polyuria/nocturia) and decreased sodium reabsorption (salt losing nephropathy).

**5. How useful is the presence of eosinophiluria in establishing a diagnosis of acute (allergic) interstitial nephritis (AIN)?**

Not very. Eosinophiluria (up to 30%) has been seen in many other disorders (acute glomerulonephritis [GN], crescentic GN, transplant rejection, infectious interstitial nephritis, acute prostatitis).

Conversely, the urinalysis can be normal in patients with biopsy-proven severe AIN. The presence of about 50% or more eosinophiluria is, however, highly associated with AIN. Assessing for the presence of eosinophiluria with a Hansel stain is more sensitive than the Wright stain.

### 6. What are some of the more common interstitial renal diseases?

1. **AIN** most commonly occurs as an idiosyncratic reaction to medications. It was first described with methicillin. The classic presentation is an allergic reaction to the drug with low-grade fever, arthralgias, myalgias, rash, and eosinophilia. The renal manifestations include acute renal failure typically over a few weeks, eosinophiluria, sterile pyuria, and mild proteinuria. Treatment consists of stopping the offending drug and, generally, administering a short course of a corticosteroid. When AIN occurs in association with nonsteroidal anti-inflammatory drugs (NSAIDs), the allergic features are usually absent. Interestingly, patients with AIN caused by NSAIDs sometimes present with nephrotic-range proteinuria due to minimal change disease.

2. **Analgesic nephropathy (AN)** accounts for upwards of 25% of patients with end-stage renal disease (ESRD) in parts of Australia. In some regions of the United States (especially the southeast), it is responsible for about a third of all cases of chronic interstitial nephritis. AN is seen in individuals who ingest combination analgesics that contain, at the very least, acetaminophen and aspirin. In some regions of the U.S., these medications were packaged as headaches powders. A history of consuming these analgesics three to four times a day for several years is generally present in patients so afflicted. In patients with significant azotemia, the estimated amount of analgesics ingested over a mean of about 15 years is 10 kg; the minimum amount required to be associated with renal insufficiency is at least 1 gm/day for more than 3 years. AN is much more common in women. The incidence of malignancies of the uroepithelial tract is increased in patients with AN. Stopping the drugs is key. Data are still lacking that establish a relationship between non-phenacetin combination analgesics and nephropathy. The mechanism of injury appears to be dose dependent and prolonged negative free water clearance that serves to further concentrate the metabolites of acetaminophen. The metabolism of acetaminophen via the cytochrome P-450 system produces toxic reactive oxygen metabolites that deplete glutathione and covalently bind to cellular sulfhydryl groups resulting in cell death. Aspirin is hypothesized to further reduce the already low renal blood flow, thus further concentrating the toxic metabolites and compromising the ongoing production of glutathione.

3. **Papillary necrosis** represents ischemic infarcts that subsequently result in atrophy of the overlying cortex. The lesion is nonspecific. In adults, it is most commonly seen as a complication of long-standing analgesic use (especially aspirin), diabetes mellitus (with or without obstruction), sickle cell disease (SS, SC, or sickle-thalassemia), or chronic lower urinary tract obstruction. The presentation can range from being asymptomatic to symptoms of renal colic. Urinalysis may show sloughed papillary. Papillary necrosis can be best diagnosed with an intravenous pyelogram (IVP) or computed tomography (CT) scan.

4. **Sickle cell nephropathy** occurs within the first decade of life with defect in concentrating ability. Blood transfusion at this early age will reverse this defect. With time, repeated sickling of red blood cells in the microcirculation (in either sickle cell disease or trait) within the relatively hypoxic, hypertonic, acidotic, and low-flow medullary region of the kidney results in edema, focal scarring, interstitial fibrosis, and tubular atrophy. Impaired concentrating ability (with preservation of diluting ability), distal RTA, renal tubular hyperkalemia, and papillary necrosis (in up to a one-third of patients) are the common tubular manifestations of sickle cell nephropathy. Hematuria is the most common manifestation of sickle cell nephropathy. It usually responds to hypotonic fluid administration to increase urine flow and bed rest. More significant bleeding that requires transfusions and

fails conservative therapy may require epsilon-amino caproic acid therapy or selective renal artery embolization. Proteinuria occurs in up to 25% of patients. Nephrotic range proteinuria due to sickle cell glomerulopathy occurs in less than 5% of patients. Renal failure is not uncommon in patients with long-standing sickle disease.

    5. **Lead nephropathy**, or **plumbism**, most commonly occurs from occupational exposure (iron ore smelting) but can be caused by chronic exposure to lead in old water pipes, lead-based paints from old homes, homemade alcohol (moonshine or white lightning), and the manufacture of ceramic and crystal. Because lead rapidly deposits in bone and soft tissue, blood levels are generally normal. Chronic exposure can be assessed by measuring 24-hour urinary lead content after lead mobilization by ethylenediamine tetraacetic acid (EDTA). Lead affects the S3 portion of the proximal tubule and therefore may present with isolated tubule defects or complete Fanconi syndrome. These patients most commonly present with gout. Hypertension is not always present. Improvement in renal failure has been noted in patients after lead mobilization and normalization of total body lead stores when treated with EDTA.

    6. **Chinese herb nephropathy** due to *Aristolochia fangchi* in dietary herbal regimens was first described as a disorder causing progressive tubulointerstitial disease and renal failure in middle-aged women in 1992. It is also associated with an increased incidence of uroepithelial tumors. There is no treatment for this irreversible disorder.

    7. **Myeloma kidney** results from the uptake of nephrotoxic light chains by the proximal tubule and distal tubule and from obstruction by cast formation. These casts are found in both the proximal and distal tubules and are typically associated with multinucleated giant cells. Interestingly, 75% of patients with multiple myeloma have kappa light chains, whereas 75% of patients with primary amyloid have lambda light chains. Multiple myeloma is associated with a number of other renal syndromes, which are summarized in Chapter 39.

## BIBLIOGRAPHY

1. Batuman V, Landy E, Maesaka JK, et al: Contribution of lead to hypertension with renal impairment. N Engl J Med 309:17–21, 1983.
2. Diedrich D: The kidney and sickle cell disease. In Jacobson HR, Striker GE, Klahr S (eds): The Principles and Practice of Nephrology, 2nd ed. St. Louis, Mosby, 1995, pp 246–253.
3. Paller MS: Drug-induced nephropathies. Med Clin North Am 74:909–917, 1990.
4. Pirani CL, Valeri A, D'Agati V, et al: Renal toxicity of nonsteroidal anti-inflammatory drugs. Contr Nephrol 55:159–175, 1987.
5. Reginster F, Jadoul M, van Ypersele de Strihou C: Chinese herbs nephropathy presentation, natural history and fate after transplantation. Nephrol Dial Transplant 12:81–86, 1997.
6. Rota S, Mougenot B, Baudouin B, et al: Multiple myeloma and severe renal failure: A clinicopathologic study of outcome and prognosis in 34 patients. Medicine 66:126–137, 1987.

# 36. REFLUX NEPHROPATHY

*Beth A. Vogt, M.D.*

### 1. What is vesicoureteral reflux?

Vesicoureteral reflux is defined as retrograde propulsion of urine into the upper urinary tract during bladder contraction. Currently, vesicoureteral reflux is believed to result from ectopic insertion of the ureter into the bladder wall, which results in a shorter intravesicular ureter that acts as an incompetent valve during micturition.

### 2. How common is vesicoureteral reflux?

The exact incidence and prevalence of vesicoureteral reflux is not known. Population studies show a less than 1% incidence of reflux in healthy children without a history of urinary tract infection. However, at least one third of children evaluated for their first urinary tract infection have vesicoureteral reflux.

### 3. What is the difference between primary and secondary vesicoureteral reflux?

**Primary** vesicoureteral reflux refers to reflux that is not associated with other abnormalities of the urinary tract. **Secondary** vesicoureteral reflux refers to reflux associated with dysfunctional voiding syndromes (e.g., detrusor instability, detrusor-sphincter dyssynergia), obstructive uropathy (e.g., posterior urethral valves), or neurogenic bladder (e.g., myelodysplasia).

### 4. Is there a genetic basis for primary vesicoureteral reflux?

Although a gene for primary vesicoureteral reflux has not been described, a genetic predisposition clearly is present in some patients. For example, there is a 30% chance that a sibling of a child with vesicoureteral reflux will also have the disorder. Furthermore, 60–70% of offspring of individuals with a history of vesicoureteral reflux also will exhibit evidence of reflux.

### 5. How is vesicoureteral reflux discovered?

Vesicoureteral reflux most commonly is discovered by a cystogram performed as part of the evaluation of a patient with urinary tract infection. Screening identifies a smaller number of patients who have a family history of vesicoureteral reflux. Occasionally, reflux is discovered in patients evaluated by cystography for voiding dysfunction. Recently, an increasing number of cases have been discovered during evaluation of hydronephrosis detected in the antenatal period.

### 6. What tests can be performed to detect vesicoureteral reflux?

Both radiographic (using contrast dye and x-rays) and radionuclide (using a radioisotope and nuclear scanning) voiding cystourethrograms (VCUGs) can detect the presence or absence of vesicoureteral reflux. Both tests involve catheterization of the bladder, a procedure that causes discomfort and anxiety, especially in children. To date, ultrasound-based tests to evaluate patients for vesicoureteral reflux have not been reliable.

### 7. What are the advantages and disadvantages of radiographic VCUG?

The radiographic VCUG offers the ability to accurately grade reflux (see question 10). In addition, the radiographic VCUG allows visualization of the urethra, an advantage particularly important for boys in whom the diagnosis of posterior urethral valves must be excluded. The primary disadvantage of this procedure is increased exposure to radiation compared with the radionuclide VCUG.

## 8. What are the advantages and disadvantages of radionuclide VCUG?

The primary advantage to radionuclide VCUG is reduction in radiation exposure ($\frac{1}{100}$ of the radiation associated with the radiographic VCUG). In addition, radionuclide VCUG is more sensitive at detecting intermittent reflux. Disadvantages of this procedure include the inability to grade reflux accurately or to image the urethra.

## 9. Which VCUG should be used to evaluate vesicoureteral reflux?

In general, radiographic VCUG should be used for the first assessment of vesicoureteral reflux in an infant or child following urinary tract infection. This test allows careful grading of reflux and good visualization of the urethra in boys. The radionuclide VCUG is most useful as a follow-up study and as a screening test for siblings and children of patients with vesicoureteral reflux. Some clinicians advocate the use of the radionuclide VCUG for evaluation of first urinary tract infections in girls because visualization of the urethra is less important than in boys.

## 10. How is vesicoureteral reflux graded?

Vesicoureteral reflux is graded on a I–V scale (see figure) according to the International Reflux Study Committee.

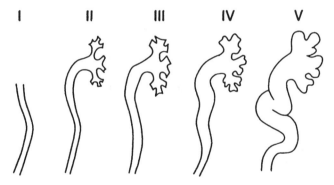

Classification of vesicoureteral reflux based on the degree of dilatation affecting the ureter and renal collecting system.

## 11. What is intrarenal reflux?

Intrarenal reflux refers to retrograde flow of urine from the renal pelvis into the papillary collecting ducts and renal tubules. Intrarenal reflux occurs primarily in specific renal papillae ("refluxing papillae") that are present in many, but not all, human kidneys and tend to be most common at the upper and lower poles. In patients with vesicoureteral reflux, cortical scarring tends to occur in association with areas of intrarenal reflux.

## 12. What are the complications of vesicoureteral reflux?

Vesicoureteral reflux may be associated with renal scarring, hypertension, and chronic renal failure. At least 30% of patients have renal scarring at the time of diagnosis. The risk of progressive scarring is greatest in children younger than 5 years. Hypertension is present in up to 20% of patients with renal scarring and may be more frequent in patients with bilateral, high-grade reflux and extensive scarring. Reflux nephropathy accounts for about 25% of cases of end-stage renal disease in children and for 5–15% of cases in adults.

### 13. What is the natural history of primary vesicoureteral reflux?

Primary vesicoureteral reflux tends to resolve over time as the intravesical segment of the ureter elongates with growth. The incidence of spontaneous resolution is greatest in patients with the lowest grades of reflux (80% of grade I; 60% of grade II, 50% of grade III). In contrast, rates of spontaneous resolution are quite low in patients with grade IV or grade V reflux. In general, 20% of patients with low-grade reflux will experience spontaneous resolution per year, although complete resolution may not occur until adolescence.

### 14. How should vesicoureteral reflux be managed?

In the past, surgical therapy was offered to most patients diagnosed with vesicoureteral reflux. With the recognition that spontaneous resolution commonly occurs, a more conservative approach is now recommended. All patients with reflux should be treated with daily prophylactic antibiotics to prevent urinary tract infection. Many clinicians obtain surveillance urine cultures every 3–4 months to ensure sterility of the urine. VCUGs should be performed every 12–18 months to assess for spontaneous resolution of reflux.

### 15. What is the current recommendation for antibiotic prophylaxis?

Most clinicians advocate the use of oral amoxicillin (10 mg/kg/dose twice a day) for infants younger than 2 months of age. For infants older than 2 months of age and children, trimethoprim-sulfamethoxazole (2.5 mg/kg/dose at bedtime) is recommended.

### 16. When should surgical ureteral reimplantation be considered?

Surgical ureteral reimplantation should be considered in children with high-grade (grade IV or V) reflux because of the lower probability of spontaneous resolution. Children with breakthrough urinary tract infections despite antibiotic prophylaxis may be considered for surgical treatment to reduce the risk of further renal scarring. Adolescents with unresolved reflux also may be considered for surgery because of the lower probability of spontaneous resolution.

### 17. Are there any new treatments for vesicoureteral reflux on the horizon?

Endoscopic injections of material (e.g., Teflon, collagen) into the ureterovesicular junction have been used to impede retrograde propulsion of urine. With further testing, such injections may emerge as a nonsurgical treatment for vesicoureteral reflux.

### BIBLIOGRAPHY

1. Elder JS, Peters CA, Arant BS, et al: Pediatric Vesicoureteral Reflux Guidelines Panel summary report on the management of primary vesicoureteral reflux in children. J Urol 157:1846–1851, 1997.
2. Elder JS: Guidelines for consideration for surgical repair of vesicoureteral reflux. Curr Opin Urol 10:579–585, 2000.
3. Garin EH, Campos A, Homsy Y: Primary vesicoureteral reflux: Review of current concepts. Pediatr Nephrol 12:249–256, 1998.
4. Greenfield SP, Wan J: The relationship between dysfunctional voiding and congenital vesicoureteral reflux. Curr Opin Urol 10:607–610, 2000.
5. Kamil ES: Recent advances in the understanding and management of primary vesicoureteral reflux and reflux nephropathy. Curr Opin Nephrol Hypertens 9:139–142, 2000.
6. Smellie JM, Prescod NP, Shaw PJ, et al: Childhood reflux and urinary infection: A follow-up of 10–41 years in 226 adults. Pediatr Nephrol 12:727–736, 1998.

# 37. RENAL VASCULITIS

*Marcia R. Silver, M.D., and Linda Zarif, M.D.*

**1. List the major types of vasculitis.**
The vasculitides are a group of diseases in which tissue ischemia and necrosis occur as a consequence of inflammation of blood vessels, either as a primary event or secondary to a systemic disease. Different vasculitides have predilections for vessels of different sizes (see table).

| VESSEL SIZE | VASCULITIDES | INVOLVEMENT |
|---|---|---|
| Large-vessel | Giant cell vasculitis | Granulomatous arteritis of aorta and major branches. Temporal artery involvement is common. Headache and polymyalgia rheumatica common in patients older than 50 years. |
| | Takayasu's arteritis | Involves aorta and major branches in patients younger than 50 years. |
| Medium-vessel | Polyarteritis nodosa | Necrotizing inflammation of medium-sized vessels. Affects renal arteries but not capillaries. No glomerulonephritis on biopsy. Often involves visceral vessels such as hepatic and mesenteric arteries. |
| | Kawasaki syndrome | More common in young children. Associated with mucocutaneous lymph node syndrome. |
| Small-vessel | **Pauci-immune vasculitis with ANCA** | |
| | Wegener's granulomatosis | Necrotizing granulomatous inflammation of upper and lower respiratory tract. Sinusitis, nasal ulcers, and hemoptysis are common, often associated with glomerulonephritis. |
| | Churg-Strauss syndrome | Eosinophil-predominant inflammation of respiratory tract. Asthma and blood eosinophilia are common. Rarely involves the kidneys. |
| | Microscopic polyangiitis | Necrotizing glomerulonephritis. Necrotizing arteritis of small- and medium-sized vessels is common. |
| | **Immune complex vasculitis** | |
| | Henoch-Schönlein purpura | IgA deposits typically identified in small vessels of skin, gut, and glomeruli. |
| | Essential cryoglobulinemic vasculitis | Cryoglobulin immune deposits of small vessels. Skin and glomeruli most commonly affected. |
| | Systemic lupus erythematosus | |
| | Other vasculitides related to connective tissue diseases | |

ANCA = antineutrophil cytoplasmic antibody.
Adapted from Jennette JC, Falk RJ, Rassy K, et al: Nomenclature of systemic vasculitides: The proposal of an international consensus conference. Arthritis Rheum 37:187–192, 1994.

## 2. What are the distinctive features of the common vasculitides?

Clinical criteria based on the size of the vessel involved were defined at the Chapel Hill Consensus Conference on the Nomenclature of Systemic Vasculitis (see above table). Patients with large-vessel vasculitis usually present with signs and symptoms of tissue ischemia. In contrast, evidence for inflammation (purpura, hemoptysis, red cell casts, and hematuria) is more commonly identified in patients with small-vessel vasculitis.

## 3. How does primary vasculitis differ from secondary vasculitis?

Primary vasculitis is a distinct group of diseases in which the blood vessels are the primary site of injury. Vasculitis also may occur as a secondary response to infection or in association with a multisystem autoimmune disease. Viral infections with hepatitis B and C (see Chapter 30, Hepatitis-associated Glomerulonephritis), human immunodeficiency virus (see Chapter 31, HIV-associated Renal Disorders), Epstein-Barr virus, cytomegalovirus, and parvoviruses have been associated with vasculitides and cause medium- or small-vessel vasculitis. Streptococcal and staphylococcal infections also may cause secondary vasculitis. Infections with methicillin-resistant *Staphylococcus aureus* (MRSA) are associated with vasculitic lesions of the lower extremities. Thorough evaluation of infection as a cause of vasculitis is critical, because immunosuppressive therapy is the mainstay of treatment for the primary forms of vasculitis and could be lethal in a patient with an underlying infection.

## 4. What is the usual clinical presentation of a patient with vasculitis?

Vasculitis should be considered in a patient who presents with dysfunction of multiple organ systems and with constitutional symptoms such as fever, fatigue, weakness, myalgias, and arthralgias. Varying degrees of renal insufficiency may be present if the renal parenchyma is involved. The presence of mononeuritis multiplex and palpable purpuric skin lesions are important clues to vasculitis.

## 5. What are the characteristic urinalysis findings in patients with vasculitis involving the kidney?

The urinalysis generally demonstrates an active sediment with microscopic hematuria and red blood cell casts. However, even with severe vasculitic involvement of the kidney, red blood cell casts may not be seen. Proteinuria is common but usually modest (< 3 gm per day).

## 6. Which of the vasculitides have a predilection for renal involvement?

Kidney involvement in small-vessel vasculitis is quite common. However, polyarteritis nodosa, a medium-size vessel vasculitis, often involves renal arteries. In contrast, Kawasaki syndrome, another vasculitis that affects medium-size vessels, rarely involves renal arteries. Large-vessel vasculitides rarely may affect renal blood vessels.

## 7. Can complement levels be helpful in establishing a diagnosis of vasculitis?

Yes. After exclusion of infection-associated vasculitic syndromes, vasculitis with low complement levels is most likely associated with systemic lupus erythematosus, cryoglobulinemia, or another autoimmune disease. Complement levels are generally normal in antineutrophil cytoplasmic antibody (ANCA)–associated small-vessel vasculitides, Henoch-Schönlein purpura, and polyarteritis nodosa. Complement levels also can be depressed in patients with atheroembolic disease, a multisystem disorder that results from dislodged microscopic emboli derived from atherosclerotic plaques (see Chapter 38, Other Vascular Renal Disorders).

## 8. What are ANCAs?

ANCAs are autoantibodies directed against intracellular neutrophil antigens. These antibodies produce one of two distinct indirect immunofluorescence patterns when serum is incubated with ethanol-fixed neutrophils: **cytoplasmic (C-ANCA)** or **perinuclear (P-ANCA)** staining. Using specific immunochemical assays, it has been shown that C-ANCAs are directed against a neutrophil and monocyte protease, proteinase 3 (PR3), whereas P-ANCAs are specific for myeloperoxidase (MPO). ANCAs are commonly detected in patients with pauci-immune small-vessel vasculitis. Indirect immunofluorescence patterns are not specific, especially for P-ANCA, and must be confirmed by enzyme immunoassays for anti-PR3 (C-ANCA) and anti-MPO (P-ANCA).

**9. What vasculitides cause pulmonary-renal syndrome?**

Pulmonary-renal syndrome refers to the constellation of nephritis and hemoptysis or infiltrates on chest x-ray and can be caused by a number of disorders:

| | |
|---|---|
| Microscopic polyangiitis | Goodpasture's syndrome |
| Wegener's granulomatosis | Henoch-Schönlein purpura |
| Churg-Strauss syndrome | Behçet's disease |
| Systemic lupus erythematosus | Rheumatoid vasculitis |

Pulmonary-renal syndrome can be caused by both primary and secondary vasculitides. However, other multisystem diseases can present with concurrent pulmonary and renal involvement and need to be considered in the differential diagnosis. These include:

- Congestive heart failure (causing hemoptysis from pulmonary edema) with associated renal failure
- Renal failure complicated by pneumonia (especially with *Legionella* infection)
- Nephrotic syndrome with renal vein thrombosis and pulmonary embolism

**10. What is pauci-immune glomerulonephritis?**

The term *pauci-immune glomerulonephritis* refers to an often rapidly progressive glomerular inflammatory disease with prominent crescent formation seen on light microscopy and in which immune deposits are not detected on immunofluorescence microscopy. Eighty percent to 90% of patients with pauci-immune glomerulonephritis are ANCA-positive.

**11. How do ANCAs differentiate the etiologies of pauci-immune glomerulonephritides?**

Eighty percent to 95% of patients with Wegener's granulomatosis have positive tests for C-ANCA or PR3-ANCA. Five percent to 20% are positive for P-ANCA or MPO-ANCA. Forty percent to 80% of patients with microscopic polyangiitis have positive tests for P-ANCA or MPO-ANCA. Patients with Churg-Strauss syndrome may have positive tests for either C-ANCA or P-ANCA. A number of other diseases, such as rheumatoid arthritis, Behçet's disease, systemic lupus erythematosus, and Sjögren's syndrome, may be associated with a positive P-ANCA on indirect immunofluorescence but will be P-ANCA–negative using the specific enzyme immunoassay for MPO. Differentiating between specific ANCA-associated small-vessel vasculitides in an individual patient is not possible using only ANCA assays, although a positive C- or P-ANCA by indirect immunofluorescence and enzyme immunoassay strongly suggests a diagnosis of small-vessel vasculitis. A tissue biopsy may be needed to differentiate between the ANCA-associated small-vessel vasculitides, and biopsy confirmation of vasculitis is prudent prior to initiation of immunosuppressive therapy.

**12. Are there prognostic markers of renal survival in pauci-immune ANCA-related vasculitis?**

Yes. The best predictors of renal survival are serum creatinine (high serum creatinine on presentation predicts worse prognosis), race (blacks have a worse prognosis than whites), and presence of arterial sclerosis on kidney biopsy. Age, ANCA pattern, the presence of pulmonary renal involvement, glomerular necrosis, and percent of glomeruli with crescents do not correlate with long-term renal survival. Immunosuppressive therapies appear to have improved the prognosis of some forms of severe vasculitis, including renal vasculitis. For example, in Wegener's granulomatosis, the 1-year patient survival described before the use of cyclophosphamide was ~20%. With the use of cytotoxic agents, the 1-year patient survival is now ~80%.

Patients with ANCA-associated systemic vasculitis who develop end-stage renal disease (ESRD) and require dialysis or renal transplantation do as well as other nondiabetic ESRD patients overall. However, they are subject to flares of their vasculitis, and vigilance is required to diagnose and treat these flares early and effectively.

## 13. What is the therapy for vasculitis?

Therapy should be guided by the severity of illness. Underlying infection needs to be ruled out before initiating immunosuppressive therapy. Giant cell arteritis and Takayasu's disease are usually treated with high doses of corticosteroids. Steroids are contraindicated in Kawasaki syndrome, which is usually treated with aspirin and high-dose gamma globulin. Henoch-Schönlein purpura is often mild and self-limited and may be treated with supportive care. If intestinal involvement or azotemia complicates Henoch-Schönlein purpura, corticosteroid therapy may be indicated. Patients with ANCA-associated vasculitis (Wegener's granulomatosis and microscopic polyangiitis) usually are treated with a combination of corticosteroids and cytotoxic drugs. Evidence supporting use of plasmapheresis is limited, but it may be beneficial when vasculitis is associated with rapidly progressive glomerulonephritis and dialysis dependence or with hemoptysis.

## 14. Do ANCAs play a pathogenic role or are they an epiphenomenon?

The pathogenic role of ANCAs remains controversial. In support of their pathogenic role, several in vitro studies have demonstrated degranulation of neutrophils and production of oxygen free radicals after incubation with ANCA. These activated neutrophils can then attach to vascular endothelial cells and cause damage. If this theory is correct, circulating (extracellular) ANCAs would need to interact with their target proteins, all of which are intracellular. It has been suggested that these target proteins (e.g., MPO) are translocated to the cytoplasmic membrane in apoptotic or cytokine-primed neutrophils. An alternate hypothesis proposes that release of antigenic proteins from neutrophils at the site of vascular injury occurs secondary to an underlying infection or an immune complex disease in which immune complexes are rapidly cleared from the vascular bed. The latter theory may explain why some patients with mild to moderate Wegener's granulomatosis may respond to antibiotics such as trimethoprim-sulfamethoxazole.

### BIBLIOGRAPHY

1. Allen A, Pusey C, Gaskin G: Outcome of renal replacement therapy in antineutrophil cytoplasmic antibody-associated systemic vasculitis. J Am Soc Nephrol 9:1258–1263, 1998.
2. Falk RJ, Jennette JC: ANCA are pathogenic: Oh yes they are! J Am Soc Nephrol 13:1977–1979, 2002.
3. Hagen EC, Daha MR, Hermans J, et al: Diagnostic value of standardized assays for anti-neutrophil cytoplasmic antibodies in idiopathic systemic vasculitis. Kidney Int 53:743–753, 1998.
4. Herbert LA, Cosio FG, Neff JC: Diagnostic significance of hypocomplementemia. Kidney Int 39:811–821, 1991.
5. Hogan SL, Nachman PH, Wilkman S, et al: Prognostic markers in patients with ANCA-associated microscopic polyangiitis and GN. J Am Soc Nephrol 7:23–32, 1996.
6. Jennette JC, Falk RJ: Renal involvement in systemic vasculitis. In Greenberg A (ed): Primer on Kidney Diseases, 2nd ed. San Diego, Academic Press, 1998, pp 200–207.

7. Jennette JC, Falk RJ: Small-vessel vasculitis. N Engl J Med 337:1512–1523, 1997.
8. Johnson RJ: The mystery of the antineutrophil cytoplasmic antibodies. Am J Kidney Dis 26:57–61, 1995.
9. Kamesh L, Harper L, Savage CO: ANCA-positive vasculitis. J Am Soc Nephrol 13:1953–1960, 2002.
10. Langford CA, Klippel JH, Balow JE, et al: Use of cytotoxic agents and cyclosporine in the treatment of autoimmune disease. Ann Intern Med 129:49–58, 1998.
11. Rees AJ: Vasculitis and the kidney. Curr Opin Nephrol Hypertension 5:273–281, 1996.
12. Westman KWA, Bygren PG, Olsson H, et al: Relapse rate, renal survival and cancer morbidity in patients with Wegener's granulomatosis or microscopic polyangiitis with renal involvement. J Am Soc Nephrol 9:842–852, 1998.

# 38. OTHER VASCULAR RENAL DISORDERS

*Donald E. Hricik, M.D.*

**1. What are the renal manifestations of scleroderma?**
- Hypertension, sometimes malignant (i.e., scleroderma renal crisis)
- Renal insufficiency
- Varying degrees of proteinuria and hematuria

**2. How common is renal disease in patients with scleroderma?**
Thirty percent to 50% of patients with scleroderma ultimately develop evidence of renal involvement. Up to 15% of patients develop scleroderma renal crisis.

**3. What are risk factors for renal disease in patients with scleroderma?**
- Diffuse skin involvement
- African ethnicity
- Female gender (especially in the age range between 20 and 50 years)
- Cold exposure

**4. What is the clinical course of patients with scleroderma renal disease?**
Renal manifestations typically develop about 4 years following the onset of other systemic manifestations of the disorder. Severe hypertension and abrupt onset of renal failure characterize scleroderma renal crisis. If left untreated, end-stage renal disease usually develops within 1–2 months. Early, aggressive control of hypertension may prevent the development of renal crises and slow the progression of renal insufficiency.

**5. What are the pathologic findings in patients with scleroderma renal crisis?**
The acute phase comprises fibrinoid necrosis characterized by intravascular deposition of platelet-fibrin thrombi. With healing, there is progressive intimal thickening and concentric hypertrophy of interlobular arteries, leading to an onion-skin appearance. The histopathology is similar to that seen in patients with other forms of malignant hypertension, thrombotic thrombocytopenic purpura, radiation nephritis, and chronic renal allograft rejection.

**6. What is the treatment for renal disease in scleroderma?**
The malignant hypertension that occurs in patients with scleroderma is mediated by activation of the renin-angiotensin system resulting from progressive vascular sclerosis. Thus, angiotensin inhibitors are the treatment of choice for both the prevention and treatment of hypertension complicating this disorder.

**7. What is atheroembolic renal disease?**
Atheroembolic renal disease results from dislodgment of microscopic cholesterol emboli from atherosclerotic plaques leading to occlusion of the lumina of small renal blood vessels, ischemia, and renal dysfunction. The presence of atherosclerotic plaques is obviously the main predisposing factor. Spontaneous atheroembolic disease has been described; however, most cases occur after vascular manipulation (e.g., aortic surgery, arteriography, cardiac catheterization, or angioplasty).

### 8. What are the clinical features of atheroembolic renal disease?

Renal failure may be the sole manifestation or part of a systemic presentation characterized by ischemia of multiple organs. Renal involvement is characterized by a slow progressive decline in renal function within days or weeks of vascular manipulation. Beyond the site of plaque dislodgment, bluish discoloration of the extremities, palpable purpura, and livedo reticularis are common. Proteinuria has been reported, and up to 15% of patients exhibit eosinophiluria; however, the urinalysis is more often relatively unremarkable. Peripheral eosinophilia and hypocomplementemia sometimes are observed but are nonspecific findings. In severe cases, signs of ischemia or infarction in other organ systems can be observed (e.g., intestinal infarction). Although the syndrome of atheroembolic renal disease is most often recognized as a catastrophic disorder resulting in irreversible renal failure, it has been recognized recently as a cause of occult and sometimes reversible renal insufficiency.

### 9. Describe the pathologic findings in atheroembolic renal disease.

The pathologic hallmark consists of obstruction of small- to medium-sized vessels (ranging from 50 to 900 μm in diameter) with atheromatous debris. During routine fixation of tissues in formalin, cholesterol dissolves, and cholesterol crystals cannot be observed unless special fixatives are used. However, characteristic needle-shaped clefts, previously occupied by the crystals, can be seen within vascular lumina with routine microscopy (see figure). The deposition of cholesterol crystals leads to vascular and perivascular inflammation that can ultimately result in fibrosis.

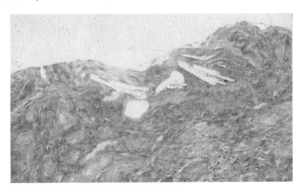

Micrograph showing intravascular needle-shaped clefts in a patient with acute renal failure due to atheroembolic disease.

### 10. What are the diagnostic and treatment measures in patients with suspected atheroembolic renal disease?

Most cases are diagnosed on clinical grounds. In some cases, biopsies of the kidney, skin, or muscle may be necessary to confirm the diagnosis. There is no specific therapy for this disorder, and management is entirely supportive. Some experts suggest that anticoagulation is contraindicated because it may prevent healing of exposed atherosclerotic plaques.

### 11. What are the common causes of renal vein thrombosis?

Renal vein thrombosis can occur in severely dehydrated neonates or children. It also can occur as a complication of trauma or malignancy (especially in cases of renal cell carcinomas that have a proclivity for renal vein invasion). The majority of cases occur in patients with heavy proteinuria and the nephrotic syndrome, usually reflecting a hypercoagulable state (see Chapter 17, Nephrotic Syndrome).

**12. What is the clinical presentation of a patient with renal vein thrombosis?**

Most cases are occult and asymptomatic. In severe cases, patients may present with flank pain, microscopic or gross hematuria, high lactate dehydrogenase levels (reflecting renal infarction), or signs of associated pulmonary emboli.

**13. What imaging studies are helpful in the diagnosis of renal vein thrombosis?**

Computed tomography (CT) scan, magnetic resonance imaging (MRI), and duplex ultrasound have all been used to diagnose renal vein thrombosis noninvasively. However, inferior vena cava venography or the venous phase of arteriography remains the gold standard for diagnosis.

**14. What are the clinical characteristics of hemolytic uremic syndrome (HUS) and thrombotic thrombocytopenic purpura (TTP)?**

HUS and TTP are disorders characterized by thrombotic microangiopathy. The syndromes differ somewhat with respect to etiology, natural history, and clinical characteristics (see table).

*Clinical Manifestations of Renal Thrombotic Microangiopathies*

| HEMOLYTIC UREMIC SYNDROME | THROMBOTIC THROMBOCYTOPENIC PURPURA |
| --- | --- |
| Microangiopathic hemolytic anemia | Microangiopathic hemolytic anemia |
| Thrombocytopenia | Thrombocytopenia |
| Renal failure | Renal failure |
| | Fever |
| | Neurologic manifestations |

**15. What are the causes of HUS?**

Fifty percent to 90% of cases in children are preceded by diarrhea, often caused by toxigenic *Escherichia coli*. More than half of cases in adults are not associated with diarrheal illness and may be idiopathic, related to nonenteric infections (including pneumonia, meningitis, and human immunodeficiency virus [HIV] infection), or secondary to malignant hypertension, connective tissue disease, or preeclampsia. HUS has been associated with a number of drugs including oral contraceptives, mitomycin C, cyclosporine, and tacrolimus.

**16. What causes TTP?**

It has long been recognized that TTP is associated with the release into the circulation of unusually large multimers of von Willebrand factor, providing evidence of endothelial dysfunction. Recently, a severe deficiency in von Willebrand–cleaving protease activity (< 5% of that in normal plasma) or a deficiency in the inhibitor of this protease has been observed in most patients with TTP but not in patients with HUS. Measurement of protease activity, therefore, may be helpful diagnostically. However, further studies are needed to determine whether the level of protease activity correlates with response to treatment or prognosis.

**17. What therapies are available for patients with HUS and TTP?**

HUS is often managed with supportive care, including dialysis when necessary. In contrast, plasma therapies are beneficial in patients with TTP. Plasma exchange using fresh frozen plasma as the initial replacement fluid is associated with a good response in more than 70% of patients. Corticosteroids, vincristine, antiplatelet agents, and splenectomy have each been used in patients with both HUS and TTP, but the absence of controlled trials makes it difficult to ascertain the benefit of these modalities.

## BIBLIOGRAPHY

1. Bell WR, Braine HG, Ness PM, Kickler TS: Improved survival in thrombotic thrombocytopenia purpura-hemolytic uremic syndrome: Clinical experience in 108 patients. N Engl J Med 325:398–403, 1991.
2. Bianchi V, Robles R, Alberio L, et al: Von Willebrand factor-cleaving protease (ADAMTS13) in thrombocytopenic disorders: A severely deficient activity is specific for thrombotic thrombocytopenia purpura. Blood 100:710–713, 2002.
3. Donohoe J: Scleroderma and the kidney. Kidney Int 41:462–477, 1992.
4. Mannesse CK, Blankenstijn PJ, Man int Veld AJ, Schalekamp MADH: Renal failure and cholesterol embolization: A report of 4 surviving cases and a review of the literature. Clin Nephrol 36:240–245, 1991.
5. Rabelink TJ, Zwaginga JJ, Koomans HA, Sixma JJ: Thrombosis and hemostasis in renal disease. Kidney Int 46:287–296, 1994.
6. Remuzzi G, Ruggenenti P: The hemolytic uremic syndrome. Kidney Int 47:2–19, 1995.
7. Steen VD, Costantino JP, Shapiro AP, Medsger TA: Outcome of renal crisis in systemic sclerosis: Relation to availability of angiotensin-converting enzyme (ACE) inhibitors. Ann Intern Med 113:352–357, 1990.
8. Tadhani RI, Carmago CA, Xavier RJ, et al: Atheroembolic renal failure after invasive procedures. Natural history based on 52 histologically proven cases. Medicine 74:350–358, 1995.

# 39. RENAL DISEASE DUE TO DYSPROTEINEMIAS

*Edmond Ricanati, M.D.*

**1. List the different types of dysproteinemias associated with renal disease.**
* Multiple myeloma
* Amyloidosis
* Cryoglobulinemia
* Light chain nephropathy
* Waldenström's macroglobulinemia. This produces renal disease only rarely because the monoclonal immunoglobulin M (IgM) paraprotein characteristics of this disorder are generally too large to be trapped by the glomeruli. However, a small percentage of patients with Waldenström's macroglobulinemia (about 20% of cases) have light chains in their urine. These patients are prone to developing renal disease.

**2. What is the pathogenesis of renal disease in multiple myeloma?**
An estimated 25% of patients with multiple myeloma develop renal failure. The renal injury in multiple myeloma results from overproduction of monoclonal light chains by the rapid proliferation of plasma cells derived from a single clone. These abnormal proteins are freely filtered by the glomeruli and produce extensive renal tubular damage leading to chronic progressive renal disease by:
* Formation of intratubular casts by precipitation of aggregated light chains forming large molecules, which obstruct the tubular lumen. Experimental evidence does show that light chains have an affinity to bind with specific sites on the Tamm-Horsfall glycoprotein, which is locally secreted by the tubular cells of the ascending limb of the loop of Henle. Binding of light chains to this protein causes the formation of intratubular casts.
* Tubular injury due to the reabsorption of the filtered light chains, which are toxic to the tubular cells

**3. How are light chains detected in the urine?**
The urinary dipstick does not detect light chains; it primarily detects albumin. Sulfosalicylic acid (SSA), which precipitates all proteins in the urine, is the simple test of choice. A positive SSA test with a negative dipstick test is highly suggestive of the presence of light chains. The electrophoretic pattern of urine proteins is characteristic of multiple myeloma and usually shows a sharp monoclonal light chain peak. Patients with multiple myeloma often excrete large quantities of light chains, sometimes exceeding 1 gm per day. Not all light chains are nephrotoxic. Patients excreting lambda chains generally have a more severe form of renal disease than those excreting kappa chains.

**4. Patients with multiple myeloma can develop acute renal failure. What predisposing factors can cause this complication?**
1. **Hypercalcemia**, which is commonly found in multiple myeloma and is due to increased bone reabsorption (see Chapter 71, Hypocalcemia and Hypercalcemia). This results from the overproduction of cytokines such as interleukin 6, which directly stimulates

osteoclasts. Hypercalcemia can precipitate acute renal failure by causing vasoconstriction and by precipitating with light chains in the tubules, causing intratubular obstruction.

2. **Use of radiocontrast agents in the presence of dehydration**. The mechanism for the acute renal failure is not clear; the high concentration of urinary light chains that are excreted may combine with the contrast agent to produce intratubular obstruction. Hydration is strongly recommended in such patients before use of radiocontrast agents.

3. **Acute urate nephropathy**. The rapid breakdown of abnormal plasma cells, especially following chemotherapy, and the release of large quantities of uric acid lead to the formation of intratubular urate casts.

5. **What are the principal treatments for multiple myeloma with renal failure?**
   1. **Chemotherapy**
      • In patients with small to moderate tumor burdens, an alkylating agent (e.g., melphalan) and steroids are used.
      • In patients with extensive tumor burdens, treatment regimens include:
      VAD (vincristine, Adriamycin, and dexamethasone)
      ABCM (Adriamycin, carmustine [BCNV], cyclophosphamide, and melphalan)
   2. **Plasmapheresis** in combination with chemotherapy to remove more rapidly circulating myeloma proteins. This approach is not very effective in patients with histologic evidence of advanced renal disease (e.g., interstitial fibrosis or amyloidosis). Plasmapheresis is most effective when started early in the course of myeloma kidney disease.
   3. **Dialysis** when uremia occurs

6. **How does amyloidosis cause renal disease?**
   Two types of amyloidosis exist: (1) primary amyloidosis (AL amyloidosis) and (2) secondary or reactive amyloidosis (AA amyloidosis). In **AL amyloidosis**, renal disease results from the deposition of amyloid fibrils, derived from immunoglobulin light chains, in the glomeruli, blood vessels, and tubules. In **AA amyloidosis**, amyloid fibrils are derived from an acute phase reactant serum protein, amyloid AA, which is a protein produced by the liver in chronic inflammatory conditions. Renal disease due to amyloid AL tends to be more severe than renal disease due to amyloid AA. The amyloid fibrils in AL amyloidosis tend to coalesce and have a characteristic ability to bind to Congo red, producing an intense yellow-green fluorescence under polarized light. It is not clear what stimulates the formation of beta-pleated fibrils from normal plasma proteins.

7. **What are the renal manifestations of primary amyloidosis?**
   The renal manifestations of AL amyloidosis depend on the site of deposition of amyloid fibrils in the kidney. Most commonly, amyloid deposits occur in the glomeruli (both in the mesangium and capillary loops). Such patients usually present with nephrotic-range proteinuria, hypoalbuminemia, and peripheral edema. Initially, plasma creatinine is normal, but with progression of the disease, the plasma creatinine rises and renal failure ensues. In some cases, amyloid fibrils deposit primarily in the blood vessels, leading to progressive renal failure without significant proteinuria. This type of renal disease is apparently more common in secondary amyloidosis (amyloid AA renal disease). Tubular deposits of amyloid fibrils also can occur and may lead to tubular dysfunction such as distal renal tubular acidosis and nephrogenic diabetes insipidus.

8. **What is the treatment for amyloidosis?**
   In secondary amyloidosis, treatment is primarily directed to the underlying inflammatory process (such as osteomyelitis, rheumatoid arthritis, regional enteritis, chronic bronchiectasis with repeated infections), successful treatment of which can arrest the pro-

gression of the renal disease. In primary amyloidosis, the renal disease progresses relentlessly, and there is no proven effective therapy for this disease. Survival time is short, and death usually is due to cardiovascular complications resulting from the deposition of amyloid fibrils in the myocardium and blood vessels. Prednisone and melphalan have been used with equivocal results. The addition of colchicine (which has been shown experimentally to decrease amyloid formation) to the prednisone and melphalan regimen has been found to prolong survival in some series.

### 9. What are cryoglobulins?

Cryoglobulins are immunoglobulins that precipitate when plasma is cooled and redissolve when plasma is warmed. Three types of cryoglobulinemia have been identified. In type I cryoglobulinemia, a single monoclonal immunoglobulin is present. Types II and III cryoglobulinemias are characterized by mixed types of immunoglobulins. In type II cryoglobulinemia, a mixture of polyclonal immunoglobulins and a monoclonal immunoglobulin, usually IgM, is directed against the IgG immunoglobulins. In type III cryoglobulinemia, a mixture of polyclonal antibodies have anti-IgG and anti-IgM (rheumatoid factor) activity.

### 10. What renal diseases are associated with cryoglobulinemia?

All types of cryoglobulinemias can be associated with glomerular disease. The pattern of glomerular disease depends on the site of immunoglobulin deposition and the types of immunoglobulins involved. The glomerular lesions in type I and III are variable and nonspecific; however, type II cryoglobulinemia results in a well-characterized form of membranoproliferative glomerulonephritis, now recognized to be a manifestation of hepatitis C in most cases (see Chapter 30, Hepatitis-associated Glomerulonephritis).

### 11. What is light chain nephropathy?

Light chain nephropathy is a renal disease characterized by the deposition of monoclonal light chains in renal glomeruli or the tubulointerstitium. In contrast to patients with multiple myeloma or amyloidosis, patients with light chain nephropathy exhibit no skeletal evidence of plasma cell overgrowth, and the light chains do not form amyloid fibrils. The characteristic histologic lesion is a nodular glomerulopathy with negative Congo red stains. Patients present either with nephrotic syndrome or with evidence of tubular dysfunction (e.g., Fanconi syndrome). Anecdotal reports have shown improvement following treatment with melphalan and prednisone.

### BIBLIOGRAPHY

1. D'Amico G, Fornasieri A: Cryoglobulinemic glomerulonephritis: A membranoproliferative glomerulonephritis induced by hepatitis C virus. Am J Kidney Dis 25:361–369, 1995.
2. Ganeval D, Rabian C, Guérin V, et al: Treatment of multiple myeloma with renal involvement. Adv Nephrol 21:347–370, 1992.
3. Gertz MA, Kyle RA, Greipp PR: Response rates and survival in primary systemic amyloidosis. Blood 77:257–262, 1991.
4. Heilman RL, Velosa JA, Holley KE, et al: Long-term follow-up and response to chemotherapy in patients with light-chain deposition disease. Am J Kidney Dis 20:34–41, 1992.
5. Sanders PW, Herrera GA: Monoclonal immunoglobulin light chain–related renal diseases. Semin Nephrol 13:324–341, 1993.

# VI. End-Stage Renal Disease: Causes and Consequences

## 40. EPIDEMIOLOGY AND OUTCOMES OF END-STAGE RENAL DISEASE

*Ashwini R. Sehgal, M.D.*

**1. What is end-stage renal disease?**

End-stage renal disease (ESRD) is irreversible, severe kidney failure for which patients require treatment with dialysis or kidney transplantation in order to survive.

**2. How many people have end-stage renal disease?**

About 1 of every 1000 Americans receive treatment for ESRD, for a total of nearly 350,000 affected individuals. The prevalence of treated ESRD is increasing at a rate of about 8% per year. It is unclear how many patients with ESRD are untreated (and die as a result). The prevalence of treated ESRD in Canada and Western Europe is about half that in the United States.

**3. Name the most common causes of ESRD.**

The major causes of ESRD are diabetes mellitus (one-third of patients) and hypertension (one-fourth of patients). Other common causes include glomerulonephritis and polycystic kidney disease. In at least 5% of patients, the cause is unknown.

**4. What demographic factors are associated with ESRD?**

Advanced age, black race, male sex, and low socioeconomic status are associated with an increased likelihood of ESRD. For example, blacks account for nearly one-third of ESRD patients but only one-eighth of the general population.

**5. How is ESRD treated?**

In the United States, ESRD currently is treated by:
- Hemodialysis (60%)
- Peritoneal dialysis (10%)
- Kidney transplantation (30%)

**6. How long do dialysis patients survive?**

The death rate among dialysis patients in the United States is approximately 23% per year. A 45-year-old dialysis patient has a life expectancy of about 7 years compared with 35 years for someone from the general population. This marked difference may be because of comorbid conditions, failure of dialysis to completely replace normal kidney function, or adverse effects of dialysis treatment.

**7. List the factors that influence mortality in dialysis patients.**

Demographic factors associated with increased mortality include advanced age, white race, male gender, and low socioeconomic status. Medical factors associated with increased mortality include diabetes mellitus as a cause of renal failure, other comorbid conditions such as cardiovascular disease, and poor nutritional status. A treatment factor associated with increased mortality is inadequate dose of dialysis (see Chapter 47, Hemodialysis: Assessing Adequacy).

**8. What are the common causes of death in patients with ESRD?**

The most common causes of death are **cardiovascular disease** and **infection**. Withdrawal of dialysis also is a common cause of death, especially among elderly patients. Dialysis most often is withdrawn when new medical complications occur or when patients simply become so tired of treatment that death is preferable to ongoing dialysis.

**9. How much does it cost to treat dialysis patients?**

Because of congressional legislation, virtually all patients with ESRD in the United States are eligible for Medicare coverage. Total annual Medicare costs for ESRD are about $15 billion. Outpatient and inpatient Medicare costs per dialysis patient are approximately $50,000 per year. This amount includes care for dialysis-related conditions as well as for other medical conditions.

### BIBLIOGRAPHY

1. Daugirdas JT, Blake PG, Ing TS: Handbook of Dialysis. Philadelphia, Lippincott Williams & Wilkins, 2001.
2. Greenberg A (ed): Primer on Kidney Diseases, 3rd ed. San Diego, Academic Press, 2001.
3. Ifudu O: Care of patients undergoing hemodialysis. N Engl J Med 339:1054–1062, 1998.
4. U.S. Renal Data Systems: USRDS 2000 Annual Data Report. Bethesda, MD, National Institutes of Health, 2000.

# 41. RENAL OSTEODYSTROPHY

*Lavinia A. Negrea, M.D.*

### 1. What is renal osteodystrophy?
Renal osteodystrophy refers to several bone diseases that occur as a complication of chronic renal insufficiency. In many cases, two or more of these disease processes occur simultaneously.

### 2. How are renal bone diseases classified?
- High-turnover bone disease (due to persistently high levels of parathyroid hormone [PTH])
- Low-turnover bone disease (generally associated with relatively low levels of PTH)

### 3. Name the factors contributing to sustained increases in PTH secretion, parathyroid hyperplasia, and ultimately high-turnover bone disease.
The factors responsible for secondary hyperparathyroidism associated with renal failure are hyperphosphatemia due to diminished renal phosphorus excretion, hypocalcemia, impaired renal production of active 1,25-dihydroxyvitamin D, alterations in the control of PTH gene transcription, and skeletal resistance to the calcemic action of PTH.

### 4. Describe the bone lesion associated with hyperparathyroidism and high-turnover.
The clinical symptoms of **osteitis fibrosa cystica** include nonspecific bone pain and proximal myopathy. The serum-intact PTH level is usually above 250–300 pg/ml. Radiologic features are subperiosteal erosions of the phalanges and erosions at the proximal end of the tibia, the neck of the femur or humerus, and the inferior surface of the distal end of the clavicle. The skull has a mottled and granular salt-and-pepper appearance. The histologic features include increased numbers of osteoclasts and osteoblasts, increased amounts of woven osteoid, and peritrabecular fibrosis.

### 5. How is osteitis fibrosa cystica treated?
Treatment of this disorder entails prevention and correction of the factors leading to secondary hyperparathyroidism. This includes phosphorus control (dietary restriction, phosphate binders, dialysis), calcium control (oral supplements, dialysis, vitamin D), and suppression of PTH by vitamin D administration. Parathyroidectomy might be required eventually.

### 6. What bone lesions are classified as low-turnover bone disease?
- Osteomalacia
- Adynamic or aplastic bone disease

### 7. What causes osteomalacia and how does it manifest in dialysis patients?
The most common cause of osteomalacia in patients on dialysis in the United States is aluminum intoxication. Abnormalities of vitamin D metabolism and metabolic acidosis may contribute to the development of osteomalacia. Aluminum-associated osteomalacia presents with severe bone pain and increased incidence of fractures. Serum PTH is, in general, normal or low, and hypercalcemia is common. Looser zones or pseudofractures are radiologic characteristics. Osteomalacia is characterized by excess osteoid (unmineralized bone

collagen), due to impaired mineralization. Deposits of aluminum can be seen in aluminum-related osteomalacia along trabecular bone surfaces using histochemical staining.

### 8. What are the main risk factors for aluminum toxicity?

Aluminum ingested with the diet undergoes renal excretion. As renal function deteriorates, aluminum excretion decreases, resulting in an increased total aluminum body burden. Diabetes mellitus, prior parathyroidectomy, failed renal transplant, and consumption of aluminum-based phosphate binders over long periods of time are considered the main risks for aluminum toxicity. Citrate markedly enhances intestinal aluminum absorption. Therefore, concomitant use of citrate-containing medications (calcium citrate, Shohl's solution) along with aluminum-containing medications (Amphojel, Carafate) can lead to aluminum accumulation.

### 9. What are the ABCs of aluminum toxicity?

- **M**icrocytic **a**nemia
- **B**one disease
- **C**entral nervous system abnormalities (dialysis encephalopathy)

### 10. What strategies are used to treat aluminum bone disease?

Discontinue all aluminum-based medications and ensure that the dialysis water has a minimal amount of or no aluminum. For symptomatic patients, deferoxamine administered in dialysis will be necessary.

### 11. What is adynamic bone disease?

An adynamic bone lesion is associated with nonspecific bone pain and increased incidence of fractures. Low levels of PTH (< 100 pg/ml) and hypercalcemia are common features. On histology, there is normal or decreased osteoid volume and decreased mineralization.

### 12. What are the risk factors for adynamic bone disease?

Peritoneal dialysis
Diabetes mellitus
Advanced age
Vitamin D therapy

### 13. How is adynamic bone disease treated?

Avoid oversuppression of PTH by limiting the use of vitamin D therapy, and discontinue all aluminum sources. PTH stimulation is actually desired by inducing hypocalcemia during dialysis with low calcium dialysate.

### 14. What is mixed renal osteodystrophy?

Mixed renal osteodystrophy entails histologic findings of both osteitis fibrosa cystica and osteomalacia on bone biopsy. It may be seen in patients with established osteitis fibrosa who are developing aluminum-related bone disease.

### 15. What is calciphylaxis?

Calciphylaxis is a syndrome characterized by skin necrosis that is attributed to medial calcifications of the small and medium-sized arteries. It usually occurs in the setting of uncontrolled hyperparathyroidism. It manifests as painful violaceous lesions with *peau d'orange* appearance that progress to superficial ulceration and necrosis. It is usually symmetric and may involve the trunk and extremities. The lesions have a tendency to become infected. In general, calciphylaxis carries a very poor prognosis.

### 16. What is dialysis-related amyloidosis?

Dialysis-related amyloidosis refers to the clinical manifestations that result from the deposition of a unique, amyloid fibril protein derived from $beta_2$-microglobulin in bony structures and synovial tissue of patients who have been on dialysis for long periods of time (generally > 7 years). Radiographically, bone cysts occur at the end of long bones, particularly the femoral head and proximal humerus. Metacarpal, carpal, and tarsal bones also may be involved. Multiple bone cysts suggest amyloid, whereas brown tumors of osteitis fibrosa are isolated, usually in the rib or jaw.

### 17. Name the most common clinical manifestations of dialysis-related amyloidosis.

Carpal tunnel syndrome is the most frequent clinical feature. Scapulohumeral involvement is common and is manifested as shoulder pain. Characteristically, pain is worse at night or at rest and improves with motion. Other affected sites are metacarpophalangeal and interphalangeal joints, shoulders, wrists, and knees. The cervical spine is the most common site of destructive spondyloarthropathy. Bone cysts from amyloid deposition also occur, especially in long bones, and can be associated with pathologic features.

### 18. What bone lesion is typical after kidney transplantation?

Osteopenia is common following renal transplantation, with evidence of reduced bone mass found in some patients as early as 6 months after transplantation and in nearly all patients within 5 years. The use of corticosteroids for immunosuppression is considered to be the major contributor.

BIBLIOGRAPHY

1. Danesh F, Ho LT: Dialysis-related amyloidosis: History and clinical manifestations. Semin Dial 14:80–85, 2001.
2. Goodman WG, Coburn JW, Slatopolsky E, Salusky IB: Renal osteodystrophy in adults and children. In Favus MJ (ed): Primer on the Metabolic Bone Diseases and D Disorders of Mineral Metabolism, 3rd ed. Philadelphia, Lippincott-Raven, 1996, pp 341–360.
3. Hruska KA, Teitelbaum SL: Renal osteodystrophy. N Engl J Med 333:166–174, 1995.
4. Salusky IB, Goodman WG: Adynamic renal osteodystrophy: Is there a problem? J Am Soc Nephrol 12:1978–1985, 2001.
5. Sprague SM, Moe SM: Clinical manifestations and pathogenesis of dialysis-related amyloidosis. Semin Dial 9:360–369, 1996.

# 42. UREMIC PERICARDITIS

*Marcia R. Silver, M.D.*

### 1. What is uremic pericarditis?

Uremic pericarditis is an inflammation of the pericardium occurring in patients with advanced acute or chronic renal failure. The condition generally is diagnosed by the presence of characteristic chest pain, a pericardial friction rub, typical electrocardiographic (ECG) changes, and sometimes fever, general malaise, and pericardial effusion. Uremia is probably the most common cause of pericarditis. In 1987, patients with end-stage renal disease (ESRD) were hospitalized for pericarditis at a rate 200 times that of the general population.

### 2. What is the difference between pericarditis and pericardial effusion?

**Pericarditis** is inflammation of the pericardium. **Pericardial effusion** refers to the presence of abnormal amounts of fluid in the pericardial space and may occur without signs or symptoms of inflammation. Up to 40% of stable dialysis patients studied with echocardiography have pericardial effusions, but most of these patients do not have signs or symptoms of pericarditis.

### 3. What is pericardial tamponade?

Pericardial tamponade refers to compression of the heart by the pericardium or its contents (fluid or blood) that impedes the inflow of blood into the right and left ventricles. Clinical signs suggesting tamponade include hypotension, tachycardia, jugular venous distention, and pulsus paradoxicus. The ECG may show decreased voltage and electrical alternans. Echocardiography demonstrates compromise of cardiac filling and the presence of a pericardial effusion. Cardiac catheterization usually shows equalization of pressures in the right and left heart chambers.

### 4. What is dialysis pericarditis and how does it differ from uremic pericarditis?

**Uremic pericarditis** usually occurs in patients not yet treated with dialysis and tends to resolve with dialytic therapy, suggesting that uremia per se is important in the pathophysiology. By contrast, **dialysis pericarditis** most often occurs in patients who have been on dialysis for some time. Although some cases may occur as a consequence of uremia resulting from inadequate dialysis, clusters of dialysis pericarditis suggest that this disorder may sometimes be caused by viral infection. Compared with classic uremic pericarditis, dialysis pericarditis is more often hemorrhagic in character and more often associated with large pericardial effusions and tamponade.

### 5. What clinical findings suggest uremic pericarditis?

Typically, the patient complains of chest pain that is worse in the supine position and that is relieved by sitting up and forward. On physical examination, a two- or three-component pericardial friction rub is characteristic; however, such rubs tend to wax and wane over time. As an effusion increases in size, the rub may disappear because a fluid cushion develops between the walls of the pericardial sac. Precipitous hypotension may be the first sign of pericarditis, usually indicating the presence of tamponade. The ECG typically reveals widespread ST segment elevations.

The above findings are not *specific* for uremic pericarditis, however. Other causes of pericarditis must be considered, including trauma, aortic dissection, infections (viral, bacterial, mycobacterial), malignancies, and myocardial infarction (Dressler's syndrome). Ultimately, the diagnosis of uremic pericarditis is a diagnosis of exclusion.

### 6. How common is uremic pericarditis?

Older reports suggest a cumulative incidence of 5–40% in patients with chronic renal failure. However, such data were generated in an era when dialysis was often postponed until patients were severely uremic and when less attention was paid to parameters of dialysis adequacy. In addition, variations in the reported incidence reflect differences in the definition of the disorder—some older studies included all patients with pericardial effusions, even in the absence of other clinical signs and symptoms of pericardial inflammation. Dialysis pericarditis is less common among peritoneal dialysis patients than among hemodialysis patients, and the incidence in all dialysis patients seems to be decreasing.

### 7. What is the treatment for uremic pericarditis?

Whereas patients with pericardial tamponade clearly require urgent therapy that may include either pericardiocentesis or surgery for creation of a "pericardial window," the management of patients with uremic or dialysis pericarditis in the absence of tamponade is less certain. Uremic pericarditis is treated promptly with dialytic therapy performed on a daily basis until there is clear resolution of pericarditis. Heparin use is kept to a minimum in order to minimize the risk of bleeding into the pericardial space. Dialysis pericarditis is treated similarly, with institution of daily dialysis without heparin and with careful examination of all aspects of the dialysis procedure to reveal any problems leading to underdialysis. Volume removal should be attempted if there is evidence of fluid overload. Improvement is usually seen in 1–2 weeks. If there is no evidence of underdialysis, and other causes have been excluded, a viral etiology may be presumed and the dialysis schedule may not need to be altered. Persistent chest pain may be treated with nonsteroidal anti-inflammatory drugs, although these agents may increase the risk of pericardial hemorrhage and should be used cautiously. Patients with slowly evolving tamponade physiology or persistent, large pericardial effusion despite weeks of daily dialysis may require either simple pericardiocentesis or a few days of continuous catheter drainage with instillation of nonabsorbable steroids into the pericardial space. Rarely, pericardial window or even pericardiectomy may be required.

### 8. What is the prognosis of patients with uremic or dialysis-related pericarditis?

In the setting of acute renal failure, complete resolution of pericarditis is the rule in patients who recover from the underlying renal failure. Mortality rates of up to 5% have been reported in patients with dialysis-associated pericarditis. However, data from serial reports of the United States Renal Data System suggest that mortality rates from this complication of ESRD have decreased with time (see table).

*Death Rates (from Pericarditis) per 1000 Patient Years*

| TIME PERIOD | DEATH RATE |
|---|---|
| 1987–1989 | 1.6 |
| 1988–1990 | 1.4 |
| 1989–1991 | 1.0 |
| 1991–1993 | < 1 |
| 1994–1996 | 0.3 |

## BIBLIOGRAPHY

1. Comty CM, Cohen SL, Shapiro FL: Pericarditis in chronic uremia and its sequels. Ann Intern Med 75:173–183, 1971.
2. DePace NL, Nestico PF, Schwartz AB, et al: Predicting success of intensive dialysis in the treatment of uremic pericarditis. Am J Med 76:38–46, 1984.
3. Gunukula SR, Spodick DH: Pericardial disease in renal patients. Semin Nephrol 21:52–56, 2001.
4. Silverberg S, Oreopoulos DG, Wise DJ, et al: Pericarditis in patients undergoing long-term hemodialysis and peritoneal dialysis. Am J Med 63:874–880, 1977.
5. Silver MR, Logue E, McCord G: Rates of pericarditis associated with various treatment modalities for end-stage renal disease [abstract]. J Am Soc Nephrol 3:394, 1992.
6. Wray TM, Stone WJ: Uremic pericarditis: A prospective echocardiographic and clinical study. Clin Nephrol 6:295–301, 1976.

# 43. ANEMIA ASSOCIATED WITH RENAL FAILURE

Jay B. Wish, M.D.

**1. What causes anemia in patients with renal disease?**

The anemia of chronic renal disease is caused primarily by deficiency of erythropoietin. The kidneys are the major source of erythropoietin, and, as renal function declines, production of erythropoietin declines proportionately. As a result, there tends to be a linear relationship between hematocrit and creatinine clearance in patients with renal insufficiency, although a wide range of hematocrit levels may be observed for any degree of renal disease.

A number of other factors tend to decrease red cell life span from the normal of 120 days to approximately 70–80 days in patients with chronic renal failure. These include red cell trauma due to microvascular disease from diabetes or hypertension, blood loss due to the hemodialysis procedure, an increased incidence of gastrointestinal bleeding due to peptic ulcer disease and angiodysplasia of the bowel, and increased oxidative stress leading to shortened red cell survival.

**2. How does one evaluate anemia in a patient with chronic renal disease?**

Erythropoietin deficiency is a diagnosis of exclusion, and determination of erythropoietin levels in patients with chronic renal disease is generally not indicated. The routine evaluation of such patients should include measurement of red blood cell indices, reticulocyte count, transferrin saturation, and serum ferritin and a test for occult blood in the stool. If these tests reveal no easily correctable cause of anemia, such as gastrointestinal bleeding or iron deficiency, it can be presumed that the anemia is due primarily to erythropoietin deficiency.

**3. How are the tests of iron status in patients with chronic renal disease interpreted?**

The two most commonly used tests of iron status are transferrin saturation and serum ferritin. **Transferrin saturation** is computed by dividing the serum iron level by the total iron-binding capacity. The total iron-binding capacity correlates with circulating transferrin, which is the major iron-binding protein in plasma. Transferrin saturation correlates with the amount of iron available for erythropoiesis because only circulating iron is available to the bone marrow for incorporation into newly synthesized red blood cells. The **serum ferritin** level correlates with storage iron located primarily in the reticuloendothelial system. Interpretation of serum ferritin levels is confounded by the fact that ferritin will rise as an acute phase reactant in the setting of acute or chronic inflammation. In patients with chronic renal disease, a serum ferritin level less than 100 ng/ml correlates with a deficiency in storage iron; such patients will almost invariably respond to supplemental iron therapy. Patients with a transferrin saturation of less than 20% have decreased iron delivery to the erythroid marrow, but supplemental iron may or may not correct this problem, depending on whether storage iron can effectively be released to the transferrin carrier protein.

A newer test, **reticulocyte hemoglobin content** (cHr), measures the amount of hemoglobin in the youngest red blood cells and is a useful marker of current iron availability to the bone marrow. The cHr test is available on some hematology analyzers that perform complete blood counts. A cHr value of < 29 pg correlates with functional iron deficiency.

**4. What is functional iron deficiency?**

Functional iron deficiency is a phenomenon that occurs in patients treated with pharmacologic doses of erythropoietin when the bone marrow is stimulated to produce red blood cells faster than the transferrin carrier protein can deliver adequate iron substrate. In such patients, the transferrin saturation tends to be low or low-normal, while the serum ferritin level may be normal or even high. The operative definition of functional iron deficiency is based on a response to intravenous iron supplementation characterized by either an increase in hematocrit or a decrease in erythropoietin requirements to achieve the same hematocrit. Studies have demonstrated that functional iron deficiency is common in patients with end-stage renal disease who are treated with erythropoietin and that intravenous iron supplementation will decrease erythropoietin requirements by approximately 30–35%. Because of the risk of fatal anaphylactic reactions, iron dextran has fallen out of favor as an intravenous iron supplement and has been replaced by sodium ferric gluconate and iron sucrose.

### 5. Why are oral iron supplements often ineffective in treating the iron deficiency in patients on chronic hemodialysis?

Oral iron absorption tends to be inversely proportional to serum ferritin levels. In patients with a serum ferritin of 100 ng/ml or higher, oral iron absorption is approximately 1–2% of the administered load. A patient taking ferrous sulfate, 325 mg three times daily, will consume 200 mg of elemental iron, of which 2–4 mg will be absorbed daily. The iron requirements in anemic patients undergoing hemodialysis are often enormous. Increasing the hematocrit from 25% to 35% in a 70-kg patient requires the incorporation of 600 mg of elemental iron into the newly synthesized red blood cells. In addition, the estimated daily iron losses in hemodialysis patients are approximately 4–7 mg. Thus, the 2–4 mg of oral iron absorbed daily would barely keep pace with ongoing iron losses let alone repair the accumulated iron deficit. Compounding this problem is the phenomenon of functional iron deficiency, which often results in the need for high levels of storage iron to facilitate release of iron to transferrin and delivery of that iron to the erythroid marrow. As a result, most hemodialysis patients receiving erythropoietin require intravenous iron supplements.

### 6. How is erythropoietin administered?

Human recombinant erythropoietin is a polypeptide hormone that, like insulin, must be given parenterally through a subcutaneous or intravenous route. A number of studies have demonstrated that subcutaneously administered erythropoietin, because of its slower absorption and longer half-life, is more effective than a comparable dose administered intravenously. Several studies have demonstrated a 30–35% reduction in the erythropoietin dose required to achieve the same hematocrit when patients are switched from the intravenous to the subcutaneous route of administration.

For patients receiving erythropoietin intravenously on hemodialysis, the recommended starting dose is 50 U/kg of body weight three times weekly, with the dose titrated at monthly intervals depending on the hematocrit response. For patients receiving erythropoietin therapy subcutaneously, the recommended starting dose is 30 U/kg administered three times weekly (as is typically done in hemodialysis facilities) or 50 U/kg administered twice weekly (which is typical for predialysis and peritoneal dialysis patients). Again, the dose would be titrated at monthly intervals depending on the hematocrit response. **Darbepoetin alfa**, an analogue of human erythropoietin with two extra carbohydrate side-chains, has a longer duration of action when compared with both native and recombinant hormone. The recommended starting dose for darbepoetin alfa is 0.45 µg/kg once weekly for both intravenous and subcutaneous administration, with subsequent titration based on the hemoglobin concentration.

### 7. What is the target hematocrit or hemoglobin for patients receiving erythropoietin therapy?

The practice guidelines prepared by the National Kidney Foundation's Dialysis Outcomes Quality Initiative (DOQI) recommend a target hematocrit of 33–36% or a target hemoglobin of 11–12 gm/dl. This is supported by a number of studies that demonstrate that this hematocrit and hemoglobin level is associated with improved functional and cognitive status, improved quality of life, regression of left ventricular hypertrophy, and decreased morbidity and mortality when compared with patients with chronic renal failure and lower hematocrit and hemoglobin levels. Whether patients with chronic renal failure would benefit from having hematocrit and hemoglobin levels closer to those of the normal population remains a subject of some controversy. As of 1999, medical justification is required for reimbursement from Medicare or Medicaid for erythropoietin administered to patients with a 3-month rolling average hematocrit greater than 37.5.

## BIBLIOGRAPHY

1. Fishbane S, Frei GL, Maesaka J: Reduction in recombinant human erythropoietin doses by the use of chronic intravenous iron supplementation. Am J Kidney Dis 26:41–46, 1995.
2. Foley RN, Parfrey PS, Harnett JD, et al: The impact of anemia on cardiomyopathy, morbidity, and mortality in end-stage renal disease. Am J Kidney Dis 28:53–61, 1996.
3. Macdougall IC, Gray SJ, Elston O, et al: Pharmacokinetics of novel erythropoiesis-stimulating protein compared with epoetin alfa in dialysis patients. J Am Soc Nephrol 10:2392–2395, 1999.
4. Mittman N, Sreedhara R, Mushnick R, et al: Reticulocyte hemoglobin content predicts functional iron deficiency in hemodialysis patients receiving rHuEPO. Am J Kidney Dis 30:912–922, 1997.
5. National Kidney Foundation: DOQI clinical practice guidelines for anemia of chronic kidney disease, 2000. Am J Kidney Dis 37(suppl 1):S182–S238, 2001.
6. Wingard RL, Parker RA, Ismail N, Hakim RM: Efficacy of oral iron therapy in patients receiving recombinant human erythropoietin. Am J Kidney Dis 25:433–439, 1995.

# 44. OTHER MANIFESTATIONS OF UREMIA

*Donald E. Hricik, M.D.*

### 1. What is the cause of and treatment for uremic pruritus?

The cause is unknown. Some, but certainly not all, cases are associated with secondary hyperparathyroidism or a high calcium $\times$ phosphorus product and respond to appropriate measures (see Chapter 41, Renal Osteodystrophy). Itching often persists despite otherwise adequate dialysis. Antihistamines constitute the mainstay of therapy. In severe cases, ultraviolet phototherapy can be helpful.

### 2. What are the neurologic effects of uremia?

| *Central nervous system* | *Peripheral nervous system* |
|---|---|
| Lethargy | Symmetric sensorimotor polyneuropathy |
| Irritability | Restless legs syndrome |
| Alterations in memory | |
| Coma (severe cases) | |
| Seizures (rare) | |
| Myoclonus or asterixis | |

### 3. How does uremia affect sexual function?

In men, erectile dysfunction and decreased libido are common and related, in part, to hypogonadism and low testosterone levels. Women may exhibit signs and symptoms of hyperprolactinemia but generally show signs of hypogonadism manifested either by dysfunctional uterine bleeding or amenorrhea. Fertility is not always impaired, but term pregnancy is rare in women with end-stage renal disease (see Chapter 21). Spontaneous abortion is the rule in women who become pregnant. Fertility can be fully restored after successful kidney transplantation.

### 4. What is the nature of the bleeding diathesis in patients with uremia?

Uremic patients commonly exhibit platelet dysfunction best assessed by measurement of a bleeding time. At best, only a crude correlation exists between the degree of azotemia and the degree of platelet dysfunction.

### 5. What is the clinical significance of uremic platelet dysfunction?

Spontaneous or surgically induced bleeding is common in patients with uremia. In the absence of risk factors such as heart failure, obesity, and immobilization, thromboembolic events are less common in patients with renal failure than in the general population.

### 6. What pharmacologic agents have been used to prevent or treat uremic bleeding?

1. Desmopressin (DDAVP)
2. Cryoprecipitate
3. Conjugated estrogens (particularly for chronic gastrointestinal bleeding)

### 7. What is uremic serositis?

Akin to uremic pericarditis (see Chapter 42), uremia can be associated with inflammation of other serous membranes leading, for example, to noninfectious pleuritis or peritonitis. In addition, uremia has been named as an occasional cause of gastritis, enteritis, and even pancreatitis.

### 8. What is uremic cardiomyopathy?

It remains unclear whether uremia per se can suppress myocardial function. However, successful renal transplantation is sometimes associated with improved myocardial performance in patients previously deemed to have heart failure, suggesting that uremic cardiomyopathy probably occurs in some patients.

### 9. How does uremia affect glucose tolerance?

Most nondiabetic patients with uremia exhibit mild glucose intolerance that is rarely of clinical significance. Because the kidney is involved in the metabolism of insulin, patients with type 2 diabetes mellitus often exhibit reduced insulin requirements as renal failure progresses to end stage. A poorly understood syndrome of spontaneous hypoglycemia has been observed in some dialysis patients. It appears to be associated with defects in gluconeogenesis and generally is associated with a poor prognosis.

### 10. Name some other metabolic abnormalities associated with uremia.

Hypertriglyceridemia is common and related both to overproduction and decreased clearance of very low density lipoproteins. Recent studies suggest that advanced glycation end products accumulate in patients with renal failure, even in the absence of diabetes. The mechanism is unclear, but these compounds may contribute to cardiovascular disease. Abnormal glycation of beta$_2$-microglobulin is now known to cause a secondary form of amyloidosis associated with arthropathy in dialysis patients.

### 11. How does uremia influence immune function?

Inadequate production of antibodies, enhanced susceptibility to infection, and an increased incidence of certain cancers all suggest that uremia is associated with immune deficiency. Responsible factors may include iron overload, lack of circulating opsonins, and accumulation of various substances with known immune suppressant effects (e.g., indoles, phenols, parathyroid hormone). Although the number of circulating white blood cells is not altered in uremia, the function of white cells (e.g., response to chemotoxins, phagocytic function) is abnormal.

BIBLIOGRAPHY

1. Bagdade JD, Porte D, Bierman EL: Hypertriglyceridemia: A metabolic consequence of chronic renal failure. N Engl J Med 279:181–186, 1968.
2. DeFronzo RA, Alvestrand A: Glucose intolerance in uremia: Site and mechanisms. Am J Clin Nutr 33:1438–1444, 1980.
3. Lim VS, Henriquez C, Sievertsen G, et al: Ovarian function in chronic renal failure: Evidence suggesting hypothalamic anovulation. Ann Intern Med 93:21–27, 1980.
4. Manucci PM, Remuzzi G, Pusineri F, et al: Deamino-8-D-arginine vasopressin shortens the bleeding time in uremia. N Engl J Med 308:8–12, 1983.
5. Miyata T, Wada Y, Jida Y, et al: Implications of an increased oxidative stress in the formation of advanced glycation end products in patients with end-stage renal failure. Kidney Int 51:1170–1181, 1997.
6. Procci SR, Goldstein DA, Adelstein J, et al: Sexual dysfunction in the male patient with uremia: A reappraisal. Kidney Int 19:317–323, 1981.
7. Shemin D, Elnour M, Amarantes B, et al: Oral estrogens decrease bleeding time and improve clinical bleeding in patients with renal failure. Am J Med 89:436–440, 1990.
8. Vanholder R, Ringoir S: Infectious morbidity and defects of phagocytic function in end-stage renal disease: A review. J Am Soc Nephrol 3:1541–1554, 1993.

# VII. Renal Failure: Management

## 45. MANAGEMENT OF PATIENTS WITH PROGRESSIVE RENAL FAILURE

Jay B. Wish, M.D.

### 1. What is chronic kidney disease and how is it classified?

Chronic kidney disease (CKD) includes conditions that affect the kidney for ≥ 3 months with the potential to cause either progressive loss of kidney function or complications resulting from decreased kidney function. CKD may be present with or without a decrease in glomerular filtration rate (GFR) and is manifested either by pathologic abnormalities of the kidney or by markers of kidney damage, such as abnormalities in the composition of the blood or urine and abnormalities in imaging tests. CKD also includes all patients with GFR < 60 ml/min/1.73 m$^2$ for 3 months, with or without kidney damage. The National Kidney Foundation (NKF) Kidney Disease Outcomes Quality Initiative (K/DOQI) Clinical Practice Guidelines for CKD Evaluation, Classification, and Stratification divides CKD into five stages:

| STAGE | DESCRIPTION | GFR (ml/min/1.73 m$^2$) | ACTION |
|---|---|---|---|
| 0 | At increased risk | > 90 (with CKD risk factors) | Screening, CKD risk reduction |
| 1 | Kidney damage with normal or increased GFR | ≥ 90 | Diagnosis and treatment, treatment of comorbid conditions, slowing progression, cardiovascular risk reduction |
| 2 | Kidney damage with mildly decreased GFR | 60–90 | Estimating progression |
| 3 | Moderately decreased GFR | 30–59 | Evaluating and treating complications |
| 4 | Severely decreased GFR | 15–29 | Preparation for renal replacement therapy (dialysis or transplantation) |
| 5 | Kidney failure | < 15 (or dialysis) | Replacement (if uremia present) |

GFR = glomerular filtration rate; CKD = chronic kidney disease.

### 2. What are the major causes of chronic kidney disease in the United States?

*Major Causes of CKD in the United States\**

| CAUSE | INCIDENCE |
|---|---|
| Diabetes mellitus Type 1 (7%) Type 2 (37%) | 44% |

*Table continued on next page*

*Major Causes of CKD in the United States\* (continued)*

| CAUSE | INCIDENCE |
|---|---|
| Hypertension and large-vessel disease | 27% |
| Glomerulonephritis | 10% |
| Interstitial nephritis | 4% |
| Cystic and hereditary/congenital diseases | 3% |
| Systemic diseases (e.g., lupus and vasculitis) | 2% |
| Neoplasms | 2% |
| Miscellaneous conditions | 4% |
| Uncertain etiology | 4% |

*Based on data gathered from incident dialysis patients from 1995 to 1999.

### 3. What are the actions necessary for the evaluation and management of CKD, regardless of the diagnosis?

The approach to the patient with CKD requires that the clinician understand the separate but related concepts of diagnosis, comorbid conditions, severity of disease, and risks for loss of kidney function and cardiovascular disease. Patients with CKD should be evaluated to determine the etiology of the kidney disease so that specific therapy can be applied, if available. Comorbid conditions can be classified into those that cause the kidney disease (e.g., diabetes and hypertension), those that cause cardiovascular disease (which is highly associated with CKD and the major cause of death in these patients), and those that are unrelated to the CKD (therapy of which will often improve patient well-being and can be integrated into the management of the CKD). Treatment and prevention of cardiovascular disease in patients with CKD include risk factor reduction (e.g., control of blood pressure exercise, smoking cessation, treatment of hyperlipidemia) as well as specific therapies for the cardiovascular manifestations; both should begin as early as possible. It has been demonstrated that dialysis patients in their 20s have the same risk of death from cardiovascular disease as patients without CKD in their 80s.

Assessment of the severity of CKD should be done periodically with calculation of GFR from validated formulas that do not require 24-hour urine collections, which are notoriously inaccurate. Once the severity of the CKD is established, complications such as anemia, malnutrition, and bone disease, which tend to correlate with the degree of renal insufficiency, can be anticipated and addressed. Many drugs require dosage modifications that are based on the level of residual renal function. The risk and rate of loss of kidney function is determined by the diagnosis and by modifiable and nonmodifiable factors. The rate of decline in GFR should be assessed to predict the interval until the onset of kidney failure and to assess the effect of interventions. Interventions to slow the rate of decline in GFR should be considered in all patients with CKD and include treatment of the underlying disease (e.g., strict glucose control in diabetics), strict blood pressure control, the use of angiotensin-converting enzyme (ACE) inhibitors or angiotensin-2 receptor blockers (ARBs), and the avoidance of insults to the kidneys, such as volume depletion or administration of radiocontrast agents, nonsteroidal anti-inflammatory agents (including cyclooxygenase 2 [COX-2] inhibitors), and other nephrotoxic agents (e.g., aminoglycoside antibiotics).

### 4. What is the relationship between blood pressure control and the progression of kidney disease?

High blood pressure is both a cause and a complication of kidney disease. High blood pressure is associated with adverse outcomes including more rapid loss of kidney function and cardiovascular disease, so blood pressure should be monitored closely and treated aggressively in patients with CKD. The Modification of Diet in Renal Disease study demonstrated that CKD patients with proteinuria > 1 gm/day had a slower rate of renal disease progression with a target blood pressure of 125/75 compared with the conventional target of 140/90. Because of the close correlation among blood pressure control, CKD progression, and cardiovascular risk, many authors recommend a target blood pressure of 130/80 in CKD patients with < 1 gm/day proteinuria and a target blood pressure of 125/75 in patients with > 1 gm/day proteinuria.

Blood pressure control should be achieved through nonpharmacologic and pharmacologic approaches. Nonpharmacologic approaches include dietary sodium restriction, weight loss in the obese, and a regular exercise program. A number of studies have demonstrated that ACE inhibitors and ARBs are superior to other classes of antihypertensive agents in slowing the rate of progression in patients with CKD, especially those with diabetic nephropathy. Recent data suggest that these agents are beneficial even in the absence of hypertension. Because ACE inhibitors and ARBs can produce an acute decline in renal function by decreasing glomerular hydrostatic pressure (which is the mechanism by which they preserve renal function over the long term), renal function should be monitored frequently, especially in patients also receiving diuretics. Many nephrologists will accept a slight initial increase in serum creatinine as a result of ACE inhibitor or ARB therapy as a trade-off for their long-term renal protective effect. Serum potassium levels also should be monitored closely in CKD patients receiving ACE inhibitors or ARBs, and hyperkalemia or a severe acute decline in renal function may necessitate decreasing the dose or discontinuing these agents. Other classes of antihypertensive agents, including calcium channel blockers, central and peripheral adrenergic blockers, vasodilators, and diuretics, can be used in combination with ACE inhibitors and ARBs (or without ACE inhibitors or ARBs if they are contraindicated) to bring the blood pressure of the CKD patient to the target level, because the success of blood pressure control has a greater impact on outcomes than the class(es) of agents used. Some studies have suggested that dihydropyridine calcium channel blockers should not be used in patients with CKD unless they are also receiving an ACE inhibitor or ARB, because these calcium channel blockers have been shown to increase proteinuria when used as monotherapy.

### 5. When should a patient with CKD be referred to a nephrologist?

The Institute of Medicine has recommended that female patients with CKD be referred to a nephrologist for initial consultation when their serum creatinine is 1.5 mg/dl and male patients be referred when their serum creatinine is 2.0 mg/dl. Unfortunately, this practice is not widely employed; the United States Renal Data System reported that 39% of patients with CKD were not referred to a nephrologist until ≤ 3 months before initiation of dialysis. Late nephrology referral is associated with increased morbidity (longer and more expensive hospitalization) at the time of and 6 months following dialysis initiation, increased use of hemodialysis over peritoneal dialysis, increased use of temporary vascular access, poorer nutritional status, and poorer patient rehabilitation. A partnership between the primary care physician (PCP) and nephrologist should be established so that the PCP continues to provide day-to-day patient management, and the nephrologist makes recommendations regarding care strategies to slow renal disease progression, address comorbid conditions and systemic complications, and ultimately prepare the patient for renal replacement therapy (dialysis or transplantation). It is expected that the nephrologist will assume significantly more responsibility when the creatinine clearance falls below 30 ml/min/1.73 $m^2$, at which time the patient is likely to demonstrate more of the systemic complications of CKD (anemia, bone disease, nutritional abnormalities) and will need to start considering renal replacement therapy modality options and undergoing placement of vascular access if hemodialysis is preferred.

## 6. What is the role of dietary protein restriction in patients with CKD?

Although a number of animal models and small studies have suggested that dietary protein restriction (< 0.8 gm/kg/day) slows the progression of CKD, the largest prospective, randomized study to address this issue, the Modification of Diet in Renal Disease, failed to demonstrate a significant impact of moderate or severe (with ketoacid supplements) dietary protein restriction in patients with various levels of renal dysfunction caused by a variety of renal diseases. On the other hand, because uremia may produce anorexia and a distaste for meats, malnutrition in patients approaching dialysis is a common problem, and mortality during the first year on dialysis is highly correlated with the serum albumin level at the time of dialysis initiation. There remain many proponents of dietary protein restriction in patients with CKD who cite the fact that a meta-analysis of 13 studies of dietary protein restriction involving 1919 patients found that a low-protein diet reduced the rate of GFR decline by 0.53 ml/min/year and the fact that a low-protein diet may delay the need for dialysis because many uremic signs and symptoms are thought to be related to the accumulation of nitrogenous waste products of dietary protein catabolism. Opponents of dietary protein restriction note that the higher cost, inconvenience, and nonpalatability of low-protein diets may hinder patient adherence and promote risk of protein malnutrition if the diet is not closely supervised by a renal dietitian. The compromise position is not to recommend dietary protein restriction but to recommend against dietary protein excess, with a daily protein intake of 0.8–1.0 gm/kg under the supervision of a renal dietitian.

## 7. When and how is anemia treated in patients with CKD?

Because erythropoietin (EPO), which stimulates the bone marrow to make red blood cells, is made primarily in the kidneys, erythropoietin and red blood cell production inevitably decline as renal function worsens. However, there is a tremendous variability in the level of anemia in patients with a given level of renal dysfunction, with some patients developing anemia early and some patients developing anemia late in the course of their CKD. Once anemia (hemoglobin < 12 gm/dl) develops, the patient should be evaluated with red blood cell indices (the anemia of CKD is normochromic, normocytic), iron studies (serum ferritin and transferrin saturation), reticulocyte count, and a test for occult blood in the stool to rule out causes of anemia other than CKD EPO deficiency. The treatment of choice for anemia due to EPO deficiency is, obviously, EPO replacement. Unfortunately, EPO replacement is expensive, and many insurers will not pay for it until the patient's hemoglobin is < 10 gm/dl. Medicare will pay for EPO only if the patient receives the injection in a health care facility. As a result of the inconvenience of self-injection or the necessity of a trip to a health care facility, most CKD patients who receive recombinant human EPO injections do so subcutaneously once per week, as opposed to the three times per week frequency of intravenous EPO injections for hemodialysis patients. Recent data suggest that recombinant human EPO can be effective when given every 2 weeks in some patients with CKD. Darbepoetin alfa, a synthetic analog of EPO, has two extra carbohydrate side chains, which give it a longer duration of action. Studies with darbepoetin alfa in patients with CKD suggest that it is effective when given every 2–4 weeks. Iron studies should be monitored periodically in all patients with CKD, especially if they are receiving an EPO product, because they may consume all their available iron stores in the synthesis of new red blood cells, develop functional iron deficiency, or develop absolute iron deficiency due to poor dietary intake or losses from uremic platelet dysfunction. Oral iron supplements should be administered routinely in patients receiving EPO products. If iron deficiency persists despite oral supplements of 200 mg of elemental iron per day, intravenous iron therapy should be considered.

The treatment of anemia in patients with CKD is important because it improves quality of life (exercise capacity, cognitive function) and because it is associated with a lower incidence and regression of left ventricular hypertrophy, which is a significant risk factor for subsequent cardiovascular morbidity and mortality.

## 8. How and when should patients with CKD be prepared for renal replacement therapy?

Preparation for hemodialysis takes time, both in terms of the patient's acceptance of its inevitability and in terms of placing a permanent vascular access that is ready to use when the patient needs dialysis. When the patient's GFR is < 30 ml/min/1.73 m$^2$, it is time to discuss with the patient and those close to the patient the fact that renal replacement therapy will be required in the future and that the patient needs to prepare for this by learning about the modalities available (hemodialysis, peritoneal dialysis, and transplant) and choosing the modality best suited to the patient's condition and lifestyle. Not all patients will be suited for all modalities, and the nephrologist should provide some guidance regarding the appropriateness of each modality for the patient. All patients who appear to be headed for hemodialysis should be instructed to "save" an upper extremity for permanent vascular access by refusing venipunctures and IVs in that arm. Even if a patient expresses a preference for peritoneal dialysis or transplant, it may be appropriate to instruct the patient to "save" an upper extremity anyway, because the patient may eventually require hemodialysis. The evaluation of a patient for transplantation may take many months, especially if living donors are involved. Therefore, even though the United Network for Organ Sharing does not allow patients to be placed on the waiting list for cadaveric transplants until the GFR is < 20 ml/min/1.73 m$^2$, the evaluation should be initiated when the GFR is around 30 ml/min/1.73 m$^2$, in anticipation of the lengthy evaluation process. If the patient chooses hemodialysis as the preferred modality, the patient should be referred for placement of permanent vascular access as soon as possible, because the patient may require vascular studies to assess the arterial and venous circulation and because arteriovenous fistulas, the preferred vascular access, may take 3–6 months to develop adequately to be used for hemodialysis. If the patient is not a candidate for an arteriovenous fistula, the surgeon may choose to wait until about 2 months before hemodialysis is anticipated to place an arteriovenous graft; grafts take about 3–4 weeks to develop but have a limited life span because of the development of myointimal hyperplasia at the venous anastomosis.

## 9. When should a patient with CKD be started on dialysis?

The decision to start a patient with CKD on dialysis is based on both the level of residual renal function and the effects of the renal dysfunction on the patient in terms of symptoms, degree of disability, nutritional status, and biochemical abnormalities. The most common uremic symptoms that prompt the initiation of dialysis are fluid overload, gastrointestinal symptoms (anorexia, nausea, vomiting), and neurologic symptoms (fatigue, sleep abnormalities, cognitive dysfunction). The more comorbid diseases a CKD patient has (especially diabetes and heart disease), the higher the GFR at which the patient is likely to develop symptoms. Some patients develop uremic symptoms at a GFR of 20 ml/min/1.73 m$^2$, but some do not develop uremic symptoms until the GFR is < 5 ml/min/1.73 m$^2$, so establishing a universal GFR "trigger" for dialysis is impossible. The mean ± standard deviation (SD) of GFR for incident dialysis patients in the United States in 2001 was 9.6 ± 7.6 ml/min/1.73 m$^2$. The NKF guideline cited in question 1 suggests that patients should be considered for dialysis when their GFR is < 15 ml/min/1.73 m$^2$, but this is a benchmark for clinical dialysis indications, not an indication on its own. Although a patient with a GFR in this range may not report symptoms, the symptoms of uremia can be insidious, may be attributed by the patient to another cause, or may be consciously or unconsciously withheld because the patient is not ready to start dialysis. In this setting, monitoring the serum albumin is important because it is a marker of the patient's nutritional status that may indicate anorexia that the patient does not report. Because the serum albumin at the time of dialysis initiation is directly associated with survival during the first year on dialysis, patients with advanced CKD and hypoalbuminemia should be considered for dialysis before the albumin level falls further, even if they are relatively asymptomatic.

BIBLIOGRAPHY

1. Kasiske BL, Lakatua JD, Ma JZ, et al: A meta-analysis of the effects of dietary protein restriction on the rate of decline of renal function. Am J Kidney Dis 31:954–961, 1998.
2. Levin A, Singer J, Thompson CR, et al: Prevalent left ventricular hypertrophy in the predialysis population: Identifying opportunities for intervention. Am J Kidney Dis 27:347–354, 1996.
3. Lewis EJ, Hunsicker LG, Clarke WR, et al: Renoprotective effect of the angiotensin-receptor antagonist irbesartan in patients with nephropathy due to type 2 diabetes. N Engl J Med 345: 851–860, 2001.
4. National Kidney Foundation: K/DOQI clinical practice guidelines for chronic kidney disease: Evaluation, classification, and stratification. Am J Kidney Dis 39(suppl 1):S1–S266, 2002.
5. National Kidney Foundation: K/DOQI clinical practice guidelines for nutrition in chronic renal failure. Am J Kidney Dis 35(suppl 2):S1–S140, 2000.
6. Obrador GT, Ruthazer R, Arora P, et al: Prevalence of and factors associated with suboptimal care before initiation of dialysis in the United States. J Am Soc Nephrol 10:1793–1800, 1999.
7. Periera BJ: Optimization of pre-ESRD care: The key to improved dialysis outcomes. Kidney Int 57:351–365, 2000.
8. Peterson JC, Adler S, Burkart JM, et al: Blood pressure control, proteinuria, and the progression of renal disease: The Modification of Diet in Renal Disease Study. Ann Intern Med 123:754–762, 1995.
9. Praga M: Slowing the progression of renal failure. Kidney Int 61(suppl 80):S18–S22, 2002.
10. Sarnak MJ, Levey AS: Cardiovascular disease and chronic renal disease: A new paradigm. Am J Kidney Dis 35(suppl 1):S117–S131, 2000.

# 46. TECHNICAL ASPECTS OF HEMODIALYSIS

*Jay B. Wish, M.D.*

### 1. What is the technical basis for dialysis?

*Dialysis* refers to the diffusion of small molecules down their concentration gradient across a semipermeable membrane. In hemodialysis, blood is withdrawn from the patient's body and passed by a membrane that separates the blood from a dialysate solution on the other side. The dialysate solution contains electrolytes and glucose. Small molecules such as urea, potassium, and phosphorus diffuse down their concentration gradients from the blood into the dialysate solution. In the dialysate solution, small molecules such as calcium and bicarbonate move down their concentration gradients from the dialysate solution into the blood. The effect is to remove low–molecular-weight toxins from the blood while increasing the plasma concentration of molecules that may be deficient in the patient with renal failure.

### 2. What are the two components of hemodialysis?

The process of hemodialysis consists of **diffusion** and **ultrafiltration**. Diffusion refers to the movement of small molecules down their concentration gradients. Urea is most commonly chosen as the marker for small-molecule diffusion during dialysis. Urea itself is not a uremic toxin, but its blood level and clearance by dialysis seem to correlate with that of other uremic toxins. Diffusive clearance of urea by hemodialysis is a function of three factors:

1. **Blood flow rate:** More urea diffusion will occur if more blood is exposed to the dialysis membrane per unit of time.

2. **Membrane surface area:** The larger the surface area of the membrane, the more urea diffusion can occur per unit of time.

3. **Time:** The longer the dialysis treatment, the more urea diffusion will occur.

Ultrafiltration refers to the removal of water from the patient's circulation during the dialysis treatment. In peritoneal dialysis, the movement of water from the patient's circulation into the dialysate is propelled by an osmotic radiant caused by the high concentration of glucose in the dialysate (see Chapter 50, Technical Aspects of Peritoneal Dialysis). In hemodialysis, the movement of water from the patient's circulation to the dialysate is propelled by a transmembrane hydrostatic pressure gradient. The blood compartment is under positive pressure because the blood is being pushed by a pump through the extracorporeal circuit. Dialysate is under negative pressure, because the dialysate fluid is being pulled by a pump through the circuit. The sum of the positive pressure in the blood compartment and the negative pressure in the dialysate compartment equals the transmembrane pressure. Removal of water during the dialysis treatment is a function of three factors:

1. The transmembrane hydrostatic pressure

2. The ultrafiltration coefficient of the dialysis membrane, which is a function of its surface area, composition, thickness, and porosity

3. The duration of the dialysis treatment

### 3. What is the composition of the dialysate solution used for hemodialysis?

The dialysate solution consists of sodium, chloride, bicarbonate, calcium, magnesium, potassium, and dextrose. The concentrations of sodium and chloride approximate those in plasma. Because the concentration of bicarbonate generally exceeds that of plasma in patients with renal failure, there is net diffusion of bicarbonate from the dialysate into the plasma. Concentration of magnesium in the dialysate is generally less than that of plasma, so removal of magnesium usually occurs during the dialysis treatment. Concentration of potassium in the dialysate is variable and can be adjusted depending on the patient's serum potassium level. Concentration of calcium in the dialysate is also variable, so net removal or delivery of calcium can occur during the dialysis, depending on the clinical indications. Concentration of glucose in dialysate is generally around 200 mg/dl, so net diffusion of glucose into the patient occurs during the hemodialysis treatment.

### 4. What is the composition of the dialysis membrane?

Most dialysis membranes used in the United States are of a hollow fiber design. A typical hollow fiber artificial kidney is composed of approximately 10,000 capillary tubes arranged in parallel. The blood circulates through the lumen of the capillary tubes, and dialysate solution bathes the capillary tubes from the outside, moving in the opposite direction. A small minority of dialysis procedures in the United States are performed using parallel plate membranes, which comprise a stacked array of flat membrane envelopes. Blood circulates through the inside of the envelope, and the dialysate solution bathes the envelope from the outside.

Dialysis membranes are either cellulose-based or polymer-based. **Cellulosic membranes** cost less because of the abundance of raw cellulose in the environment. They tend to have a low ultrafiltration coefficient, can be reused frequently, and can be used with less technically sophisticated dialysis machines. A major disadvantage of cellulosic membranes is their "bioincompatibility." Some types of cellulosic membranes activate complement through the alternative pathway, leading to agglutination of white blood cells in the lungs and transient hypoxemia during dialysis. Chronic complement activation may contribute to the amyloidosis that may develop in patients who have been dialyzed for many years. Some studies suggest that the use of cellulosic membranes may be associated with higher rates of morbidity and mortality among patients with acute renal failure than those observed with the use of polymer membranes.

**Polymer membranes** cost more and must be used with more expensive dialysis machines that tightly control ultrafiltration. However, they are more biocompatible than cellulosic membranes and do not cause any complement activation. Furthermore, the high porosity of some of these membranes (termed *high-flux*) may augment the convective removal of uremic toxins through increased "solvent drag." Water purification standards for dialysate used with high-flux membranes must be extremely rigorous because of the potential for back filtration of contaminants (such as endotoxins) through the large pores in such membranes.

### 5. How is blood removed from the patient's body during hemodialysis?

Adequate access to blood circulation must be maintained in patients undergoing hemodialysis to sustain extracorporeal blood flow rates of 300 ml/min. The superficial venous circulation is inadequate for this purpose. Most chronic hemodialysis patients have an arteriovenous fistula or an arteriovenous graft. An arteriovenous fistula is a direct surgical anastomosis between an artery and a superficial vein that causes the vein to dilate and develop a thickened wall. A well-developed arteriovenous fistula is the most desirable permanent hemodialysis access because it involves no foreign body and is able to sustain the greatest extracorporeal blood flow rates. An arteriovenous graft involves the surgical interposition of a synthetic blood vessel between an artery and a vein. This artificial vessel is placed below the skin such that it can be repeatedly cannulated with a large-bore needle as necessary to sustain adequate extracorporeal blood flow rate. The major complications associated with arteriovenous grafts or fistulas are thrombosis and infection.

When hemodialysis is required in patients who do not have a functioning arteriovenous fistula or graft, temporary or semipermanent vascular access is achieved by the use of a central venous catheter with two large-bore lumens; blood is removed from the patient through one lumen and blood is returned to the patient through the other lumen. Such catheters are generally placed into the superior vena cava through the internal jugular veins or into the interior vena cava through the femoral veins. If catheter access for hemodialysis is required for a long period of time, the catheter often is placed using a cuffed subcutaneous tunnel to decrease the incidence of infection. Such catheters generally are discouraged as long-term vascular access for hemodialysis patients, however, because of their significantly higher rate of infectious complications when compared with arteriovenous fistulas and grafts. Subclavian vein dialysis catheters are discouraged because of a high rate of subsequent subclavian vein stenosis, which may impede the ability to successfully construct a fistula or graft in the affected extremity.

**6. What prevents the patient's blood from clotting while it is in the extracorporeal hemodialysis circuit?**

Hemodialysis patients are routinely given heparin during the hemodialysis treatment to prevent thrombosis in the extracorporeal circuit. Although the dose of heparin required generally correlates with the weight of the patient and the duration of the hemodialysis treatment, the heparin dose must be individualized for each dialysis patient to prevent complications. Some dialysis facilities give an initial bolus of heparin followed by an infusion of heparin administered up to the last hour of the dialysis treatment. Other facilities administer heparin in 2 boluses, with approximately two-thirds of the total dose given at the initiation of the dialysis treatment and approximately one-third of the heparin dose given about 2 hours into the dialysis treatment. The appropriate dose of heparin is generally the amount that prevents clotting in the extracorporeal circuit but, at the same time, does not lead to bleeding from the needle puncture sites for more than 10 minutes after the needles are removed at the end of the hemodialysis treatment.

### BIBLIOGRAPHY

1. Dobkin JF, Miller MH, Steigbigel NH: Septicemia in patients on chronic hemodialysis. Ann Intern Med 88:28–33, 1987.
2. Hakim RM: Clinical implications of hemodialysis membrane biocompatibility. Kidney Int 44:484–494, 1993.
3. Jannett TC, Wise MG, Shanklin NH, Sanders PW: Adaptive control of anticoagulation during hemodialysis. Kidney Int 45:912–915, 1994.
4. Ketchersid TL, van Stone JC: Dialysate potassium. Semin Dial 4:46–51, 1991.
5. National Kidney Foundation: K/DOQI clinical practice guidelines for vascular access, 2000. Am J Kidney Dis 37(suppl 1):S137–S1881, 2001.
6. Palmer BF: The effect of dialysate composition on systemic hemodynamics. Semin Dial 5:54–60, 1992.
7. Shusterman NH, Feldman HI, Wasserstein A, Strom BL: Reprocessing of hemodialyzers: A critical appraisal. Am J Kidney Dis 14:81–91, 1989.

# 47. HEMODIALYSIS: ASSESSING ADEQUACY

Jay B. Wish, M.D.

## 1. What is adequate hemodialysis?

Adequate hemodialysis can be defined as the amount of dialysis required for optimal patient survival. Patient survival, morbidity, and quality of life all have been linked to measures of hemodialysis adequacy. Thus, it is important to know what adequate hemodialysis means and to be able to prescribe it, deliver it, and monitor its influence on the dialysis patient population.

## 2. How is the dose of dialysis measured?

In hemodialysis, an artificial kidney is used to replace the natural kidney's function to eliminate waste products and endogenous toxins. The dose of dialysis therefore can be measured by the clearance of these waste products. Like any drug clearance by first order kinetics, this can be measured as:

$$\text{Clearance} = \log (C_t/C_o)^{Kt/V}$$

where $C_t$ = concentration of the drug (toxin) at time point t, $C_o$ = initial concentration prior to clearance, K = constant (value for rate of diffusion), t = time elapsed, and V = volume of distribution of the substance. Although many waste products accumulate in renal failure, by convention, clearance of urea has been used as a surrogate for clearance of "uremic" toxins.

## 3. Is urea the primary toxin that causes the signs and symptoms of uremia?

No. This is a common misconception. Urea per se is not inherently toxic and is not responsible for most of the signs and symptoms associated with uremia. It was chosen as a marker because it is easily measurable, well distributed in body tissues, elevated in renal failure, and dialyzable. The clearance of urea forms the cornerstone of measuring the efficacy and, by inference, the adequacy of dialysis therapy.

## 4. How do urea levels translate into practical and useful parameters to measure dialysis dose?

The serum urea levels before and after hemodialysis therapy are the main values considered when assessing the adequacy of treatment. Urea levels in dialysate also can be used, but this option is too cumbersome for most facilities. The National Kidney Foundation's Dialysis Outcomes Quality Initiative (DOQI) Clinical Practice Guidelines for Hemodialysis Adequacy recommend using serum levels to assess dialysis adequacy in conjunction with formal urea kinetic modeling, which uses complicated calculations to plot urea removal, urea generation, and volume of distribution. Recognizing that the parameter Kt/V is an exponent in the formula in question 2, the equation can be rearranged:

$$Kt/V = -\text{Ln} (C_t/C_o)$$

where $C_t$ = postdialysis serum urea nitrogen and $C_o$ = predialysis serum urea nitrogen level. In essence, Kt/V describes the fractional clearance of urea in relation to its distribution volume. The DOQI guidelines recommend the use of formal kinetic modeling, the natural logarithm formula, or the urea reduction ratio (see question 5) for assessment of dialysis adequacy.

**5. How can Kt/V be measured if the tools for formal kinetic modeling are unavailable?**

To further define Kt/V, one must understand that K ultimately represents the clearance coefficient of the dialyzer, t is the time on dialysis, and V is the volume of distribution of urea. Thus, Kt actually represents the volume of blood cleared of urea as it passes through the dialyzer. Because urea is also distributed in tissues, it must equilibrate with blood during dialysis so that only a certain portion of the total body urea can be cleared at any given time. Thus, the initial natural logarithm formula for Kt/V in question 4 was further refined by Daugirdas into:

$$Kt/V = -Ln\ [(R - 0.008) \times t] + [(4 - 3.5\ R)\ (UF/W)]$$

where R is the postdialysis over predialysis serum urea level ($C_t/C_o$), t = time of dialysis (in hours), UF = ultrafiltration volume in liters (amount of fluid removed by dialysis), and W = patient's postdialysis weight in kilograms. The first part of the equation represents the effects of urea generation during dialysis, and the second part represents the additional urea removed with the fluid during dialysis. Thus, even with a simple scientific calculator, one can calculate the Kt/V if one knows the predialysis serum urea level, the postdialysis serum urea level, the patient's predialysis weight, the postdialysis weight, and the duration of dialysis therapy.

**6. What about the urea reduction ratio (URR)?**

This even simpler calculation represents the drop in urea levels after dialysis in the form of a percentage. It is calculated as follows:

$$URR = 100\% \times [1 - (C_t/C_o)]$$

where $C_t$ and $C_o$ represent postdialysis and predialysis serum urea levels. However, the URR does not account for the contribution of ultrafiltration to the final delivered dose of dialysis. The inaccuracy makes it unreliable as the sole measure of the delivered dose of dialysis in individual patients. It remains a useful epidemiologic tool, however.

**7. Is Kt/V related to patient outcome?**

Yes. Results of the National Cooperative Dialysis Study (NCDS) indicated high rates of morbidity in patients with a Kt/V < 1. Subsequent studies have correlated low Kt/V with higher mortality.

**8. What is the target Kt/V for adequate hemodialysis?**

The target delivered Kt/V has been subject to debate, and the DOQI guideline has stated after a thorough review of the literature that there is insufficient evidence to set an optimal value. However, with the support of data from the NCDS and other studies, the minimum delivered Kt/V recommended for all patients is 1.2 (this would roughly correlate to an average URR of > 65%). Some centers advocate higher Kt/V values of 1.4–1.6.

**9. What is the difference between the prescribed dose and the delivered dose of hemodialysis?**

Delivered Kt/V reflects the amount of dialysis the patient is actually getting. When starting a patient on dialysis, an estimate of the Kt/V prescription can be made by establishing values for K, t, and V. The literature for most dialyzers will supply the K value as tested in vitro in milliliters per minute (ml/min) that indicates the volume cleared of urea at a given blood flow rate; t is the time (duration) of dialysis that is prescribed by the physician and thus is the variable under our control. V is the calculated volume of distribution of urea, which roughly corresponds to 0.6 ml/gm of body weight. Therefore, a 60-kg man with a time of 3 hours on a polysulfone F8 dialyzer (K = 240 ml/min at a blood flow of 300 ml/min) will have a prescribed Kt/V of:

$$(240\ ml/min) \bullet (240\ min/0.6) \bullet (60,000\ ml) = 57,600\ ml/36,000\ ml = Kt/V = 1.6$$

## 10. What Kt/V should be prescribed?

To prevent the delivered dose of hemodialysis from falling below the recommended minimum dose, the DOQI guidelines recommend a minimum prescribed Kt/V of 1.3. After all, in a random distribution falling on a bell-shaped curve, if the median is 1.2, half of the Kt/V will be less than 1.2 if it is the target. Thus, to increase the chances of most people having a delivered Kt/V of 1.2, the prescribed Kt/V should be at least 1.3.

## 11. What factors account for differences between prescribed and delivered Kt/V?

The many factors that can cause a discrepancy between the prescribed and delivered dose of dialysis can be grouped under (1) compromised urea clearance and (2) reductions in treatment time (see tables).

*Reasons for Compromised Urea Clearance*

| PATIENT-RELATED REASONS | STAFF-RELATED REASONS | MECHANICAL PROBLEMS |
|---|---|---|
| Decreased effective time on dialysis | Decreased effective time Decreased BFR | Dialyzer clotting during reuse |
| • Decreased BFR | • Less than prescribed | Blood pump calibration error |
| • Access clotting | • Difficult cannulation | Dialysate pump calibration error |
| • Use of intravenous catheters (instead of an arteriovenous graft or fistula) | Decreased dialysate flow rate • Less than prescribed • Inappropriately set | Inaccurate estimation of dialyzer performance by the manufacturer |
| • Inadequate flow through vascular access Recirculation | Dialyzer • Inadequate quality control of "reuse" | Variability in blood tubing |
| • Use of catheters | | |
| • Inadequate access for prescribed BFR | | |
| • Stenosis, clotting of access | | |

BFR = blood flow rate.
Adapted from Parker TF: Trends and concepts in the prescription and delivery of dialysis in the United States. Semin Nephrol 12:267–275, 1992.

*Reasons for Decreased Effective Time on Dialysis*

| PATIENT-RELATED REASONS | STAFF-RELATED REASONS | MECHANICAL REASONS |
|---|---|---|
| Late start (patient tardy) | Late start (staff tardy) | Clotting of dialyzer |
| Early sign off | Wrong patient taken off | Dialyzer leaks |
| • With consent (i.e., symptoms) | Time calculated incorrectly Time on/off read incorrectly | Machine malfunction |
| • Against advice (i.e., social) | Clinical deficiencies (e.g., no | |
| Medical complications (e.g., hypotension) | time registered) Premature discontinuation | |
| "No show" | for unit convenience | |
| | • Scheduling conflicts | |
| | • Emergencies | |
| | Incorrect assumptions of continuous treatment time (e.g., failure to account for interruptions of treatment such as repositioning needles or accidental removal) | |

*Table continued on next page*

*Reasons for Decreased Effective Time on Dialysis (cont.)*

| PATIENT-RELATED REASONS | STAFF-RELATED REASONS | MECHANICAL REASONS |
|---|---|---|
|  | Inaccurate assessment of effective time by using variable time pieces |  |

Adapted from Parker TF: Trends and concepts in the prescription and delivery of dialysis in the United States. Semin Nephrol 12:267–275, 1992.

### 12. How often should adequacy of hemodialysis be measured?

Because clinical signs and symptoms alone are not reliable indicators of dialysis adequacy, it is recommended that adequacy be measured using Kt/V for the delivered dose of dialysis. By convention, dialysis lab tests are drawn monthly, and it is pragmatic to do Kt/V measurements at the same time.

### 13. What are middle molecules?

These hypothetical substances, theorized to be 500–2000 daltons in molecular weight, historically were thought to affect patient outcome as they accumulated in renal failure. No middle molecular toxins have ever been specifically identified. However, the benefits of longer dialysis time on patient survival theoretically could reflect improved clearance of middle molecules. The newer high-flux membranes with larger pores theoretically are able to clear middle molecules better than regular high-efficiency or cellulosic dialysis membranes. The benefit of high-flux dialysis will need to be proven in future clinical trials.

### 14. What lies ahead for optimizing dialysis therapy?

The National Institutes of Health (NIH) recently completed the multicenter HEMO Study, a prospective, randomized trial designed to assess the effect of hemodialysis dose (small-molecule clearance) and flux (middle-molecule clearance) on morbidity and mortality. The study failed to demonstrate improved outcomes for patients whose Kt/V was 0.3 higher than the DOQI target (vs. those at the target) or for patients dialyzed with high-flux (vs. high-efficiency) membranes. Based on the remarkable health and survival of patients in Tussin, France, who are dialyzed with low blood flow rates for 8 hours three times weekly, attention has again turned to the independent role of dialysis duration for improved toxin clearance. Trials are underway in the United States and Canada examining outcomes for patients who are dialyzed for 6 or more hours 5 nights per week while sleeping or who are dialyzed for shorter treatments on a daily basis.

### BIBLIOGRAPHY

1. Collins AJ, Ma JZ, Umen A, Keshaviah P: Urea index and other predictors of hemodialysis patient survival. Am J Kidney Dis 23:272–282, 1994.
2. Consensus Conference Development Panel: Morbidity and mortality of renal dialysis: An NIH consensus conference statement. Ann Intern Med 121:62–70, 1994.
3. Daugirdas JT: Second generation logarithmic estimates of single-pool variable volume Kt/V: An analysis of error. J Am Soc Nephrol 4:1205–1213, 1992.
4. Gotch FA, Sargent JA: A mechanistic analysis of the National Cooperative Dialysis Study (NCDS). Kidney Int 28:526–534, 1985.
5. Held PJ, Levin NW, Randall R, et al: Mortality and duration of hemodialysis treatment. JAMA 265:871–875, 1991.
6. Lacson E, Wish JB: Hemodialysis adequacy. In Henrich W (ed): Principles and Practice of Dialysis, 2nd ed. Baltimore, Lippincott Williams & Wilkins, 1998.
7. National Kidney Foundation: K/DOQI clinical practice guidelines for hemodialysis adequacy, 2000. Am J Kidney Dis 37(suppl 1):S7–S64, 2001.

8. Parker TF: Trends and concepts in the prescription and delivery of dialysis in the United States. Semin Nephrol 12:267–275, 1992.
9. Sehgal AR, Snow RJ, Singer ME, et al: Barriers to adequate delivery of hemodialysis. Am J Kidney Dis 31:593–601, 1998.
10. Szczech LA, Lowrie EG, Li Z, et al: Changing hemodialysis thresholds for optimal survival. Kidney Int 59:738–745, 2001.

# 48. COMPLICATIONS OF HEMODIALYSIS

*Lavinia A. Negrea, M.D.*

### 1. How common is hypotension during dialysis? What causes it?
Hypotension occurs in 10–30% of hemodialysis treatments. Factors related to **decreases in blood volume** include:
- Target "dry weight" set too low
- Too rapid removal of water (high ultrafiltration rate)
- Low dialysate sodium concentration

**Cardiovascular** factors include:
- Dialysate that is relatively too warm
- Food ingestion during dialysis (splanchnic vasodilatation)
- Administration of short-acting antihypertensive medications prior to dialysis
- Lack of peripheral vasoconstriction due to autonomic neuropathy
- Congestive heart failure
- Acetate-containing dialysate

### 2. What life-threatening disorders should be considered in the differential diagnosis of hypotension during dialysis?

| | |
|---|---|
| Sepsis | Pericardial tamponade |
| Internal hemorrhage | Arrhythmia |
| Myocardial infarction | Air embolism |

### 3. What approaches will prevent hypotension during dialysis?
Hypotension can be prevented by frequent determinations of the **dry weight** (the weight below which the chronic hemodialysis patient has orthostatic hypotension), avoiding large interdialytic fluid gains, and holding short-acting antihypertensive medications until immediately prior to dialysis. Midodrine, an alpha-adrenergic agonist, can be administered prior to dialysis in refractory cases.

### 4. Describe the clinical manifestations of dialysis dysequilibrium syndrome.
Clinical manifestations occur during or immediately after dialysis and include headache, lethargy, nausea, muscular twitching, and malaise. Symptoms can progress to obtundation, seizures, or coma. The syndrome occurs most commonly after the first few dialysis treatments in patients with chronic renal failure and long-standing uremia.

### 5. What causes dialysis dysequilibrium, and how can it be prevented?
The syndrome occurs when the plasma solute level is rapidly lowered during dialysis. Plasma becomes hypotonic with respect to the brain tissue and water shifts in the brain, leading to cerebral edema. Acute changes in cerebrospinal fluid pH also have been incriminated. Dysequilibrium is best prevented by deliberately limiting solute removal during the first treatment session and by stepwise increases in the subsequent sessions. Administration of mannitol also may prevent shifts of water into the brain.

### 6. What are dialyzer reactions?
There are two main types of dialyzer reactions:

1. **Type A, or anaphylactic reaction**. The symptoms of this type of reaction occur during the first few minutes of dialysis and include anxiety, dyspnea, urticaria, and pruritus. These reactions are thought to be due to residual amounts of ethylene oxide, which is used to sterilize dialyzers, and can range from mild discomfort to true anaphylaxis.

2. **Type B, or nonspecific dialyzer reaction.** Symptoms occur within the first 30 minutes of dialysis, are less severe and much more common, and include chest pain, back pain, varying degrees of nausea, and pruritus. Use of unsubstituted cellulose membranes and activation of complement are the implicated etiologies.

### 7. Which processes are responsible for dialysis-associated hypoxemia?

Hypoxemia occurs commonly during hemodialysis. With bicarbonate-containing dialysis solution, rapid transfer of bicarbonate from dialysis solution to the blood can result in metabolic alkalosis and subsequent hypoventilation. Unsubstituted cellulose dialysis membranes can impair intrapulmonary oxygen diffusion through complement activation and sequestration of neutrophils within pulmonary capillaries.

### 8. Name the most important factors contributing to arrhythmias during dialysis.

The hemodialysis procedure does not increase the likelihood of arrhythmias in all patients. In patients with ischemic heart disease and those receiving cardiac glycosides, factors contributing to arrhythmias are:
- Acidosis
- Hypoxemia
- Hypotension
- Removal of certain antiarrhythmic agents during dialysis
- Hypokalemia
- Hypomagnesemia

### 9. What accounts for increased bleeding tendencies in hemodialysis patients?

Uremic bleeding (see Chapter 44, Other Manifestations of Uremia) can persist in some patients after initiation of dialysis. This can be aggravated by intradialytic administration of heparin.

### 10. What causes chest pain during hemodialysis?

Chest pain occurs in 1–4% of dialysis treatments. It is often associated with back pain when **dialyzer reaction** is the cause (see question 6). Chest pain caused by dialysis should be differentiated from other causes such as angina or hemolytic reactions.

### 11. What factors are responsible for headaches during dialysis?

Headaches can be a subtle manifestation of dysequilibrium syndrome. In patients who are coffee drinkers, headache can be a manifestation of caffeine withdrawal because the blood caffeine concentration is acutely reduced during dialysis.

### 12. What causes nausea and vomiting during dialysis?

Nausea and vomiting occur in up to 10% of dialysis treatments. Most episodes are related to hypotension. Nausea also can be a manifestation of dysequilibrium syndrome or dialyzer reaction.

### 13. What causes pruritus during dialysis?

Pruritus is experienced by many dialysis patients, sometimes with exacerbation during or immediately after dialysis. Proposed causes are dryness of the skin, secondary hyperparathyroidism, abnormal calcium-phosphorus product, and elevated plasma histamine concentration.

**14. Are fever and chills during hemodialysis always caused by infection?**

Febrile episodes in dialysis should always be evaluated aggressively, with infection-induced fevers representing the main concern. The vascular access site is the source of 50–80% of bacteremic episodes in hemodialysis patients, most often associated with temporary catheters, least often with native arteriovenous fistulas. Febrile reactions during hemodialysis also can be related to exposure to endotoxins originating from the dialyzer or dialysate. These **pyrogenic reactions** are manifested by fever, chills, nausea, and hypotension. Patients with pyrogen-related fever are afebrile prior to dialysis, and no bacteremia can be demonstrated in blood cultures.

**15. What causes hemolysis during dialysis?**

Hemolysis can be a medical emergency, presenting with chest tightness, back pain, shortness of breath, fall in hematocrit, and hyperkalemia. Acute hemolysis almost always is due to a technical problem (chloramine-T or nitrate contamination, overheated or hypotonic dialysis solutions).

**16. What is the cause of muscle cramps during dialysis?**

Muscle cramps occur in up to 20% of hemodialysis treatments and appear to be related to rapid ultrafiltration or use of low-sodium dialysate. Preventive measures include avoidance of large fluid gains between treatments and administration of quinine sulfate or oxazepam prior to dialysis. Carnitine supplementation and stretching exercises also may be beneficial.

BIBLIOGRAPHY

1. Bregman H, Daugirdas JT, Ing TS: Complications during hemodialysis. In Daugirdas JT, Blake PG, Ing TS (eds): Handbook of Dialysis, 3rd ed. Philadelphia, Lippincott Williams & Wilkins, 2001, pp 148–168.
2. Jaber BL, Pereira JG: Acute complications of hemodialysis. In Johnson RJ, Feehally J (eds): Comprehensive Clinical Nephrology. London, Mosby, 2000, pp 79.1–79.10.
3. Jameson MD, Wiegmann TB: Principles, uses, and complications of hemodialysis. Med Clin North Am 74:945–960, 1990.
4. Kaufman AM, Polaschegg H, Levin NW: Complications during hemodialysis. In Nissenson AR, Fine RN (eds): Dialysis Therapy, 2nd ed. St. Louis, Mosby, 1993, pp 109–132.
5. Schulman G, Hakim RM: Complications of hemodialysis. In Jacobson HR, Striker GE, Klahr S (eds): The Principles and Practice of Nephrology, 2nd ed. St. Louis, Mosby, 1995, pp 673–683.

# 49. CONTINUOUS RENAL REPLACEMENT THERAPY

*Jeffrey R. Schelling, M.D.*

**1. Which patients should be considered for continuous renal replacement therapy?**

In patients with acute renal failure requiring renal replacement therapy, the major therapeutic options are standard, acute intermittent dialysis or continuous renal replacement therapy (CRRT). In acute circumstances, the same general acute indications apply for both renal replacement modalities: (1) fluid volume overload that is refractory to diuretic therapy, (2) hyperkalemia that is causing cardiac arrhythmias or is refractory to medical management, (3) persistent metabolic acidosis despite aggressive medical therapy, (4) uremia, particularly uremic pericarditis, and (5) removal of ingested toxins from the blood. If criteria for acute renal replacement therapy are met, the choice of acute intermittent hemodialysis versus CRRT depends on whether the patient has adequate blood pressure to tolerate solute and fluid removal over the 3–4-hour period required for intermittent dialysis compared with the 24-hour period needed for CRRT. Although the hemodynamic criteria are somewhat arbitrary, most nephrologists would consider patients with a blood pressure less than 90/60 mmHg or patients requiring intravenous vasopressor support to maintain a blood pressure above 90/60 mmHg to be suitable candidates for CRRT. In addition to the standard indications for dialysis, CRRT has been shown to be effective for treatment of lithium toxicity and for reduction of intracranial pressure. Although it has been suggested that CRRT may be beneficial for other "nonrenal" conditions, such as cytokine removal in sepsis or hepatic or congestive heart failure, efficacy of CRRT for these conditions has not been established.

**2. What forms of CRRT are available?**

The major options are:
- Continuous venovenous hemofiltration (CVVH)
- Continuous venovenous hemodialysis (CVVHD)
- Continuous venovenous hemodiafiltration (CVVHDF) (see figure)
- Continuous arteriovenous hemofiltration (CAVH)
- Continuous arteriovenous hemodialysis (CAVHD)
- Continuous arteriovenous hemodiafiltration (CAVHDF)

Peritoneal dialysis also is a form continuous dialysis, but this topic is extensively addressed in Chapters 50 and 51. Continuous venovenous forms of CRRT require a double-lumen dialysis catheter in a large vein. Blood flow from the arterial port of the catheter to the artificial kidney (dialyzer) is aided by a pump. Blood then passes through the dialyzer and returns through the venous port of the dialysis catheter. In contrast, continuous arteriovenous forms of CRRT require a femoral arterial catheter, but no pump, because the patient's own arterial pressure drives blood flow to the dialyzer. **Hemofiltration** implies that net fluid is removed—this is achieved by removing plasma and repleting only a portion of the plasma volume with a relatively smaller amount of "replacement fluid." **Dialysis** implies that there is dialysate (containing high concentrations of $HCO_3^-$ [or $HCO_3^-$ equivalents, such as acetate] and low concentrations of potassium relative to blood) flowing in a countercurrent direction to blood, which facilitates solute removal. **Diafiltration** combines both hemofiltration and dialysis capabilities by including replacement fluid and dialysate in the circuit.

186

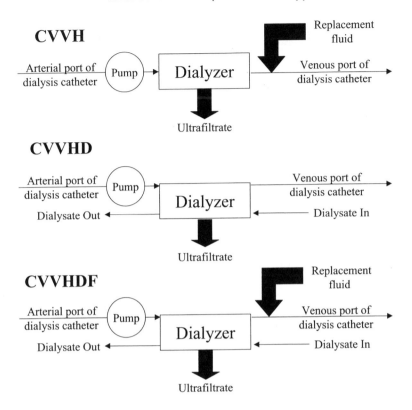

Sequence of dialysis process for continuous venovenous hemofiltration (CVVH), continuous venovenous hemodialysis (CVVHD), and continuous venovenous hemodiafiltration (CVVHDF).

### 3. What are the advantages of continuous venovenous versus arteriovenous systems?

Continuous venovenous and arteriovenous systems are both very effective for solute and fluid removal. The biggest advantage of continuous venovenous systems is elimination of the need for arterial cannulation, which is a potential source of serious complications, such as bleeding and leg and foot ischemia. For these reasons, continuous venovenous techniques have become the preferred form of CRRT at most hospitals. The advantage of the arteriovenous approach is that a pump is not required, which is therefore less expensive in terms of equipment and personnel costs.

### 4. What needs to be done to get a patient started on CVVH?

The major tasks are placing a double-lumen dialysis catheter in a large (usually femoral) vein, as described above, and preparing a machine (for venovenous CRRT), dialyzer, and solutions. Depending on the type of CRRT chosen, replacement fluid or dialysate must be ordered. Commercially available dialysate is generally used. Some commercial solutions will suffice for replacement fluid, but many institutions make their own replacement fluid, which requires some preparation time by a technician in a sterile environment. In most instances, CRRT can be initiated within 3–4 hours.

### 5. What parameters are involved to achieve fluid and solute removal by CRRT?

The major biophysical processes that permit fluid and solute removal are convection and diffusion. Fluid removal by hemofiltration is achieved primarily by **convection** and requires a blood flow rate greater than 50 ml/min. Hemodialysis is achieved primarily by **diffusion** across the semipermeable dialyzer membrane and, to a lesser extent, by convection. To achieve effective solute removal, the dialysate flow rates should be at least 1 L/hr, and recent studies indicate that patient outcomes are significantly improved with higher dialysate flow rates ($\geq$ 35 ml/kg/hr). A minimum mean arterial pressure of 60 mmHg is necessary for effective solute clearance, but clearances are enhanced when mean arterial pressures exceed 80 mmHg.

### 6. How is clotting of the dialyzer prevented?

Under ideal conditions, the anticipated life span of the dialyzer is about 2 days. The main reason for discontinuation of a dialyzer is that clots begin to form, which results in less available dialyzer membrane surface area. In some circumstances, the entire system (dialyzer and dialysis catheter) can thrombose. Slowing of the clotting process can be accomplished with anticoagulation therapy (usually heparin), which is administered through the proximal dialyzer port. Anticoagulation adequacy is usually monitored by the partial thromboplastin time (PTT) drawn from a sample from the dialyzer, with a target PTT of 40–60 seconds. In cases in which heparin is contraindicated, protocols using citrate or regional heparin anticoagulation have been proposed as alternatives. Another simple option is to administer hemofiltration replacement fluid through the predialyzer port at a high rate. Although this may not be as effective as pharmacologic anticoagulation, it has been the author's experience that this is usually sufficient to prevent dialyzer clotting for at least 24 hr.

### 7. What are potential complications of CRRT?

Because of the requirement for a dialysis catheter, infection or line sepsis is a major complication of CRRT. Because CRRT employs low blood flow rates, some form of anticoagulation is necessary to maintain patency of the system (see question 6), with an associated risk of bleeding. In the absence of anticoagulation, dialyzers may clot frequently, which adds considerably to the expense of the procedure. Large amounts of low–molecular-weight substances are removed with CVVH or CAVH. Many of these, such as uremic toxins, are removed by intent. However, removal of other substances, such as magnesium, calcium, and vitamins, is not desirable. Magnesium and calcium depletion can be avoided by concomitant, continuous infusions of magnesium sulfate and calcium gluconate, with close monitoring of serum magnesium and ionized calcium concentrations. The benefits of vitamin replacement are less clear.

### 8. Why is continuous dialysis *theoretically* more effective than intermittent hemodialysis in hemodynamically unstable patients?

The obvious answer is that fluid removal in a hypotensive patient is more effective and better tolerated hemodynamically if it is accomplished over a longer time period. One benefit of enhanced fluid removal by CRRT is the capacity to administer blood products or large volumes of total parenteral nutrition (TPN) to catabolic patients. Although avoidance of overt hypotension is clearly beneficial in the maintenance of blood flow to critical organs, such as the brain and heart, it is not as widely recognized that some types of acute renal failure, such as ischemic acute tubular necrosis, may result in loss of renal blood flow autoregulation. Under these circumstances, even low-normal blood pressures may result in decreased renal perfusion, which may cause additional ischemia and prolong the course of acute renal failure. Therefore, because fluid removal by CRRT should be gentler by not precipitating a diminution in cardiac output and blood pressure, CRRT theoretically should result in improved renal outcomes and mortality.

**9. What data are available comparing the efficacy of intermittent dialysis versus CRRT?**

There are many retrospective studies from the past 15 years. On balance, these studies demonstrate that the continuous dialysis group experiences a slight benefit in morbidity and mortality over those patients receiving intermittent dialysis. These data are consistent with studies demonstrating equivalent solute clearances and superior fluid removal with CRRT compared to conventional, intermittent hemodialysis. However, firm conclusions cannot be drawn from these studies primarily because of retrospective study design and, in most instances, lack of an appropriate control group. Recently, however, a well-designed randomized, prospective trial comparing continuous versus intermittent hemodialysis was published by Mehta et al. that revealed that CRRT was associated with an increase in mortality relative to intermittent dialysis. There was no difference in length of ICU stay or time to renal recovery. However, despite careful randomization, the baseline severity of illness was greater in the CRRT group, which therefore favored a better outcome in the intermittent dialysis group. Because others have not yet replicated these data, clinical outcomes in CRRT versus conventional hemodialysis remain unclear.

### BIBLIOGRAPHY

1. Bellomo R, Ronco C, Mehta RL: Nomenclature for continuous renal replacement therapies. Am J Kidney Dis 28:S2–S7, 1996.
2. Conger JD: Interventions in clinical acute renal failure: What are the data? Am J Kidney Dis 26:556–576, 1995.
3. Conger JD, Schultz MF, Miller F, Robinette JB: Responses to hemorrhagic arterial pressure reduction in different ischemic renal failure models. Kidney Int 46:318–323, 1994.
4. Ifudu O: Care of patients undergoing hemodialysis. N Engl J Med 339:1054–1062, 1998.
5. Mehta RL, McDonald B, Gabbai FB, et al: A randomized clinical trial of continuous versus intermittent dialysis for acute renal failure. Kidney Int 60:1154–1163, 2001.
6. Ronco C, Bellomo R, Homel P, et al: Effects of different doses in continuous veno-venous haemofiltration on outcomes of acute renal failure: A prospective, randomised trial. Lancet 356:26–30, 2000.
7. Swartz RD, Messana JM, Orzol S, Port FK: Comparing continuous hemofiltration with hemodialysis in patients with severe acute renal failure. Am J Kidney Dis 34:424–432, 1999.

# 50. TECHNICAL ASPECTS OF PERITONEAL DIALYSIS

*Miriam F. Weiss, M.D.*

### 1. How is a peritoneal dialysis patient like a salmon?

A canal that passes from the peritoneal cavity through the body wall to a pore on the surface of the abdomen has been identified in salmonids (*Salmo giardneri, Salmo salar, Coregonus artedii*). Peritoneal fluid, cells, and injected particles or bacteria are actually "voided" from the pore, enabling the peritoneum to function like an excretory organ. By creating an artificial abdominal pore (peritoneal dialysis catheter), the inherent "excretory" capacity of the peritoneum is made available to sustain life in patients with kidney failure.

### 2. How does peritoneal dialysis work?

Dialysate solution (containing balanced electrolytes and high concentrations of dextrose) is introduced into the peritoneal cavity. Uremic toxins diffuse across peritoneal capillaries, through the interstitium, across the peritoneal mesothelial layer, and into the peritoneal cavity. Fluid is removed by ultrafiltration when water in the blood moves across these peritoneal layers into the hypertonic dialysate along an osmotic gradient. Toxins and ultrafiltered water are removed when the dialysate is drained from the peritoneal cavity.

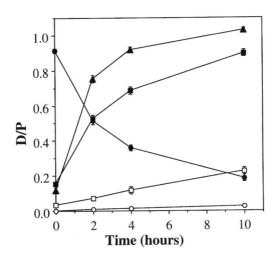

Increasing dialysate levels of urea (*closed triangle*), creatinine (*closed square*), beta$_2$-microglobulin (*open square*), and protein (*open circle*) over the course of a long dwell. results are expressed as the ratio of the level in dialysate (D) to the level in plasma (P). The decrease in the ratio of initial dialysate glucose to dialysate glucose (closed circle) is also shown (D/D0). The data represent the mean ± standard error of 38 peritoneal equilibration tests.

### 3. What is the peritoneum?

The peritoneum is a membrane lining the surface of the abdominal cavity and its organs. It includes the visceral peritoneum, lining the abdominal and pelvic walls and the diaphragm, and the parietal peritoneum, covering the stomach, intestines, and surface of the liver and spleen. In the supine position, most of the dialysate in the peritoneal cavity is distributed near the liver and spleen and between the small intestines. The peritoneum forms a closed sac in men. In women, the fallopian tubes open into the peritoneum.

### 4. Why doesn't dialysis fluid drain through the fallopian tubes and leak from the uterus in women treated by peritoneal dialysis?

The tubes are usually collapsed, so there is no free communication between the peritoneum and the exterior. On the other hand, female patients occasionally report blood in their dialysate during ovulation. In patients with endometriosis, intraperitoneal bleeding may be seen as blood-tinged dialysate during the menstrual period.

### 5. How big is the peritoneum?

The surface area of the peritoneum is equivalent to that of the skin, approximately 1.73 $m^2$ in an average-sized adult male. Peritoneal blood flow is between 75 and 200 ml/minute, compared with normal renal blood flow of ~400 ml/minute. The hypertonic dialysate instilled into the peritoneal cavity causes vasodilation, thus increasing blood flow.

### 6. What are the indications for peritoneal dialysis?

Peritoneal dialysis is a long-term treatment alternative for *any* patient with end-stage renal disease. Peritoneal dialysis has medical advantages over hemodialysis in some circumstances. It has been a successful adjuvant to the management of congestive heart failure refractory to conventional medical treatment, even in patients who do not have renal failure.

Initiation of hemodialysis in newly diagnosed end-stage kidney failure is associated with a rapid decline in what is left of kidney function. Treatment with peritoneal dialysis preserves native kidney function longer. This advantage has led several experts to recommend that peritoneal dialysis is the best modality to use early in the course of renal failure.

### 7. What are the contraindications to peritoneal dialysis?

There are few absolute contraindications to peritoneal dialysis. A patient or caregiver must be able to master the concepts and procedures necessary to perform dialysis in a safe way. Relative but major contraindications to peritoneal dialysis include (1) inguinal, umbilical, or diaphragmatic hernias, particularly if pleuroperitoneal leak and hydrothorax develop; (2) ostomies (colostomy or nephrostomy); (3) recent aortic valve prosthesis; and (4) abdominal wall abscess. Minor contraindications include morbid obesity (may necessitate omentectomy at the time of catheter placement), polycystic kidneys (increased intra-abdominal pressure), and diverticulosis. The large volume of peritoneal fluid in the abdominal cavity reduces gastric emptying time and may exacerbate underlying gastroparesis in patients with diabetes.

### 8. What are the unique design features of a chronic peritoneal dialysis catheter?

In 1968, Tenckhoff developed a silicone catheter with two Dacron cuffs. The cuffs are positioned within the abdominal wall just above the peritoneum and just below the skin (see figure). The Dacron cuffs heal with the formation of fibrosis, preventing bacteria from moving from the skin into the tunnel (which bridges the distance between the two cuffs) and the peritoneum. A patient with a well-healed peritoneal catheter is free to shower or swim without danger of bacteria entering the peritoneum around the catheter.

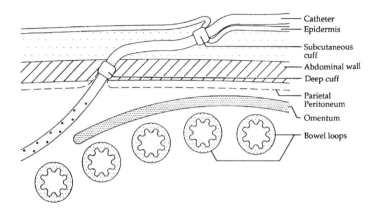

Cross-section of the proper position of a double-cuffed Tenckhoff catheter as it crosses the abdominal wall. (From Ash SR, Carr DJ, Diaz-Buxo JA: Peritoneal access devices. In Nissenson AR, Fine RN, Gentile DE (eds): Clinical Dialysis, 2nd ed. Norwalk, CT, Appleton & Lange, 1990, pp 212–239, with permission.)

**9. Compare peritoneoscopic placement with surgical placement of chronic peritoneal dialysis catheters.**

|  | ADVANTAGES | DISADVANTAGES |
|---|---|---|
| Peritoneoscopy | Outpatient procedure, local anesthesia and analgesia<br>Smaller exit-site incision | Requires specialized equipment<br>Greater risk of subcutaneous leak of dialysate, if catheter is used early<br>Greater likelihood of developing late pericatheter hernia |
| Surgical placement | Direct visualization of placement for both external and internal cuffs<br>Reduced risk of subcutaneous leak of dialysate, if catheter used early | Surgical procedure, requiring general anesthesia<br>Larger exit-site incision |

**10. How long is the healing period after catheter placement?**

A catheter break-in period of 10 days to 2 weeks is recommended to allow the cuffs to seal. To prevent increased intra-abdominal pressure that may disrupt fibroblast ingrowth into the cuffs, patients should avoid strenuous activity or heavy lifting. Physicians should avoid infusing full volumes of dialysate into the peritoneal cavity. Fluid leakage around the cuffs inhibits fibroblasts from growing into the cuffs and encourages the development of infection along the catheter tract, or peritonitis. When the need to treat uremia is urgent, patients can be started on hemodialysis through a temporary catheter. Alternatively, they can be hospitalized for low-volume exchanges while on bed rest.

**11. What is an "exchange"?**

An exchange consists of draining out dialysate that has been dwelling in the peritoneum and infusing a fresh volume of dialysate. Commercial dialysate comes in flexible plastic bags. The standard size is 2–3 L per exchange. An array of devices and systems are available to enable patients to perform sterile connection and disconnection procedures during the exchange.

### 12. What do CAPD, CCPD, and NIPD stand for?

**Chronic ambulatory peritoneal dialysis (CAPD)** consists of 4–5 exchanges using 2–3 L of dialysate with each exchange. The patient carries fluid in the abdomen 24 hours per day. Exchanges are spaced out throughout the day, usually upon awakening, at lunchtime, at dinnertime, and before bed.

In **continuous cycler-assisted peritoneal dialysis (CCPD)**, an automated cycler machine performs some of the dialysis exchanges (usually at night while the patient is asleep). When the patient is not connected to the cycler machine, the peritoneal cavity is filled with a volume of dialysate that is either drained by hand or drained when the patient connects back to the machine for another set of exchanges.

**Nocturnal intermittent peritoneal dialysis (NIPD)** is like CCPD, except the peritoneal cavity is empty of fluid when the patient is not using the cycler machine.

### 13. What is the composition of peritoneal dialysate?

Current commercially available dialysate solutions contain dextrose, in concentrations of 1.5%, 2.5%, or 4.25%, as the main osmotic solute. Maximal ultrafiltration occurs by 3–4 hours using 1.5% dextrose (see figure). By 8–10 hours, most patients will have absorbed a significant amount of dextrose or diluted the dextrose content with ultrafiltrate. As a result, the osmotic gradient will be dissipated. At this point, dialysate can be absorbed, resulting in a net positive fluid balance. Using 4.25% dextrose dialysate, maximal ultrafiltration occurs about 5 hours after infusion, and net positive ultrafiltration is not dissipated for 12–15 hours. Therefore, higher concentrations of dialysate glucose are useful in CAPD for the overnight dialysis exchange and in CCPD for the long diurnal dwell. Polyglucose solutions that are not absorbed are currently undergoing testing as alternative osmotic agents. These solutions will have the advantage of providing continuous ultrafiltration without dissipation of the osmotic gradient.

The major bicarbonate-generating base used in peritoneal dialysate is lactate (35–40 mEq/L). Although only L-lactate is normally present in the body, DL-lactate is used. The liver can generate bicarbonate from both isomers. Some loss of bicarbonate into the dialysate occurs early in the exchange but is compensated by the metabolism of the administered lactate. The sodium concentration of the dialysate, 132 mEq/L, is slightly lower than serum (135–142 mEq/L) to allow net removal of $Na^+$ and $Cl^-$ to take place across the dialysate. Commercial dialysate contains no potassium. Peritoneal dialysis is effective at controlling hyperkalemia in most patients treated with peritoneal dialysis, in part, through constant removal of $K^+$ across the peritoneum. In fact, hypokalemia can become a problem in patients who have poor dietary intake and are receiving maximally effective dialysis clearance.

Standard dialysate solutions contain 3.5 mEq/L of calcium. Thus, the ionized calcium concentration is much higher than normal blood ionized calcium, causing a net positive calcium balance. Over time, the increased absorption of calcium from dialysate, concurrent with the routine use of calcium-containing phosphate binders, can result in excessive suppression of hyperparathyroidism, a form of renal osteodystrophy called **hypoplastic bone disease**, and hypercalcemia. Dialysate solutions containing 2.5 mEq/L of calcium are also available and may mitigate this problem.

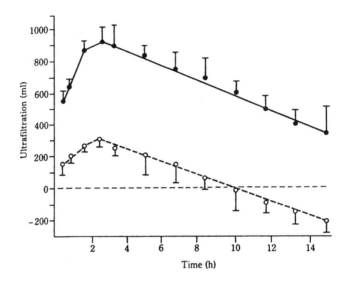

Net ultrafiltration (volume drained versus volume instilled) as a function of time after infusion of dialysate. The figure compares 1.5% dextrose (*open circles*) with 4.25% dextrose (*closed circles*). (From Sorkin MI, Diaz-Buxo JA: Physiology of peritoneal dialysis. In Daugirdas JJ, Ing TS (eds): Handbook of Dialysis, 2nd ed. Boston, Little, Brown, 1994, pp 245–261, with permission.)

### 14. Are there any dialysate formulations that do not contain dextrose?

Icodextrin, a long-chain polymer derived from starch, has been tested extensively in the United States and is used widely in Europe. Because of its high molecular weight, icodextrin is not absorbed across the peritoneal membrane as rapidly as dextrose-based dialysate. Therefore, ultrafiltration is increased over the course of a long dwell. Icodextrin-based dialysate is particularly useful in patients with large fluid weight-gains, to help control fluid balance.

Amino acid–based, dextrose-free dialysate solutions have been shown to be useful in patients with malnutrition. Several formulations are available. Particular benefit may come from the use of essential amino acids. Enrichment with L-glutamine, which has antioxidant properties, may confer unique benefits.

### 15. What is a peritoneal dialysis prescription, and how is it determined?

The dialysis prescription encompasses the volume of dialysate, the osmolality of the dialysate, and the frequency of exchanges—three factors that determine solute clearance in peritoneal dialysis. Peritoneal permeability is a major factor in determining the rate of fluid and solute removal during peritoneal dialysis. Norms have been established that enable the nephrologist to categorize patients' permeability patterns (see question 16). Patients with high peritoneal permeability (rapid transporters) have an early loss of osmotic gradient because glucose is quickly absorbed across the peritoneum. To prevent fluid overload, such patients must have decreased dwell time in order to drain dialysate when the osmolality of the fluid is still high. These patients respond best when treated with CCPD or NIPD.

### 16. What is the peritoneal equilibration test?

Although several standardized tests to determine the function of the peritoneal membrane have been developed, the fast peritoneal equilibration test is most widely used. This test is reproducible and accurate. The test starts with drainage of the previous night's dialysis bag. A fresh bag of 2.5% dextrose is infused over 10 minutes. A blood sample is taken during the equilibration period. After 4 hours, the dialysate is drained, and a sample of it is taken. The volume of the drained dialysate is ascertained. Both dialysate and blood are assayed for creatinine. The 4-hour dialysate-to-plasma ratio (D/P creatinine) and the net ultrafiltration (volume drained minus volume exchanged) are compared with standards that allow the nephrologist to classify the patient's peritoneal function as low, low-average, high-average, or high in its transport characteristics. Patients with high transport characteristics do better with relatively short dwells. These rapid transporters will have optimal clearance of uremic toxins and removal of fluid with frequent short exchanges, such as can be provided by an automatic cycling device. Patients with low transport characteristics need to allow the dialysate to dwell for longer periods of time to optimize removal of uremic toxins and excess water.

**17. How is adequacy of treatment determined in patients on peritoneal dialysis?**

In contrast to the experience with hemodialysis (see Chapter 47, Hemodialysis: Assessing Adequacy), no large, multicenter study has been performed to determine the optimal amount of peritoneal dialysis. It is difficult to compare peritoneal dialysis and hemodialysis, because one is a continuous therapy and the other intermittent. Peritoneal dialysis patients seem to get by on about half the urea clearance of hemodialysis patients. This may be because the peritoneum is removing more large uremic toxins than the hemodialysis membrane. Alternatively, patients treated by peritoneal dialysis may tolerate a constant level of uremic toxins better than the peaks and valleys experienced by patients treated by hemodialysis.

Whereas the formula Kt/V (K = clearance coefficient of the dialyzer, t = time on dialysis, and V = volume of distribution of urea) is a very good way of assessing if adequate hemodialysis is being given to a patient, the best method for assessing adequacy for peritoneal dialysis has not been determined. Many centers ask patients to collect all of their dialysate (and any urine they have made) for a 24-hour period and to bring these volumes of fluid for testing every 6 months. The volume of urine and dialysate and the urea and creatinine concentrations are then measured, along with blood levels of these solutes, and total clearance of urea and creatinine are calculated by standard formulas. Mathematical approximations of Kt/V in peritoneal dialysis may be particularly inaccurate because they are based on assumptions about the patient's weight and the volume of distribution of urea that are probably incorrect. Nonetheless, it is recommended that patients on peritoneal dialysis reach an average weekly Kt/V target of 1.7–2.2. The total weekly creatinine clearance should be greater than 60 L/week, corrected for body surface area.

**18. Why do patients treated with peritoneal dialysis require a high-protein diet?**

Patients treated by hemodialysis are given a low-protein diet to reduce the intake of urea precursors. By contrast, patients treated by peritoneal dialysis lose between 10 and 40 gm of protein across the peritoneal membrane each day. As a result, high-protein diets (1.8–2.5 gm/kg body weight/day) are prescribed to replace these losses. Amino acid dialysate solutions are also available for malnourished patients treated by peritoneal dialysis. Amino acids not only contribute to the hypertonicity of the dialysate, but also are absorbed across the peritoneal membrane and through the peritoneal lymphatics.

**19. How does peritoneal dialysis compare to hemodialysis?**

The usual peritoneal dialysis prescription does not provide as much clearance of low–molecular-weight solutes as the usual hemodialysis regimen does. However, peritoneal dialysis removes high–molecular-weight substances better than hemodialysis. In theory, increased clearance of high–molecular-weight solutes may improve long-term control of the uremic syndrome. However, recent studies have raised the concern that patients treated by peritoneal dialysis may not exhibit adequate clearance of uremic toxins over long periods of time. The current standard of care is to increase clearance by using the maximum volume of dialysate tolerated by the patient and by increasing the frequency of dialysis exchanges consistent with the patient's underlying transport characteristics, as determined by the peritoneal equilibration test (see Chapter 51, Complications of Peritoneal Dialysis).

## BIBLIOGRAPHY

1. Ash SR: Peritoneal access devices and placement techniques. In Nissenson AR, Fine RN (eds): Dialysis Therapy, 3rd ed. Philadelphia, Hanley & Belfus, 2002, pp 45–51.
2. Blake PG, Daugirdas JT: Physiology of peritoneal dialysis. In Daugirdas JT, Blake PG, Ing TS (eds): Handbook of Dialysis, 3rd ed. Philadelphia, Lippincott Williams & Wilkins, 2000, pp 281–296.
3. Dobbie JW: From philosopher to fish: The comparative anatomy of the peritoneal cavity as an excretory organ and its significance for peritoneal dialysis in man. Perit Dial Int 8:1–3, 1988.
4. Golper TA: A summary of the 2000 update of the NKF-K/DOQI clinical practice guidelines on peritoneal dialysis adequacy. Perit Dial Int 21(5):438–440, 2001.
5. Lim VS, Flanigan MJ: Protein intake in patients with renal failure: Comments on the current NKF-DOQI guidelines for nutrition in chronic renal failure. Semin Dial 14:150–152, 2001.
6. Newman LN, Weiss MF, Berger J, et al: The law of unintended consequences in action: Increase in incidence of hypokalemia with improved adequacy of dialysis. Adv Perit Dial 16:134–137, 2000.
7. Pastan S, Bailey J: Dialysis therapy. N Engl J Med 338:1428–1437, 1998.
8. Teixeira A, Pecoits-Filho RF, Romao JJE, et al: The relationship between ultrafiltrate volume with icodextrin and peritoneal transport pattern according to the peritoneal equilibration test. Perit Dial Int 22:229–233, 2002.
9. Yatzidis H: A new superior, single and stable, amino acid and bicarbonate-based, glucose-free solution for peritoneal dialysis. Dial Transplant 31:143–150, 2002.

# 51. COMPLICATIONS OF PERITONEAL DIALYSIS

*Carolyn P. Cacho, M.D.*

## 1. What is peritonitis?

The presence of more than 100 white blood cells per cubic millimeter in the peritoneal fluid or greater than 50% polymorphonuclear neutrophils defines peritonitis in the peritoneal dialysis patient. Visibly cloudy effluent and abdominal pain usually herald the onset of the illness. Fever, nausea, and diarrhea are less consistently present. On examination, abdominal pain, decreased bowel sounds, guarding, and rebound tenderness are all typical findings.

## 2. What is the cause of peritonitis in patients treated with peritoneal dialysis?

About 95% of cases are caused by bacterial infection. Historically, *Staphylococcus epidermidis* infections due to touch contamination were the most common causative agents. However, with the introduction of the Y-set and double-bag peritoneal dialysis systems, touch contamination has declined as the cause of peritonitis. Currently, gram-positive infections account for 50–80% of all episodes of peritonitis in peritoneal dialysis patients. Gram-negative organisms account for 20–30% of all episodes. Unlike infections caused by gram-positive organisms, which usually result from touch contamination, gram-negative infections derive from a variety of sources including the skin, bowel, urinary tract, and contaminated water. Less than 5% of cases are caused by fungi, usually *Candida* species. Although the number of cases is relatively small, fungal peritonitis often follows repeated episodes of bacterial peritonitis and invariably necessitates removal of the peritoneal dialysis catheter. Rare cases of peritonitis are caused by anaerobic bacteria or mycobacteria. Finally, peritonitis may be caused by hypersensitivity to intraperitoneally administered drugs (e.g., vancomycin), a phenomenon characterized by a high number of eosinophils in the dialysis effluent.

## 3. What is the appropriate diagnostic work-up of peritonitis in a peritoneal dialysis patient?

The appearance of cloudy dialysis effluent should prompt the simultaneous initiation of the diagnostic evaluation and treatment of peritonitis. A dialysate cell count and differential are obtained to provide quick confirmation of the diagnosis. The Gram stain is often negative early in the course of infection. However, when organisms are seen, the results can be used to tailor therapy. Bacterial, fungal, and mycobacterial cultures should be obtained and are positive in more than 80% of cases. Because it is unusual for peritonitis to cause systemic illness in this setting, blood cultures are indicated only when signs of bowel perforation or sepsis is present.

## 4. How should peritonitis be treated?

Initiation of therapy need not be delayed until results of the diagnostic work-up are available. Initial therapy should cover both gram-positive and gram-negative organisms. The emergence of vancomycin-resistant organisms and concern over the adverse effect of aminoglycosides on residual renal function have increased the controversy regarding the choice of antibiotics. A first-generation cephalosporin can be administered intraperitoneally for initial gram-positive coverage instead of vancomycin. However, this choice requires careful follow-up of culture results because gram-positive infecting agents are more likely to be resistant to a cephalosporin than to vancomycin. An alternative protocol is to use vancomycin initially with a change to a second agent when culture results are available. A third-generation cephalosporin is now the first choice for gram-negative coverage; however, recent guidelines recommend omitting a loading dose. This empiric regimen should be modified based on culture and sensitivity results. Treatment typically is continued for a total of 10–14 days.

Peritonitis in the peritoneal dialysis patient is usually a benign disease, and a response to treatment, indicated by a normalization of the cell count, clearing of the dialysate, and improvement of clinical symptoms, should occur within 48 hours. Persistent elevation of the white cell count or predominance of neutrophils, cloudy dialysate, or continued abdominal pain should increase concern about infections with *Staphylococcus aureus, Pseudomonas,* or fungal species. In comparison to patients with other gram-positive infections, those with *S. aureus* infections generally have more severe disease and may even present with toxic shock–type illness. For this reason, a longer treatment course of 21 days is recommended. Pseudomonal infections are particularly difficult to eradicate and should be treated with two antibiotics for at least 21 days. Frequently, this regimen fails, and the catheter must be removed. The diagnosis of a fungal peritonitis must be considered if the dialysate is slow to clear. On occasion, fungal elements can be seen on the Gram stain, and the organisms will grow when the peritoneal fluid is sent for fungal culture. Recent recommendations for the treatment of fungal peritonitis suggest a trial of intraperitoneal fluconazole and oral flucytosine without the removal of the catheter. A more conservative alternative is to remove the catheter and administer a prolonged course of amphotericin B (total dose of about 1 gm) on hemodialysis. Once the infection has cleared, the peritoneal dialysis catheter can be reinserted. As is often the case after severe or repeated episodes of peritonitis, peritoneal scarring may prevent successful resumption of peritoneal dialysis.

Treatment of peritonitis often fails when the disease is caused by an abdominal catastrophe such as bowel perforation. The mortality rate in such cases is as high as 50%. Diagnostic studies such as computed tomography (CT) scans or contrast enemas are helpful when they confirm the presence of a perforated viscus or bowel interruption. However, a negative study does not rule out the presence of an abdominal catastrophe. The approach to such cases includes broadening of antibiotic coverage to include gram-negative organisms and antianaerobic coverage, consideration of empiric antifungal therapy, and early exploratory laparotomy. At least one study has found a correlation between mortality and time to surgical intervention.

### 5. What is an exit site infection?

Unlike peritonitis, which has a well-established and accepted definition, criteria for establishing diagnosis of an exit site infection are somewhat unsettled. Bacteria colonize most healed exit sites. These bacteria can cause infection if the exit site is traumatized, improperly anchored, or subjected to prolonged soaking. An infected exit site is often erythematous, indurated, and tender. It may bleed or exude pus. In most cases the infecting organism can be determined from a swab culture. If left untreated, the infection may extend into the tunnel and eventually cause peritonitis.

### 6. How is an exit site infection treated?

The treatment of exit site infection ranges from the use of astringent soaks to the administration of parenteral antibiotics. In cases of mild erythema and a negative bacterial culture, hypertonic saline or dilute solutions of bleach and hydrogen peroxide may reverse the condition. Induration, tenderness, or a positive culture warrants the use of antibiotics. Topical vancomycin, tobramycin, or gentamicin, in combination with an astringent soak, often will cure exit site infections. When topical treatment fails or in the case of *Pseudomonas* exit site infection, parenteral antibiotics should be used. For gram-positive infections, vancomycin may be given intraperitoneally. For persistent infections, the addition of oral rifampin is helpful. Gram-negative infections usually respond to the intraperitoneal administration of an aminoglycoside or a third-generation cephalosporin. Infections due to *Pseudomonas* also should be treated with a second agent such as ciprofloxacin. Failure to respond to parenteral antibiotics or the occurrence of relapsing exit site infections should prompt catheter replacement.

### 7. How can exit site infections be prevented?
The most important step in the prevention of exit site infection occurs at the time of catheter implantation. The use of a catheter with a swan-neck, which drains downward, and two cuffs, which serve as barriers to bacteria, has been shown to decrease the rate of exit site infection. Perioperative antibiotics, catheter immobilization, and perioperative eradication of nasal *S. aureus* are additional helpful measures. A long-term strategies for prevention of exit site infection includes daily care with a nonirritating cleansing agent.

### 8. What is the approach to inflow and outflow pain?
Pain with instillation of dialysate occasionally occurs, especially in patients who have recently started peritoneal dialysis. The pain is caused by the jet of fluid striking the viscera. Catheters with a curled intraperitoneal segment distribute the fluid over a wider area and therefore are less likely to cause this problem. However, these catheters may be more prone to kinking. Lowering the bag of dialysate decreases the rate of flow and is usually enough to stop the pain. Laparoscopic manipulation and laxation may also allow the catheter to migrate to a more comfortable position.

Outflow pain most commonly occurs at the end of drain when the abdomen is empty. It is caused by the tip of the catheter irritating the bladder or intestine. Like inflow pain, it is observed less often with curled catheters. The problem can be improved by instructing the patient to start filling with the onset of the pain and to avoid an empty peritoneum. A tidal program that leaves a small (200 ml) volume of dialysate in the peritoneum with each drain may relieve symptoms in patients who experience pain during cycling.

### 9. What causes poor dialysate drainage?
Poor outflow is one of the most common problems encountered in peritoneal dialysis practice. Recall that net ultrafiltration is determined by the osmotic tonicity of the dialysate, the length of the dwell time, the peritoneal kinetics of the patient, and any internal or external impediments to outflow. All of these factors should be considered when presented with a patient whose inflow volume is greater than outflow volume. In general, hypotonic dialysate, long dwell times, or rapid kinetics result in small net negative balances that can slowly lead to fluid overload. By comparison, mechanical impediments lead to fluid overload more rapidly.

If maneuvers such as increasing the tonicity of the dialysate, shortening the dwell time, checking for kinked tubing, and changing positions with draining have failed to solve the problem, the most likely cause of the outflow failure is an internal impediment to flow. The most common internal cause of decreased flow is constipation, which decreases the effective area available for ultrafiltration and can mimic external compression on the catheter. A fibrin clot may obstruct inflow or outflow and usually responds to the instillation of heparin in the dialysate. Rarely, dissolution of the clot with streptokinase may be necessary.

Outflow failure also may occur when the catheter becomes encased in omentum. Fortunately, this problem can be recognized by the ease of inflow and normal initial rate of outflow, which, after a few hundred milliliters of drainage, abruptly stops. Partial omentectomy through a small midline incision with catheter repositioning solves the problem. Catheter malposition is another cause of outflow failure that often occurs shortly after catheter placement. This can avoided by testing inflow and outflow at the time of catheter implantation and by checking the catheter position on plain films of the abdomen. Poor outflow also may be seen when the dialysate becomes loculated, as in cases of leaks into the abdominal or pleural cavity (see question 11).

**10. What is the approach to the peritoneal dialysis patient with a hernia?**

Hernias occur in about 10% of peritoneal dialysis patients. The prevalence of this complication appears to be related to the increase in intra-abdominal pressure, which rises with increasing volume of dialysate instilled in the abdomen. The intra-abdominal pressure may increase four- to sixfold with the instillation of standard dialysate volumes. With cough and straining at stool, these pressures may increase 100 times above normal. Hernias occur most commonly in the umbilical, inguinal, and pericatheter regions and at sites of earlier surgical incisions.

The best approach to pericatheter hernias in the peritoneal dialysis patient is to prevent formation by allowing the catheter to mature for 10–14 days prior to instilling full volumes in the peritoneal cavity. If the patient must undergo peritoneal dialysis during this break-in period, keeping the patient in a supine position keeps the intra-abdominal pressure as low as possible. Depending on the location of the hernia, the patient may present with swelling at the hernia site, genital edema, intestinal obstruction, and, in the most severe cases, strangulation with peritonitis due to bowel infarction. Because of the high intra-abdominal pressure, hernias in this patient population tend to enlarge over time and so should be repaired when they become clinically significant. Following hernia repair, it is advisable to resume peritoneal dialysis with smaller volumes of dialysate in the first 7 days after surgery.

**11. Can peritoneal dialysis patients develop leaks?**

Yes. Sometimes peritoneal dialysis patients present with abdominal or genital edema of unclear origin. This complication likely is due to dialysate seeping through the peritoneal dialysis membrane into the adjacent tissues under the influence of increased intra-abdominal pressure. If a hernia cannot be palpated, a CT scan with intraperitoneal injection of contrast dye may pinpoint the source of the leak. An alternative course is to temporarily reduce daytime volumes. If that is not successful, temporary discontinuation of peritoneal dialysis may allow the path of the leak to heal. Recurrent leaks probably should be explored surgically to find and repair the breach.

**12. Is a pleural effusion in a peritoneal dialysis patient cause for concern?**

A pleural effusion in a peritoneal dialysis patient usually is due to fluid overload and can be treated by increasing ultrafiltration through use of dialysate with higher tonicity. Occasionally, however, fluid in the pleural cavity is due to leaking of dialysate from the peritoneal space. This problem can occur at any time and may develop either rapidly and dramatically or so slowly that it is discovered only on routine x-ray examination. It is more common in females and more frequently involves the right side. The finding of a high glucose concentration in the pleural fluid is diagnostic. In equivocal cases, demonstration of contrast dye in the pleural space following injection into the peritoneum confirms the diagnosis. Treatment of this condition begins with temporary transfer to hemodialysis because cases of spontaneous remission have been reported. Unfortunately, reinitiation of peritoneal dialysis often leads to reaccumulation of dialysate in the pleural cavity. In this situation, stimulation of adhesion formation with irritants such as talc, tetracycline, and autologous blood or surgical closure of the pleural space have at times been successful.

### 13. What are the other mechanical complications of peritoneal dialysis?

Peritoneal dialysis patients may suffer from compromised respiratory function, back pain, dyspepsia, and early satiety as a direct result of the dialytic method. The large amount of instilled fluid may cause impairment of respiratory function similar to that seen in obese or pregnant patients. Symptoms are worse in the supine position, and, therefore, patients with this difficulty should carry larger volumes when ambulatory. The dialysate volume and the increased intra-abdominal pressure also can precipitate or exacerbate back pain syndromes. Patients with back pain usually are more symptomatic with large volumes while ambulatory and, therefore, are best treated with large-volume cycling at night and smaller daytime volumes. Peritoneal dialysis can result in early satiety and even dyspepsia because of large-volume dialysis and increased intra-abdominal pressure. Strategies to ameliorate this problem include eating while empty or at the beginning of a dwell, decreasing the volume of daytime dwells, and using intestinal propulsants and antireflux medications.

### 14. What are the indications for catheter removal?

The three major indications for removal of a peritoneal dialysis catheter are intractable infection of the exit site, tunnel, or peritoneum; failure to effect adequate fluid removal; and failure to support adequate clearance. Persistent leaks or inflow pain also may prompt catheter removal. In the past, removal of the catheter has usually meant at least transient transfer to hemodialysis. More recently, simultaneous removal and replacement has been shown to be successful in noninfectious indications for catheter removal such as leaks and inflow pain and in infectious cases such as nonpseudomonal exit site and tunnel infections. Furthermore, repositioning of the catheter and partial omentectomy through a midline mini-laparotomy incision are now used to treat outflow obstruction, which used to be treated with catheter removal. Peritoneal dialysis can be restarted with low fill volumes after 48 hours. If the catheter was removed for *Pseudomonas* exit site or tunnel infection or for persistent peritonitis, the catheter should be replaced after the infection has been eradicated completely. Patients with ultrafiltration failure and inadequate dialysis are transferred permanently to hemodialysis.

### BIBLIOGRAPHY

1. Burkhart J, Nolph K: Peritoneal dialysis. In Brenner B (ed): The Kidney, 5th ed. Philadelphia, W.B. Saunders, 1996, pp 2507–2575.
2. Gokal R, Alexander S, Ash S, et al: Peritoneal catheters and exit-site practices toward optimum peritoneal access: 1998 update. Perit Dial Int 18:11–33, 1998.
3. Golper T: Intermittent versus continuous antibiotics for PD-related peritonitis. Perit Dial Int 17:11–12, 1997.
4. Harwell CM, Newman LN, Cacho CP, et al: Abdominal catastrophe: Visceral injury as a cause of peritonitis in patients treated by peritoneal dialysis. Perit Dial Int 17:586–594, 1997.
5. Piraino B: Peritonitis as a complication of peritoneal dialysis. J Am Soc Nephrol 9:1956–1964, 1998.
6. Ramon RG, Carrasco AM: Hydrothorax in peritoneal dialysis. Perit Dial Int 18:5–10, 1998.
7. Vychytil A, Lorenz M, Schneider B, et al: New strategies to prevent *Staphylococcus aureus* infections in peritoneal dialysis patients. J Am Soc Nephrol 9:669–676, 1998.

# 52. NUTRITION IN DIALYSIS PATIENTS

*Ashwini R. Sehgal, M.D.*

### 1. How is the nutritional status of dialysis patients assessed?

There is no single all-purpose measure of nutritional status. Instead, a number of complementary nutritional parameters (see table) must be assessed and integrated. The most commonly used parameters are the serum albumin concentration and the protein catabolic rate.

| NUTRITIONAL PARAMETER | INTERPRETATION |
|---|---|
| Serum albumin | Reflects visceral protein stores |
| Protein catabolic rate | Measure of protein breakdown; assumed to equal protein intake when patient is in a steady state |
| Serum prealbumin | Shorter half-life than albumin; therefore, reflects changes in nutritional status more quickly |
| Body composition | Amount of metabolically active lean tissue (muscle, internal organs, extracellular water) and metabolically less active adipose tissue (fat) |
| Intake | Dietary energy and protein intake |
| Subjective global assessment | Brief nutrition-related history and physical examination that categorizes patient as well-nourished, mildly malnourished, or severely malnourished |

### 2. Why is nutrition in dialysis patients important?

Hypoalbuminemia has been identified as the strongest independent risk factor for death in several studies. Hypoalbuminemia also is associated with frequent hospitalizations, increased health care costs, and poor quality of life. Other nutritional parameters have been examined less extensively but also appear to be important predictors of mortality and morbidity.

### 3. What are optimal values for nutritional parameters in dialysis patients?

An albumin concentration of ≥ 4.0 gm/dl, measured with the bromcresol green method (or ≥ 3.7 gm/dl using the bromcresol purple method), is considered optimal. A concentration ≥ 3.5 but ≤ 4.0 gm/dl is intermediate, and a concentration ≤ 3.5 gm/dl is inadequate. Compared to hemodialysis patients with optimal albumin levels, those with inadequate levels have a three- to fivefold higher risk of death, whereas patients with intermediate levels have a twofold higher risk of death. A protein catabolic rate of ≥ 1.2 gm/kg/day is considered optimal. Optimal values for other nutritional parameters are not as well established.

### 4. What is the prevalence of malnutrition among hemodialysis patients?

About one-fifth of hemodialysis patients have inadequate albumin levels, and one-half have intermediate levels. A similar fraction of patients have suboptimal protein catabolic rates.

### 5. How do hemodialysis and peritoneal dialysis patients differ in their nutritional needs?

Peritoneal dialysis patients lose 7–16 gm of protein into their dialysate on a daily basis. This loss is even higher during episodes of peritonitis. By contrast, protein losses during hemodialysis are much smaller. Nearly half of peritoneal dialysis patients have inadequate albumin levels and over one-third have intermediate levels.

### 6. Why are some dialysis patients malnourished?

Malnutrition can result from insufficient nutrient intake, increased nutrient expenditure, or inability to utilize ingested nutrients. Insufficient intake of protein and calories appears to be the most important cause of malnutrition in dialysis patients.

### 7. How can malnutrition be treated in dialysis patients?

Several studies have examined the use of oral supplements, appetite stimulants, increased dose of dialysis, intradialytic nutrition, anabolic compounds, and patient education. Results of these studies have been mixed. Recent efforts to use essential amino acid supplements and to address specific nutritional barriers appear to be more promising.

### 8. What is the effect of inflammation on nutritional parameters?

Many dialysis patients exhibit an inflammatory state evidenced by elevated levels of inflammatory markers such as C-reactive protein. Inflammation in dialysis patients may occur in response to acute illnesses such as infection. However, in most cases the inflammation is chronic and of unclear cause. Postulated explanations include subclinical infections, interactions between the patient's blood and the dialyzer membrane, and renal failure itself. The acute-phase response that accompanies inflammation results in suppression of albumin synthesis and contributes to the development of hypoalbuminemia.

### BIBLIOGRAPHY

1. Eustace JA, Coresh J, Kutchey C, et al: Randomized double-blind trial of oral essential amino acids for dialysis-associated hypoalbuminemia. Kidney Int 57:2527–2538, 2000.
2. Ikizler TA, Hakim RM: Nutrition in end-stage renal disease. Kidney Int 50:343–357, 1996.
3. Kaysen GA, Dubin JA, Muller HG, et al: The acute-phase response varies with time and predicts serum albumin levels in hemodialysis patients. Kidney Int 58:346–352, 2000.
4. Leon JB, Majerle AD, Soinski JA, et al: Can a nutrition intervention improve albumin levels among hemodialysis patients? A pilot study. J Renal Nutr 11:9–15, 2001.
5. Mitch WE, Klahr S: Handbook of Nutrition and the Kidney. Philadelphia, Lippincott-Raven, 1998.
6. National Kidney Foundation: K/DOQI clinical practice guidelines for nutrition in chronic renal failure. Am J Kidney Dis 35:S1–S400, 2000.
7. Owen WF, Lew NL, Liu Y, et al: The urea reduction ratio and serum albumin concentration as predictors of mortality in patients undergoing hemodialysis. N Engl J Med 329:1001–1006, 1993.
8. US Renal Data Systems: USRDS 2000 Annual Data Report. Bethesda, MD, National Institutes of Health, 2000.

# 53. RENAL TRANSPLANTATION: EPIDEMIOLOGY AND OUTCOMES

*Donald E. Hricik, M.D.*

### 1. How are patients selected for kidney transplantation?

All patients with end-stage renal disease (ESRD) are considered candidates for kidney transplantation unless they have a systemic malignancy, chronic infection, severe cardiovascular disease, or neuropsychiatric disorder (including drug addiction) that precludes compliance with an immunosuppressive drug regimen. Renal transplantation can be performed before a patient requires dialysis. However, a patient cannot be listed for a cadaveric kidney transplant until his or her creatinine clearance has fallen below 20 ml/minute. Ultimately, the patient is responsible for choosing between dialysis and transplantation as options for renal replacement therapy.

### 2. Is age a consideration?

Extremes of age are considered *relative* contraindications to renal transplantation. In neonates and children younger than 2 years, technical difficulties related to the small size of the recipient often preclude successful transplantation. Advanced age is no longer considered an absolute contraindication. In fact, high rates of success have been reported in patients between 60 and 70 years of age. For patients older than 70 years, transplantation should be considered only if the patient exhibits superb extrarenal health.

### 3. How many kidney transplants are being performed these days?

In recent years, between 12,000 and 14,000 kidney transplants have been performed annually in the United States. The growth rate has been minimal during the past 10 years, primarily because of the relatively fixed number of available donors. Although there has been steady growth in the number of kidney transplants performed using living donors during the same time period, heart-beating, brain-dead cadavers still serve as donors for more than 70% of the transplants performed in the United States. Growth in the number of transplants performed has not kept pace with the 6–8% annual increase in the number of patients with ESRD. As a consequence, the number of patients waiting for cadaveric renal allografts and the waiting times for these organs have increased dramatically, as shown in the figure below.

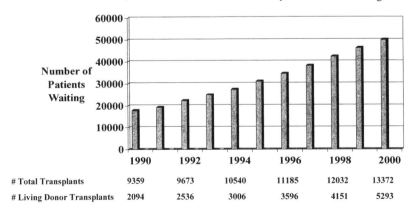

| | 1990 | 1992 | 1994 | 1996 | 1998 | 2000 |
|---|---|---|---|---|---|---|
| # Total Transplants | 9359 | 9673 | 10540 | 11185 | 12032 | 13372 |
| # Living Donor Transplants | 2094 | 2536 | 3006 | 3596 | 4151 | 5293 |

Patients waiting and kidney transplant performed.

## 4. Can anything be done to increase the donor pool?

The pool of living donors recently has been expanded by increased use of living, *unrelated* donors (e.g., spouses and friends). To increase the pool of cadaver donors, some centers have advocated acceptance of donors previously considered marginal. Examples include the use of non–heart-beating cadavers and transplantation of two kidneys from donors who previously would have been excluded from single kidney donation on the basis of advanced age or renal impairment. Because family refusal to allow organ donation from otherwise suitable cadavers remains a common problem, public education continues to play an important role in maintaining or increasing rates of cadaveric organ donation.

## 5. How successful is kidney transplantation?

Short-term success (defined by 1-year allograft survival rates) has steadily increased during the past decade (see figure). For the cohort of U.S. patients transplanted in 1994, 1-year allograft survival was 85.6% for recipients of cadaver donor allografts and 92.4% for recipients of living donor allografts.

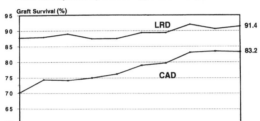

**One-Year Adjusted Medicare *Graft Survival*, First Transplant, by Donor Type and Year, 1984-1993**

One-year allograft survival, first transplants adjusted for age, sex, race, by donor type, and year, 1985–1994. (From U.S. Renal Data Systems: 1997 Annual report: VII: Renal transplantation: Access and outcomes. Am J Kidney Dis 30(suppl 1):S118–S127, 1997, with permission.)

## 6. How long do kidney transplants last?

The projected half-lives of kidney transplants have steadily improved over time as shown in the table. Because death with a functioning graft is now a common cause of graft loss, it is important to consider graft longevity both with and without death censoring.

*Projected Half-life (Years) of Kidney Transplants*

|  | 1989 | 1991 | 1993 | 1995 |
|---|---|---|---|---|
| **Without death censoring** | | | | |
| Living donor | 15.0 | 14.8 | 16.7 | 21.6 |
| Cadaver donor | 8.7 | 9.7 | 10.3 | 13.8 |
| **With death censoring** | | | | |
| Living donor | 20.8 | 21.5 | 22.9 | 35.9 |
| Cadaver donor | 12.0 | 14.5 | 15.1 | 19.5 |

## 7. How does kidney transplantation compare to dialysis in terms of patient survival?

Annual mortality rates for patients on dialysis in recent years have ranged from 21% to 25%. In contrast, mortality rates are now less than 8% per year for cadaveric transplant recipients and less than 4% per year for living-related transplant recipients. Any comparison of outcomes in patients treated with transplantation or dialysis must take into consideration that healthier patients generally are selected for transplantation. The fact that mortality rates of successfully transplanted patients are lower than those of patients maintained on dialysis while awaiting a kidney transplant suggests, however, that transplantation is associated with a clear-cut survival advantage. The benefit of transplantation is most notable in young people and in those with diabetes mellitus. For example, for *nondiabetic* dialysis patients between the ages of 20 and 39 years, projected years of life are 31 years with a kidney transplant and only 20 years without a transplant. For *diabetic* dialysis patients in the same age group, projected years of life are 25 years with a transplant and only 8 years without a transplant.

**8. What constitutes a good match between donor and recipient?**

A person's "tissue type" is determined by cell surface antigens encoded for by the family of human leukocyte (HLA) genes located on the short arm of the sixth chromosome. The HLA-A and HLA-B loci encode for class I antigens expressed on the surface of most nucleated cells. The HLA-DR (D-related) locus encodes for class II antigens expressed on selected antigen-presenting cells and activated lymphocytes. With a complement of two chromosomes, each individual expresses 6 HLA antigens. Because disparities in the HLA antigen composition of the recipient and host may trigger the immunologic events leading to allograft rejection, these 6 antigens are referred to as major transplantation antigens. The "match" between two individuals can range from 0 to 6. Six is good!

Matching based on tissue typing should not be confused with crossmatching, a laboratory test that determines whether a potential transplant recipient has preformed antibodies against the HLA antigens of the potential donor. A potential kidney transplant recipient may have a relatively good match but still exhibit a positive crossmatch against the donor that precludes transplantation. Keep in mind that, generally speaking, potential kidney transplant recipients and donors must exhibit blood group ABO compatibility in order to allow successful transplantation.

**9. What is the effect of HLA-matching on the outcome of kidney transplantation?**

Data from large registries indicate that, the better the HLA-match, the better the long-term survival of the allograft. The benefits of matching are particularly noteworthy in recipients of kidneys from donors who match for 6 HLA antigens (or who exhibit no HLA antigen mismatches). The benefits of lesser degrees of matching have become less obvious with the use of newer and more potent immunosuppressive drugs. For any number of HLA matches, the long-term survival of allografts tends to be better in recipients of living unrelated transplants compared to recipients of cadaveric allografts, suggesting that elimination of "cold" ischemia required for the preservation of cadaveric organs may outweigh the influence of matching on long-term outcome (see figure on next page).

**10. How are cadaveric renal allografts allocated to patients on the waiting list?**

In the United States, organ allocation policies are dictated by the United Network for Organ Sharing (UNOS), a government-appointed agency that maintains a computerized list of all potential kidney transplant recipients and a post-transplant database that provides a source of information about outcomes after transplantation. Currently, the allocation of cadaveric kidneys is dictated by a point system that assigns organs harvested within regional organ procurement areas. The point system is most heavily weighted by the degree of HLA-matching between the potential recipient and donor and, to a far lesser extent, by other factors such as time on the waiting list. Current UNOS policy dictates that kidneys from 6-antigen–matched donors are exported within the continental U.S. to the recipient irrespective of

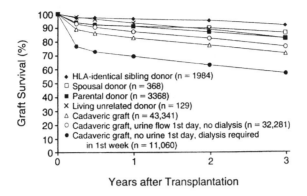

Survival of first kidney grafts. (From Terasaki PI, Cecka JM, Gjerston DW, Takemoto S: High survival rates of kidney transplants from spousal and living unrelated donors. N Engl J Med 333:333–336, 1995, with permission.)

the recipient's waiting time. This policy accounts for the occasional patient who receives a cadaveric kidney transplant after a relatively short period of waiting.

**11. What factors influence the longevity of renal allografts?**

Aside from HLA matching, factors that have been associated with decreased long-term allograft survival include the number of acute rejection episodes experienced by the recipient, delayed allograft function (defined by the need for at least one dialysis treatment after transplantation because of initially poor allograft function), and African-American ethnicity. Donor factors associated with poor long-term outcomes include extremes of age (< 5 or > 65 years of age), prolonged cold ischemia, and possibly African-American ethnicity.

**12. What are the major causes of long-term renal allograft failure?**
- Chronic rejection (see Chapter 55, Renal Transplantation: Classification and Consequences of Rejection)
- Death with a functioning allograft

**13. What are the most common causes of death after kidney transplantation?**
- Cardiovascular disease (e.g., myocardial infarction, stroke, complications of peripheral vascular disease)
- Infection

**14. What about kidney transplants from animals?**

Xenotransplantation (the transplantation of organs from one species to another) may become a reality before pigs fly. Until recently, the major barrier to transplantation between species was the presence of preformed antibodies directed against glycosylated cell surface proteins of the animal donor, which lead to immune destruction of the transplanted organ within minutes of revascularization. It is now known that this form of hyperacute rejection is mediated by complement. Genetic engineering has allowed for the procreation of animals that either express nonimmunogenic glycosylated cell surface proteins or overexpress molecules capable of preventing complement activation. Although this major hurdle has been overcome, the more traditional forms of rejection mediated by activated T cells tend to be severe after xenotransplantation and may not be prevented by currently available immunosuppressive drugs. In addition, there are serious concerns about the possibility that xeno-transplants will result in the transmission of new infectious diseases to humans. Finally, it is not clear whether proteins (e.g., enzymes, hormones) synthesized by organs transplanted from different species will be capable of sustaining their physiologic functions in humans over long periods of time.

## BIBLIOGRAPHY

1. Hariharan S, Johnson CP, Brenahan BA, et al: Improved graft survival after renal transplantation in the United Sates, 1988 to 1996. N Engl J Med 342:605–612, 2000.
2. Platt JL: Approaching the clinical application of xenotransplantation. Am J Med Sci 313:315–321, 1997.
3. Schulak JA, Mayes JT, Johnston KH, Hricik DE: Kidney transplantation in patients aged sixty years and older. Surgery 108:726–733, 1990.
4. Terasaki PI, Cecka JM, Gjerston DW, Takemoto S: High survival rates of kidney transplants from spousal and living unrelated donors. N Engl J Med 333:333–336, 1995.
5. Troppmann C, Gillingham KT, Benedetti E, et al: Delayed graft function, acute rejection, and out-come after cadaveric renal transplantation. Transplantation 59:962–968, 1995.
6. U.S. Renal Data Systems: 1997 Annual report: VII: Renal transplantation: Access and outcomes. Am J Kidney Dis 30(suppl 1):S118–S127, 1997.
7. Wolfe RA, Ashby VB, Milford EL, et al: Comparison of mortality in all patients on dialysis, patients on dialysis awaiting transplantation, and recipients of a first cadaveric transplant. N Engl J Med 341:1725–1730, 1999.

# 54. RENAL TRANSPLANTATION: DONOR AND RECIPIENT EVALUATION

*Thomas C. Knauss, M.D.*

**1. What are the current sources of donor kidneys in the United States?**
- Living related donors
- Living unrelated donors: Most often spouses or significant others
- Cadaveric donors: The majority of these donors are brain-dead individuals who are taken to the operating room with artificial life support systems intact.

Some transplant programs also use "non–heart-beating donors." These are usually individuals who do not meet criteria for brain death but are felt to have profound irreversible neurologic damage leading a family to request discontinuation of life support. The subject is taken to the operating room, and life support is discontinued. The organs are harvested after the development of asystole.

**2. Does a signed donor card ensure that a brain-dead individual is legally approved to be an organ donor?**
No. Currently, in the United States, organ donor cards express the wishes of the individual, but approval is always obtained from family members before organs are donated.

**3. What are some of the exclusion criteria for cadaveric organ donation?**
*Absolute contraindications*
- Systemic infection
- Malignancy
- Chronic kidney disease
- Long-standing diabetes mellitus
- Positive serologic test for human immunodeficiency virus (HIV)

*Relative contraindications*
- Extremes of age (< 5 years; > 65 years)
- History of risk factors for infectious diseases (e.g., intravenous drug abuse, sexual promiscuity, recent imprisonment)
- Long-standing hypertension
- Acute renal failure at the time of harvest

**4. Which infectious agents can be transferred from donor to recipient through a kidney transplant?**
- Bacteria (e.g., in bacterial pyelonephritis)
- Viruses that reside in renal tissue or passenger leukocytes (e.g., cytomegalovirus, Epstein-Barr virus, hepatitis B, hepatitis C, HIV, human herpesvirus 8)
- Fungi
- Mycobacteria

**5. What is a crossmatch?**
A crossmatch is performed by incubating donor lymphocytes (obtained from peripheral blood or from the spleen or lymph nodes) with recipient serum. The test determines whether the recipient serum contains preformed antibodies against the human leukocyte (HLA) anti-

gens of the donor. Preformed antibodies can mediate hyperacute rejection (see Chapter 55, Renal Transplantation: Classification and Consequences of Rejection), and their presence is considered a contraindication to transplantation. A final crossmatch between donor and recipient is performed routinely just prior to transplantation irrespective of whether the donor is dead or alive.

**6. Do kidney transplant donors and recipients need to have identical blood types?**

Mismatching Rh types are not important in organ transplantation. However, the donor and recipient generally must be ABO compatible. This is true under one or more of the following conditions:

- The donor and recipient are ABO identical
- The donor has blood type O (universal donor)
- The recipient has blood type AB (universal recipient)

**7. Are some HLA antigens more important than others in matching a donor and recipient for a kidney transplant?**

The major histocompatibility complex (MHC) antigens measured routinely in most HLA laboratories include the class I antigens (A, B, and C) and class II antigens (D, including the subsets DP, DQ, and DR). Practically, the antigens used clinically for matching prior to a kidney transplant are A, B, and DR. Of the individual antigens, matching for DR antigens appears to result in the most favorable long-term outcome for the allograft.

**8. What are the general principles involved in evaluating a prospective living kidney donor?**

In general, the evaluation of a potential living donor is geared to determine (1) whether there is a medical condition that will put the donor at increased risk for complications for general anesthesia and surgery and (2) whether the removal of one kidney will increase the donor's risk for developing renal insufficiency.

**9. What tests can be used to assess kidney function in potential kidney donors?**

Serum creatinine concentration
Creatinine clearance
Radionuclide glomerular filtration rate

**10. What is the minimal level of renal function required for a living kidney donor?**

Most transplant centers require a minimum glomerular filtration rate of 70 ml/min in order for a subject to serve as a living kidney donor.

**11. What other screening tests are performed routinely to rule out underlying renal disease in a prospective kidney donor?**

- Urinalysis
- Urine culture
- Measurement of urine protein (either a 24-hour collection or measurement of a protein-to-creatinine ratio in a spot urine collection)

**12. What medical conditions exclude living kidney donation?**

- Renal parenchymal disease
- Conditions that may predispose to renal disease:
    History of multiple kidney stones
    History of frequent urinary tract infections
    Hypertension

- Conditions that increase the risks of anesthesia and surgery (e.g., significant cardiac, pulmonary, or hepatic disease)
- Recent malignancy

### 13. What tests are performed as part of the living donor evaluation?
- Complete blood count
- Blood chemistries
- Urinalysis
- Urine culture
- Chest x-ray
- Electrocardiogram
- Serologic studies for past exposures to infections (cytomegalovirus, hepatitis B and C, Epstein-Barr virus, syphilis, HIV)
- Renal imaging studies

Depending on the age of the potential donor and his or her medical history, other studies (e.g., in-depth cardiac evaluation, pulmonary functions tests) may be indicated.

### 14. Why are renal imaging studies performed in evaluating living renal donors?
- To ensure that the donor has two kidneys!
- To rule out neoplasia of the urinary tract
- To rule out structural abnormalities of the urinary tract
- To assess the vascular supply of the donor kidney

### 15. Which imaging studies are done to obtain this information?
Traditionally, an intravenous pyelogram has been done followed by a renal angiogram (usually a digital subtraction angiogram). However, some transplant programs use a single study such as spiral computed tomography (CT) with three-dimensional reconstruction.

### 16. Does donation of a kidney pose a long-term renal risk for the donor?
Obviously, the living kidney donor is forever at risk for developing end-stage renal disease if the remaining kidney is damaged by unforeseen parenchymal disease or trauma. Compensatory hypertrophy and glomerular hyperfiltration occur in the remaining kidney following unilateral nephrectomy, raising the theoretical concern that the procedure may increase the long-term risk of proteinuria, hypertension, and even renal failure. Although studies from some centers have suggested a slight risk of proteinuria and hypertension, meta-analyses of data from donors followed for more than 20 years generally have shown no statistically significant increase in the incidence of these complications.

### 17. At what level of renal dysfunction is it appropriate to evaluate a patient for kidney transplantation?
Discussions regarding transplantation as a renal replacement modality should be initiated early in the course of a renal disease if it is clearly progressing to end stage. If a medically acceptable living donor has been identified, elective renal transplantation ideally is performed just before dialysis is needed. If a living-donor transplant is not an option, patients can be evaluated for transplantation at any time but cannot officially be put on the list for transplantation ("listed") until the glomerular filtration rate falls below 20 ml/min.

### 18. What are some contraindications to renal transplantation?
The only absolute contraindication is the presence of severe vascular disease that precludes the arterial and venous anastomoses required for a technically successful transplant. There are many relative contraindications (for which individualized circumstances must be taken into consideration), including:

- Recent or current malignancy
- Coronary artery disease
- Active bacterial, fungal, or viral disease
- HIV positivity
- Social conditions that prevent adherence with medical follow-up

**19. What medical evaluation is performed to determine if a patient is a suitable candidate for transplantation?**

The pretransplant evaluation varies from one transplant center to another but generally includes a complete history, physical examination, and a number of tests designed to assess overall health and to screen for occult malignancy and infection. At a minimum, this usually includes a complete blood count, blood chemistries, chest x-ray, electrocardiogram, urine culture, Pap smear, mammogram, examination of stool for occult blood, and serologic studies for cytomegalovirus, hepatitis B and C, HIV, and syphilis. The integrity of the aortoiliac circulation usually is assessed noninvasively (e.g., by duplex scanning). In many centers, a more complete cardiac evaluation (including echocardiography, stress testing, carotid studies, or myocardial perfusion scans) is performed in selected patients, including patients older than 50 years, those with diabetes mellitus, and those with symptoms suggestive of cardiovascular disease.

**20. What is the role of the social worker in evaluating a patient for renal transplantation?**

Transplantation involves a complex mix of psychosocial issues that are best evaluated by a social worker. Ability to pay for surgery, hospitalization, and immunosuppressant medications must be assessed in advance; surgical success of the transplant does not ensure overall success if the procedure leaves a patient and his or her family destitute. The psychological make-up of the potential recipient also should be assessed. The best indicator of nonadherence after a transplant is nonadherence before the transplant. Finally, family support may be critical to success, especially in the case of elderly or debilitated patients.

BIBLIOGRAPHY

1. Alexandre GPJ, Latinne D, Carlier M, et al: ABO-incompatibility and organ transplantation. Transplant Rev 5:230–241, 1991.
2. Bay WH, Hebert LA: The living donor in kidney transplantation. Ann Intern Med 106:719–727, 1987.
3. Hakim RM, Goldszer RC, Brenner BM: Hypertension and proteinuria: Long-term sequelae of uninephrectomy in humans. Kidney Int 25:930–936, 1984.
4. Jones J, Payne WD, Matas AJ: The living donor—risks, benefits, and related concerns. Transplant Rev 7:115–128, 1993.
5. Kasiske BL, Gaston RS, Bia MJ, et al: The evaluation of renal transplant candidates: Clinical guidelines. J Am Soc Nephrol 6:1–34, 1995.
6. Kasiske BL, Ravenscraft M, Ramos EL, et al: The evaluation of living renal transplant donors: Clinical practice guidelines. J Am Soc Nephrol 7:2288–2313, 1996.

# 55. RENAL TRANSPLANTATION: CLASSIFICATION AND CONSEQUENCES OF REJECTION

*Donald E. Hricik, M.D.*

### 1. What are the major forms of renal allograft rejection?

1. Hyperacute
2. Acute
3. Chronic

Older classification schemes differentiated histologic variants of rejection such as interstitial, cellular, or vascular. These latter terms have become increasingly obsolete as standardized criteria have evolved to classify allograft rejection histologically (see question 3). On the other hand, there has been increasing interest in the role of antibodies in mediating some cases of both acute and chronic rejection, such that differentiation between cellular and humoral forms of acute rejection has become increasingly relevant.

### 2. What is hyperacute rejection?

Hyperacute rejection is mediated by a transplant recipient's preformed antibodies that recognize human leukocyte (HLA) antigens in the donor organ. Preformed anti-HLA antibodies generally occur as a consequence of previous blood transfusions, pregnancy, or prior organ transplant. Occasionally, patients with autoimmune diseases may generate antibodies that cross-react with HLA antigens. In hyperacute rejection, fibrinoid necrosis typically occurs within minutes to hours leading to almost immediate destruction of the allograft. Modern crossmatching techniques are very sensitive to detecting anti-HLA antibodies and now are performed routinely prior to all kidney transplants, thus accounting for the current rarity of hyperacute rejection. A delayed form of hyperacute rejection may occur several days after transplantation. If recognized expeditiously, plasmapheresis may be beneficial in reversing the rejection process by eliminating the offending antibodies.

### 3. What is acute renal allograft rejection?

Acute rejection is mediated by activated T cells that proliferate and attack the allograft after recognizing antigens in the graft (1) directly (direct pathway) or (2) after being processed by recipient antigen-presenting cells that present donor antigens to CD4+ T cells within the grooves of surface class II HLA molecules (indirect pathway). (The cellular and intracellular events leading to T-cell activation are described in Chapter 56, Renal Transplantation: Immunosuppression.) Although subclinical cases undoubtedly occur, acute rejection in kidney transplant recipients usually is recognized clinically by the development of otherwise unexplained acute renal failure manifested by an acute rise in serum creatinine concentration and, in severe cases, by oliguria. Episodes of acute rejection can occur at any time after transplantation; however, most cases occur within the first 6 months following transplantation.

### 4. How common is acute rejection?

At least one episode of acute rejection occurs in 40–70% of cadaveric kidney transplant recipients maintained on cyclosporine, azathioprine, and steroids. Since 1994, the use of newer immunosuppressant drugs and drug combinations has been accompanied by acute rejection rates of 25% or less.

## 5. How is acute rejection treated?

Traditionally, first-line therapy of acute rejection has consisted of high doses of corti-costeroids ("pulse" steroids) administered either intravenously or orally for 3–5 days. Daily doses of methylprednisolone or its equivalent range between 250 mg and 1000 mg. Steroid-resistant rejection is usually treated with antilymphocyte antibodies including OKT3 (a monoclonal antibody directed against the CD3 complex on the surface of activated T cells) or various polyclonal antibody preparations (directed against multiple cell-surface structures on lymphocytes). Some centers use steroids or antilymphocyte antibodies for first-line ther-apy of acute rejection, depending on the severity of the rejection episode as determined by biopsy of the allograft. Some of the newer "maintenance" immunosuppressants, such as mycophenolate mofetil and tacrolimus, have proven to be effective in the treatment of acute rejection when used in high doses. Novel or unproven therapies for acute rejection include radiation of the allograft and photopheresis. Recently, high doses of human intravenous immunoglobulin (IVIG) have been used to treat acute rejection. The mechanism of action of IVIG is not well-understood. Because IVIG may inhibit the production of antibodies by plasma cells, it may be useful in treating acute rejection episodes mediated by antibodies. However, some studies have shown IVIG to be effective in more common forms of cellular rejection. Further studies are needed to determine the optimal dose of IVIG and to determine whether it should be used as first-line therapy or for acute rejection episodes that are resist-ant to standard therapy.

## 6. How successful is treatment for acute rejection?

More than 90% of acute rejection episodes occurring in the first 6 months after trans-plantation can be reversed. Treatment is less successful in patients with late acute rejection episodes (occurring more than 1 year after transplantation).

## 7. What is chronic renal allograft rejection?

Chronic rejection is manifested clinically by a slow and gradual decline in renal allo-graft function, usually beginning more than 6 months after transplantation, and typically

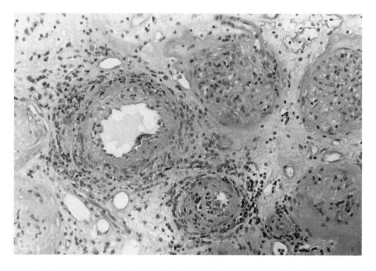

Light micrograph demonstrating the histologic changes of chronic renal allograft rejection including varying degrees of glomerulosclerosis and vascular intimal fibroplasia.

accompanied by moderate to heavy proteinuria. Histologically, chronic rejection is characterized by glomerulosclerosis, interstitial fibrosis, and obliteration of arteriolar lumina. The vasculopathy is mediated initially by lymphocytic invasion of the intima followed by infiltration of macrophages and proliferation of smooth muscle cells that ultimately lead to intimal fibrosis reminiscent of atherosclerosis (see figure). Because the pathophysiology of chronic rejection is poorly understood, treatment is unsatisfactory. Chronic rejection is currently the most common cause of long-term renal allograft failure.

**8. What is known about the pathophysiology of chronic rejection?**
Both immune and nonimmune factors play a role. Because chronic rejection is most common in patients who have experienced multiple episodes of acute rejection, it has been suggested that chronic rejection results from "smoldering" or inadequately treated acute rejection. Nonimmune factors speculated to play a role in chronic rejection include:

- Systemic hypertension
- Hyperlipidemia
- Viral infections, especially cytomegalovirus
- Drug toxicity (e.g., cyclosporine, tacrolimus)
- Ischemic injury

**9. Can immune and nonimmune forms of chronic allograft nephropathy be distinguished histologically?**
Recently, deposition of C4d in peritubular capillaries as detected by immunofluorescence microscopy has been proposed as a marker of antibody-mediated chronic allograft nephropathy. C4d is a fragment of the classical complement pathway component C4. When C4 is activated by antigen-antibody complexes, the C4d fragment is cleaved and binds covalently to tissues at the site of complement activation. A high correlation between C4d deposits and the detection of antidonor antibodies forms the basis for hypothesizing that C4d is a marker for ongoing immune injury. However, further studies are needed to determine whether therapeutic intervention in C4d-positive patients will have any impact on allograft outcome.

**10. Is there any treatment for chronic rejection?**
Because chronic rejection is characterized histologically by sclerosis and fibrosis, recently there has been interest in the possibility that the disorder is mediated by the upregulation of fibrogenic growth factors. A number of drugs, including angiotensin-converting enzyme (ACE) inhibitors, angiotensin receptor antagonists, and HMG coenzyme A (CoA)-reductase inhibitors, are capable of inhibiting these growth factors and may prove to be effective in retarding the rate of progressive renal impairment in patients with chronic rejection. As noted in question 9, further trials are needed to determine whether increasing immunosuppression will have a beneficial impact on patients with chronic allograft nephropathy and C4d deposits within the allograft.

**11. Where is Banff? What are the Banff criteria?**
A group of nephrologists and nephropathologists, apparently fond of the Canadian Rockies, has periodically convened in the lovely town of Banff, Alberta, to develop standardized histologic criteria for the diagnoses of acute and chronic renal allograft rejection. Each meeting has resulted in classification schemes that are increasingly complex. The simplified criteria for acute renal allograft rejection follow:

| BANFF GRADE | HISTOLOGY |
|---|---|
| I | Interstitial edema and tubulitis (i.e., lymphocytic invasion of tubular basement membranes) |
| II | More severe tubulitis with or without mild vasculitis characterized by intimal lymphocytic infiltrates |
| III | Severe vasculitis with fibrinoid necrosis |

## BIBLIOGRAPHY

1. Basadonna GP, Matas AJ, Gillingham KJ, et al: Early versus late acute renal allograft rejection: Impact on chronic rejection. Transplantation 55:993–998, 1993.
2. Casadei DH, Rial MD, Opelz G, et al: A randomized and prospective study comparing treatment with high-dose intravenous immunoglobulin with monoclonal antibodies for rescue of kidney grafts with steroid-resistant rejection. Transplantation 71:53–58, 2001.
3. Hariharan S, Alexander JW, Schroeder TJ, First MR: Impact of first acute rejection episode and severity of rejection on cadaveric renal allograft survival. Clin Transplant 10:538–543, 1996.
4. Hricik DE, Almawi WY, Strom TB: Trends in the use of glucocorticoids in renal transplantation. Transplantation 57:979–989, 1994.
5. Leggat JE, Ojo AD, Leichtman AB, et al: Long-term allograft survival: Prognostic implication of the timing of acute rejection episodes. Transplantation 63:1268–1272, 1997.
6. Mauiyyedi S, Pelle PD, Saidman S, et al: Chronic humoral rejection: Identification of antibody-mediated chronic renal allograft rejection by C4d deposits in peritubular capillaries. J Am Soc Nephrol 12:574–582, 2001.
7. Solez K, Axelson RA, Benediktsson H, et al: International standardization of criteria for the histologic diagnosis of renal allograft rejection: The Banff working classification of kidney transplant pathology. Kidney Int 44:411–422, 1993.
8. Tilney NL, Whitley DW, Diamond JR, et al: Chronic rejection: An undefined conundrum. Transplantation 52:389–398, 1991.

# 56. RENAL TRANSPLANTATION: IMMUNOSUPPRESSION

*Kenneth A. Bodziak, M.D.*

**1. What are the general principles underlying current immunosuppressive treatment strategies for kidney transplant recipients?**

1. The benefits of a successful transplant outweigh the risks of chronic immunosuppression.

2. Immunosuppressive therapy is required indefinitely to maintain allograft function. Although a small fraction of transplant recipients develop immunologic tolerance to their allografts, no satisfactory tests confirm this state of tolerance. Complete withdrawal of immunosuppression, whether patient- or physician-directed, is associated with a prohibitive risk of potentially irreversible allograft rejection.

3. Multidrug regimens generally are employed to prevent rejection by inhibiting T-cell immunity through disparate mechanisms.

4. Large doses of immunosuppressant drugs are used in the early post-transplant period. In patients who remain free of rejection, doses generally are tapered over time. Complete elimination of one or more drugs from multidrug regimens is possible in many stable patients.

**2. What are the risks associated with chronic immunosuppressive drug therapy?**

Each of the currently prescribed immunosuppressive agents is associated with unique side effects (see question 10). The common risks of major concern are **infection** (especially opportunistic infections) and **malignancy** (especially lymphoproliferative disease). These risks are enhanced in certain settings. For example, the risk of infection or malignancy may be increased in patients treated for acute rejection with antibody preparations. The risk of cytomegalovirus (CMV) infection is increased when a CMV-seronegative recipient receives an organ from a CMV-seropositive donor. The risk of lymphoproliferative disease is increased when an Epstein-Barr virus (EBV)–seronegative recipient receives an organ from an EBV-seropositive donor.

**3. What is induction immunosuppressive therapy?**

*Induction therapy* refers to the immunosuppressive drug therapy provided during the early post-transplant period (i.e., the first 1–3 weeks following transplant surgery). However, more commonly, the term describes the use of anti–T-cell antibodies during this early post-transplant period.

**4. What antibodies are used for induction therapy?**

**Polyclonal antibodies** (that bind to multiple cell surface molecules):
- Antithymocyte gamma-globulin (ATGAM)
- Thymoglobulin
- Other noncommercial preparations derived from injection of human thymocytes or immunoblasts into horses, rabbits, or other animals

**Monoclonal antibodies** (that bind to specific cell surface molecules):
- OKT3
- Anti-CD25 (anti–interleukin-2 [IL-2] receptor) antibodies:
    Basiliximab (Simulect)
    Daclizumab (Zenapax)

## 5. What is the rationale for induction therapy?

Theoretically, the use of induction antibodies prevents the development of acute rejection in the early postoperative period. Some, but not all, studies suggest that the use of these agents results in a lower incidence of subsequent rejection episodes and better long-term allograft survival. In addition, because perioperative use of nephrotoxic calcineurin inhibitors (i.e., cyclosporine or tacrolimus) may increase the severity and duration of delayed graft function, use of an antibody preparation may allow a delay in the introduction of the calcineurin inhibitor until adequate renal function is established. However, the benefits and risks of induction therapy have been a subject of debate. Some studies indicate that induction antibodies simply delay the time to onset of first rejection episodes. Any benefit of these expensive agents must be weighed against their potential to increase the risks of infection and malignancy. Many centers now limit use of these antibodies to transplant recipients deemed to be at high risk for rejection (i.e., African-American patients, second transplant recipients, patients who are highly sensitized as evidenced by high titers of human leukocyte [HLA] antibodies, and those with delayed allograft function following transplant surgery).

## 6. What is the immunologic basis for maintenance immunosuppression?

The T lymphocyte plays a central role in the acute rejection of allografts. Proliferation

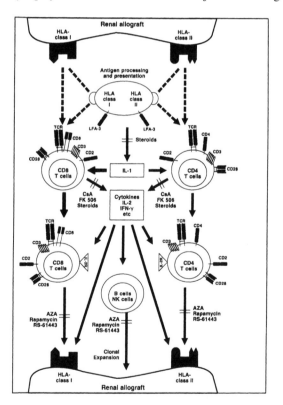

Abbreviations and drug names: HLA class I = HLA A, B, and C antigens; HLA class II = HLA DR and DQ antigens; TCR = T-cell receptor; AZA = azathioprine; IL-1 = interleukin 1; IL-2 = IFN-γ = interferon-γ; NK cells = natural killer cells; RS-61443 = mycophenolate mofetil; FK506 = tacrolimus; CsA = cyclosporine; Rapamycin = sirolimus. (Adapted from Strom TB, Suthanthiran M: Mechanisms of graft rejection. In Sayegh MH, Turka LA (eds): ASTP Lectures in Transplantation. Philadelphia, CoMed Communications, 1996, with permission.)

of T cells is initiated by recognition of antigens that are presented to the T-cell receptor–CD3 complex either directly as major histocompatibility complex (MHC) molecules on donor cells or indirectly as antigens that are processed and presented within the grooves of MHC molecules of the recipient's antigen presenting cells. Full activation of the T cell requires other costimulatory ligands between surface receptors on the lymphocyte and on antigen presenting cells. These cell surface ligands result in a cascade of intracellular events that ultimately stimulate nuclear transcription of IL-2 and other cytokines that promote the proliferation of antigen-specific clones of cytotoxic T cells that can directly injure the allograft. CD4-positive T cells are involved in the afferent antigen-recognition loop of this immune reaction, while CD8-positive T cells are cytotoxic cells that mediate the efferent cytodestructive loop of the reaction. The afferent and efferent loops of the reaction are shown schematically in the figure, which also depicts the site of action of commonly used immunosuppressive drugs.

## 7. What are the major classes of maintenance immunosuppressive drugs?

*Classes of Maintenance Immunosuppressive Drugs*

| CLASS | EXAMPLES |
|---|---|
| Immunophilin-binding agents | Calcineurin inhibitors<br>　Cyclosporine<br>　Tacrolimus (FK506)<br>Calcineurin-independent agents<br>　Sirolimus (rapamycin) |
| Glucocorticoids | |
| Antimetabolites | Purine inhibitors: nonselective<br>Azathioprine<br>Purine inhibitors: lymphocyte selective<br>Mycophenolate mofetil (RS-61443)<br>Mizoribine*<br>Pyrimidine inhibitors<br>Brequinar* |
| Poorly understood mechanisms | Deoxyspergualin*<br>Leflunomide* |

*Experimental or not yet approved by the Food and Drug Administration (FDA).

## 8. What is an immunophilin and how do immunophilin-binding agents work?

The term *immunophilin* refers to a group of cytosolic proteins that bind certain immunosuppressive agents (e.g., cyclosporine, tacrolimus, and sirolimus). The mechanism of the immunophilin-drug combination leading to inhibition of T-cell function is depicted in the figure. On stimulation with antigens, the T-cell receptor–CD3 complex and the associated CD4 or CD8 proteins activate cytosolic tyrosine kinases. Tyrosine phosphorylation and activation of phospholipase C leads to hydrolysis of phosphatidylinositol 4,5-biphosphate and generation of inositol 1,4,5-triphosphate ($IP_3$) and diacylglycerol. $IP_3$ mobilizes intracellular calcium. Calcium activates the calmodulin-dependent phosphatase, calcineurin. Diacylglycerol stimulates protein kinase C activity. Calcineurin and protein kinase C either directly or indirectly modulate regulatory molecules, such as nuclear factor of activated T cells (NF-AT) and NF-κβ, that control the production of messenger RNA for IL-2, a cytokine that plays a key role in promoting growth and proliferation.

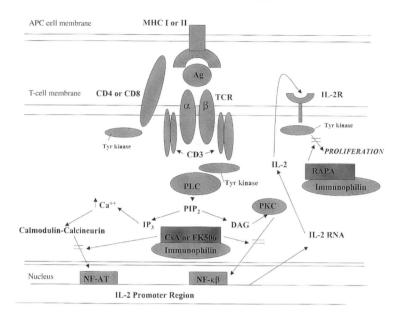

Abbreviations and drug names: Tyr kinase = tyrosine kinase; PLC = phospholipase C; TCR = T-cell receptor; PIP2 = phosphatidylinositol 4,5-biphosphate; IP3 = inositol 1,4,5-trphosphate; DAG = diacyglycerol; PKC = protein kinase C; IL-2 = interleukin-2; IL-2R = interleukin-2 receptor; NF-AT = nuclear factor of activated T cells; NF-κβ =nuclear factor-κβ; CsA = cyclosporine; FK506 = tacrolimus; RAPA = sirolimus.

Cyclosporine binds to an immunophilin called *cyclophilin*. Tacrolimus binds to a distinct immunophilin called *FK-binding protein*. The immunophilin-drug combination inhibit the actions of calcineurin and protein kinase C, thereby preventing the transcription of messenger RNA for IL-2 and other cytokines. Rapamycin (sirolimus) also binds to FK-binding protein. However, this immunophilin-drug combination does not interfere with IL-2 production but somehow blocks signal transduction that is mediated by stimulation of the IL-2 receptor and that ultimately yields cell proliferation.

**9. What are some commonly used combinations of maintenance immunosuppressive drugs?**

The recent introduction of new immunosuppressive drugs has increased the number of possible drug combinations available to prevent rejection. Currently, most centers use a combination of glucocorticoids and either cyclosporine or tacrolimus for initial maintenance immunosuppression. Many centers add either mycophenolate mofetil or azathioprine to this combination for so-called **triple therapy**. Recently, sirolimus has been used as a replacement for mycophenolate mofetil or azathioprine. Because sirolimus binds to the same immunophilin as tacrolimus, the two drugs are theoretically antagonists so that sirolimus initially was used in conjunction with cyclosporine. It is now known that the immunophilin FK-binding protein is very prevalent in the cell cytoplasm, so that sirolimus actually works synergistically with both tacrolimus and cyclosporine. Because of the long-term side effects and expense of maintenance immunosuppression, a number of clinical trials are currently testing the safety and benefits of withdrawing single drugs from multidrug regimens in stable patients.

## 10. What are the common side effects of immunosuppressive drugs?

*Side Effects of Glucocorticoids*

| | |
|---|---|
| Weight gain with cushingoid features | Dermatologic effects (acne, striae, easy |
| Hypertension | bruisability, impaired wound healing) |
| Hyperlipidemia | Impaired growth |
| Osteopenia | Glucose intolerance |
| Cataracts | |

*Side Effects of Immunophilin-binding Agents*

| SIDE EFFECT | CYCLOSPORINE | TACROLIMUS | SIROLIMUS |
|---|---|---|---|
| Nephrotoxicity | ++ | ++ | − |
| Neurotoxicity (tremor, seizures) | + | ++ | − |
| Hirsutism | ++ | − | − |
| Gingival hyperplasia | + | − | − |
| Hypertension | ++ | + | − |
| Hyperlipidemia | ++ | +/− | +++ |
| Glucose intolerance | + | +++ | − |
| Bone marrow suppression | − | − | ++ |

*Side Effects of Antimetabolites*

| SIDE EFFECT | AZATHIOPRINE | MYCOPHENOLATE MOFETIL |
|---|---|---|
| Bone marrow suppression | +++ | ++ |
| Gastrointestinal | + | ++ |

*Side Effects of Induction Antibodies*

| SIDE EFFECT | OKT3 | POLYCLONALS | ANTI-CD25 AGENTS |
|---|---|---|---|
| Fever | +++ | + | − |
| Headache | ++ | + | − |
| Myalgias | ++ | + | − |
| Gastrointestinal (diarrhea, nausea) | ++ | − | − |
| Respiratory distress | + | +/− | − |

## 11. What are the common drug interactions of concern with immunosuppressants?

The principal drug interactions involve the immunophilin-binding agents with drugs that are metabolized through cytochrome P450-3A4. Drugs that decrease metabolism of the immunophilin-binding agents include antifungals (ketoconazole, itraconazole, and fluconazole), macrolides (erythromycin and clarithromycin), calcium channel blockers (verapamil, diltiazem, and nicardipine), and metoclopramide. Grapefruit juice possesses a bioflavonoid that also interacts with these drugs to result in elevated blood levels of these immunosuppressants. Drugs that increase metabolism include anticonvulsants (e.g., carbamazepine, phenytoin, and phenobarbital) and antibiotics (e.g., rifampin, rifabutin, and isoniazid).

Azathioprine has a well-described interaction with allopurinol, a xanthine oxidase inhibitor, that can result in profound leukopenia. The rule of thumb is to reduce the azathioprine dose by 66–75% at time of initiating allopurinol. An alternative approach is to discontinue azathioprine altogether and place the patient on mycophenolate mofetil, which has no interaction with allopurinol.

## 12. What does the future hold for new immunosuppressive strategies?

Specific immunologic tolerance, that is, tolerance to an allograft without the need for immunosuppressive drugs and without loss of immunity to other exogenous antigens, would allow organ transplantation without the need for toxic immunosuppressants. To date, it has not been possible to achieve true tolerance in humans. In some animal species, specific tolerance has been achieved using some combination of bone marrow ablation, donor-specific bone marrow transplantation, and anti–T-cell antibodies following transplantation of an allograft. It remains unclear whether similar strategies will be successful in humans. Other novel approaches to achieving states of immunologic hyporesponsiveness are currently being explored and include the administration of peptides derived from MHC molecules, administration of antisense oligonucleotides, and use of antibodies that block costimulatory ligands between T cells and antigen-presenting T cells. The latter strategy has been successfully employed to induce tolerance in murine models with antibodies that block the CD40 or CD28 pathways. Somewhat surprisingly, it has been shown that concomitant administration of cyclosporine prevents tolerance induction, leading one to surmise that tolerance induction relies on active T-cell receptor to signal events that are targets of cyclosporine.

BIBLIOGRAPHY

1. de Mattos AM, Olyaei AJ, Bennett WM: Pharmacology of immunosuppressive medications used in renal diseases and transplantation. Am J Kidney Dis 28:631–637, 1996.
2. Germain RN: MHC-dependent antigen processing and peptide presentation: Providing ligands for T lymphocyte activation. Cell 76:287–299, 1994.
3. Gummert JF, Ikonen T, Morris RE: Newer immunosuppressive drugs: A review. J Am Soc Nephrol 10:1366–1380, 1999.
4. Gudmundsdottir H, Turka LA: T cell costimulatory blockade: New therapies for transplant rejection. J Am Soc Nephrol 10:1356–1365, 1999.
5. Miceli MC, Parnes JR: The role of CD4 and CD8 in T-cell activation. Semin Immunol 3:133–141, 1991.
6. Larsen CP, Elwood ET, Alexander DZ, et al: Long-term acceptance of skin and cardiac allografts after blocking CD40 and CD28 pathways. Nature 381:434–438, 1996.
7. Norman DJ: Antilymphocyte antibodies in the treatment of allograft rejection: Targets, mechanisms of action, monitoring, and efficacy. Semin Nephrol 12:315–324, 1992.
8. Strom TB, Suthanthiran M: Mechanisms of graft rejection. In Sayegh MH, Turka LA (eds): ASTP Lectures in Transplantation. Philadelphia, CoMed Communications, 1996.
9. Suthanthiran M, Morris RE, Strom TB: Immunosuppressants: Cellular and molecular mechanisms of action. Am J Kidney Dis 28:159–172, 1996.
10. Weiss A, Litman DR: Signal transduction by lymphocyte antigen receptors. Cell 76:263–264, 1994.

# 57. COMPLICATIONS OF RENAL TRANSPLANTATION

*Kenneth A. Bodziak, M.D.*

### 1. What is the incidence of post-transplant hypertension?
The reported incidence of post-transplant hypertension, defined as blood pressure values of > 140 (systolic) or > 90 (diastolic), is between 50% and 80%.

### 2. What are the common causes of post-transplant hypertension?
Common causes include treatment with the immunosuppressant medications (namely corticosteroids and the calcineurin inhibitors), preexisting essential hypertension, dysfunction of the allograft (acute or chronic rejection), diseased native kidneys, and renal artery stenosis of the allograft itself. The latter has been reported to occur in 2–12% of adult transplant recipients and should be suspected in any patient with refractory hypertension, a decline in renal function in the setting of an angiotensin-converting enzyme (ACE) inhibitor or angiotensin receptor blocker (ARB), or a diastolic bruit over the graft.

### 3. How does one diagnose and treat renal artery stenosis of the transplant kidney?
Although potentially very useful, Doppler ultrasound is also very operator-dependent. The gold standard remains angiography, with $CO_2$ angiography serving as an attractive alternative to conventional angiography, which requires administration of potentially nephrotoxic dyes. If renal artery stenosis is identified, the best treatment, if anatomically feasible, is percutaneous transluminal angioplasty with stent placement. Failing this approach, surgery may be considered. However, graft loss after surgical repair of the stenosed renal artery has been reported to be as high as 30%, reflecting the degree of difficulty in this procedure.

### 4. What, if any, are the preferred antihypertensives in the treatment of post-transplant hypertension?
Although there is no universally agreed upon regimen of antihypertensives in the treatment of post-transplant hypertension, certain classes of drugs have theoretic benefits. The dihydropyridines (e.g., amlodipine) have been shown to limit cyclosporine-induced vasoconstriction of the afferent arteriole. The non-dihydropyridines, such as verapamil and diltiazem, can not only prevent the vasoconstriction caused by cyclosporine, but also raise cyclosporine levels by inhibiting its metabolism. ACE inhibitors and ARBs can decrease proteinuria and may reduce renal fibrosis caused by the calcineurin inhibitors, but their use in this population may be complicated by hyperkalemia, anemia, or renal insufficiency.

### 5. What is the incidence of post-transplant diabetes mellitus (PTDM)?
The reported incidence of PTDM historically has varied from 2% to 46% depending on the criteria used to define DM. More recent reports have found that 4.9% of patients who had no previous history of glucose intolerance required insulin, whereas another 6.2% needed treatment with an oral agent for hyperglycemia post-transplant.

### 6. What are the risk factors for developing PTDM?
A recent multicenter study found no significant difference in the incidence of PTDM either by use of calcineurin inhibitor or by the race of the recipient. Interestingly, there was

a significant association between the absence of an antiproliferative agent (e.g., azathio-prine, mycophenolate mofetil) and the development of PTDM. The age, gender, weight at transplantation, number of transplants, and use of prednisone did not reach statistical significance for developing PTDM. Many other studies have suggested, however, that African-American ethnicity increases the risk of PTDM, and that tacrolimus is more diabetogenic than cyclosporine.

**7. What is the prevalence of hyperlipidemia post-renal transplant?**

In a report by the National Kidney Foundation Task Force on Cardiovascular Disease, over 60% of renal transplant patients had cholesterol levels of > 240 mg/dl and roughly the same percentage had low-density lipoprotein (LDL) cholesterol levels > 130 mg/dl. Triglyceride levels of > 200 mg/dl were found in approximately one-third of the patients. Corticosteroids are known to raise cholesterol levels by inducing insulin resistance, hyperinsulinemia, and increased hepatic very low-density lipoprotein (VLDL) production. Cyclosporine-treated patients have higher triglyceride and lipoprotein A levels compared with prednisone and azathioprine-treated patients. Sirolimus is associated with marked increases in triglyceride levels, as well. Withdrawal of steroids can lead to a decline in both LDL and high-density lipoprotein (HDL) cholesterol in a proportionate manner. Treatment with statins can be used, but with some caution, because synergism with the calcineurin inhibitors can lead to rhabdomyolysis; this is especially true when given in conjunction with fibric acid derivative, such as gemfibrozil.

**8. What are the most common malignancies in transplant recipients?**

The incidence of neoplasia is higher in transplant recipients than in the general population. Cancer of the skin and lip accounts for 40–53% of all malignancies in transplant recipients. Unlike the nonimmunosuppressed individual, squamous cell skin cancer is more common than basal cell cancer. Infection by human papillomavirus appears to be a risk factor for the development of skin cancer among transplant patients; it has been detected in close to 60% of nonmelanoma skin cancers in this population. Lymphoma, anogenital carcinomas, and Kaposi's sarcoma are examples of other malignancies that occur with greater frequency in transplant recipients than in the general population or in the dialysis population.

**9. What is post-transplant lymphoproliferative disease (PTLD)?**

PTLD is a neoplastic disorder that occurs as a complication of immunosuppressive therapy in solid-organ transplant recipients. Many cases result from proliferation of lymphocytes in response to reactivation of Epstein-Barr virus (EBV). The disorder sometimes presents as a mononucleosis-like syndrome with generalized lymphadenopathy. In such cases, lymph node pathology typically reveals a polyclonal proliferation of B lymphocytes that often regresses with reduction or temporary cessation of immunosuppression. More commonly, PTLD presents as frank lymphoma that demonstrates an unusual proclivity for involvement of extranodal sites such as the gastrointestinal tract or brain. In these cases, pathologic examination typically reveals a monoclonal B-cell lymphoma. Treatment usually includes chemotherapy and simultaneous reduction of overall immunosuppression.

**10. What percentage of kidney transplant patients develop PTLD?**

The overall incidence of PTLD is between 1.5% and 2.0%; however, there appears to be wide geographic variation in the reported incidence. At least half of the reported cases of PTLD are EBV-related. The incidence of lymphoma is higher in patients who have received antibody therapy (monoclonal or polyclonal) for either induction therapy or treatment of rejection and is highest during the first post-transplant year. Lymphomas represent approximately 16% of all post-transplant tumors reported to the Israel Penn Transplant Tumor Registry. Other risk factors include age (higher risk in children), transplantation between an EBV-positive donor and an EBV-negative recipient, and very high cumulative doses of immunosuppressive drugs.

**11. What bone diseases are common in transplant recipients?**
Aseptic necrosis of bone is a well-known complication of high-dose corticosteroid use. Typically, it occurs in the hips and shoulders. This often occurs in the context of preexisting renal osteodystrophy, which further weakens bone. In individuals with severe neuropathy due to uremia or diabetes, bone calcium loss may be accelerated, leading to osteomalacia. Osteopenia, largely attributable to chronic steroid therapy, occurs in many renal transplant recipients within 6 months of the transplant surgery. Osteoporosis, defined as bone density > 2.5 standard deviations below the young adult mean value, may be seen in up to 60% of renal transplant recipients who receive corticosteroids during the initial 18 months after transplantation. Risk factors other than cumulative doses of corticosteroids include female gender and postmenopausal status. For this reason, it is recommended that dual x-ray absorptiometry of the lumbar spine and hip be performed 6 months after transplant and annually thereafter.

**12. What percentage of kidney transplant recipients suffer from some type of infection (other than commonplace viral upper respiratory infections) in the first year?**
Seventy-five percent of patients experience nontrivial infections during the first post-transplant year. During the initial month, these infections are similar to those that may affect a nonimmunocompromised patient: wound infections, urinary tract infections, pneumonia, and intravenous line infections. Opportunistic infections are unusual during this time.

**13. What is the most common opportunistic infection in the first 6 months post-transplant?**
Infection with cytomegalovirus (CMV) is the most common opportunistic infection occurring during the first 6 months following kidney transplantation. Common symptoms include fever and general malaise that may accompany organ-specific symptoms of esophagitis, gastritis, hepatitis, colitis, and pneumonitis. Less common opportunistic infections include *Pneumocystis carinii, Aspergillus, Listeria monocytogenes,* and *Nocardia asteroides.*

**14. Which transplant patients are at greatest risk for clinical CMV infection?**
Individuals who are seronegative for CMV prior to the transplant and who then receive an organ from a CMV-positive donor are at highest risk (disease occurring at a rate of 56–80% in patients not treated prophylactically). These patients have no protective antibody and become infected when CMV is transmitted from the donor organ at a time of maximal immunosuppression in the early transplant period. Of course, the lowest risk group would be CMV-negative recipients receiving transplants from CMV-negative donors (disease incidence < 5%). Intermediate risk is present when the donor and recipient are both CMV-positive.

**15. What is the incidence of hepatitis C among renal transplant recipients?**
Anti-hepatitis C virus antibodies have been found in 10–40% of renal transplant recipients. Hepatitis C virus infection may be associated with an increased incidence of death resulting from liver disease and sepsis, but this remains a controversial issue.

**16. What is the incidence of post-transplant erythrocytosis among renal allograft recipients?**
Erythrocytosis, defined as a hemoglobin level of > 17–18 gm/dl or a hematocrit of > 51–52%, has been reported in 10–20% of renal allograft recipients. Complications associ-

ated with erythrocytosis include increased risk of thromboembolic events and cardiovascular disease. Methods of treatment include periodic phlebotomy and the administration of ACE inhibitors or ARBs.

### 17. What is the most common reason for failure of a kidney transplant?

Chronic rejection (see Chapter 55) is now the leading cause of renal allograft failure beyond the first post-transplant year. Among kidney transplants that function for at least 1 year, half will fail by the ninth post-transplant year. This percentage is unchanged from that seen 15 years ago, well before the availability of cyclosporine or "newer" antirejection drugs. Clinically, patients become hypertensive and moderately proteinuric and exhibit a gradual decline in renal function.

### 18. What are the most common causes of death in patients with functioning renal allografts?

Atherosclerotic vascular occlusive disease, sepsis, malignancy, and hepatic failure. Mortality from coronary artery disease is at least five times higher than that seen in the general population.

BIBLIOGRAPHY

1. Braun WE: Long-term complications of renal transplantation. Kidney Int 37:1363–1378, 1990.
2. Cohen D, Galbraith C: General health management and long-term care of renal transplant recipients. Am J Kidney Dis 38:S10–S24, 2001.
3. Curtis JJ: Hypertension following kidney transplantation. Am J Kidney Dis 23:471–475, 1994.
4. First MR, Gerber DA, Hariharan S, et al: Post-transplant diabetes mellitus in kidney allograft recipients: Incidence, risk factors, and management. Transplantation 73:379–386, 2002.
5. Fishman JA, Rubin RH: Infection in organ-transplant recipients. N Engl J Med 338:1741–1751, 1998.
6. Hill MN, Grossman RA, Feldman HI, et al: Changes in causes of death after renal transplantation: 1966 to 1987. Am J Kidney Dis 27:512–518, 1991.
7. Ho M: EBV infection and posttransplant lymphoproliferative disorders. Transplant Sci 2:88–92, 1992.
8. Julian BA, Quarles D, Niemann KM: Musculoskeletal complications after renal transplantation: Pathogenesis and treatment. Am J Kidney Dis 19:99–120, 1992.
9. Kasiske BL, Vasquez MA, Harmon WE, et al: Recommendations for the outpatient surveillance of renal transplant recipients. J Am Soc Nephrol 11:S1–S86, 2000.

# VIII. Hypertension

# 58. ESSENTIAL HYPERTENSION

*Mahboob Rahman, M.D., M.S.*

### 1. How is hypertension defined and classified?

In adults aged 18 years or older, blood pressure less than 120/80 mmHg is defined as optimal blood pressure, and readings greater than 140/90 mmHg are defined as hypertensive. Normal, high normal, and stages 1–3 of hypertension are defined below:

*Classification of Blood Pressure in Adults*

| CATEGORY | SYSTOLIC (mmHg) | | DIASTOLIC (mmHg) |
|---|---|---|---|
| Optimal | < 120 | *and* | < 80 |
| Normal | < 130 | *and* | < 85 |
| High normal | 130–139 | *or* | 85–89 |
| Hypertension | | | |
| Stage 1 | 140–159 | *or* | 90–99 |
| Stage 2 | 160–179 | *or* | 100–109 |
| Stage 3 | ≥ 180 | | ≥ 110 |

Data from National Institutes of Health: Sixth Report of the Joint National Committee on Prevention, Detection, Evaluation, and Treatment of High Blood Pressure. Bethesda, MD, NIH, 1997, NIH publication 98-4080.

### 2. What is the prevalence of hypertension in the United States? How well is blood pressure controlled in the general population?

An estimated 50 million Americans have high blood pressure. Hypertension is the leading cause of office visits to primary care physicians. Available evidence suggests that cardiovascular disease and all cause mortality increase progressively with higher blood pressure and that treatment of hypertension results in improved morbidity and mortality. However, even with widespread educational efforts, it is estimated that only 27% of patients with hypertension have blood pressure controlled to less than 140/90 mmHg.

### 3. What are the pathophysiologic mechanisms underlying essential hypertension?

Essential hypertension is a disorder of multifactorial etiologies resulting from a complex interaction of genetic factors, altered functional and structural mechanisms, and environmental factors. Most studies support the concept that inheritance of hypertension is polygenic, and a number of candidate genes are currently being investigated.

From a physiologic standpoint, all proposed mechanisms of essential hypertension have a final common pathway of increased peripheral vascular resistance. Increased sympathetic nervous system activity, alterations in the renin-angiotensin system, imbalances in the production of vasoactive metabolites such as nitric oxide and endothelins, and alterations in intracellular cation metabolism are candidate mechanisms and the focus of active investigation. A number of environmental factors such as dietary salt intake, stress, and obesity have also been implicated in the development of hypertension.

**4. What steps ensure that blood pressure is measured accurately?**

Patients should be seated in a chair with their backs supported, feet on the ground, and arms bared and supported at heart level. They should refrain from smoking or ingesting caffeine during the 30 minutes preceding the measurement and be rested for at least 5 minutes before the procedure. The appropriate-sized cuff should be used. Unless the width of the cuff is more than 40% of the circumference of the mid-upper arm, the blood pressure reading will be increased artifactually. Two or more readings separated by 2 minutes should be averaged.

**5. What is ambulatory blood pressure monitoring? When should it be used?**

Ambulatory blood pressure monitoring is a technique where several blood pressure readings are obtained over a 24-hour period while the patient goes about his usual daily activities. Some patients have "white coat" hypertension; they have high blood pressure readings at the physician's office and significantly lower blood pressure measurements at home. Ambulatory blood pressure monitoring is helpful in deciding if antihypertensive therapy is indicated in these patients. Other circumstances where ambulatory blood pressure monitoring can be useful are in the evaluation of resistant hypertension, occurrence of hypotensive episodes, episodic hypertension, and autonomic dysfunction.

**6. What are the goals of the initial evaluation of a hypertensive patient?**

The evaluation should be designed to identify known secondary causes of high blood pressure, to assess the presence of target organ damage, and to identify other cardiovascular risk factors or concomitant disorders that may affect the prognosis or choice of drug therapy.

**7. What are the key aspects of history and physical examination of the hypertensive patient?**

The history should include assessment of coexistent conditions (e.g., cardiac disease, cerebrovascular disease, peripheral vascular disease), family history of cardiovascular disease, symptoms suggestive of secondary hypertension, use of over-the-counter medications, and dietary, psychosocial and environmental factors that influence blood pressure. Physical exam should include funduscopic examination for hypertensive retinopathy, detection of bruits, assessment of the strength and symmetry of peripheral pulses, and palpation for thyromegaly.

**8. What lab tests should be ordered in the initial evaluation of a hypertensive patient?**

Laboratory tests help in determining the presence of target organ damage and other risk factors for cardiovascular disease. These include urinalysis, complete blood cell count (CBC), blood chemistry panel, total and high-density lipoprotein (HDL) cholesterol, and a 12-lead electrocardiogram (ECG). Other tests such as echocardiography and urinary microalbuminuria in patients with diabetes may be helpful in choosing antihypertensive therapy and determining goal blood pressure levels in selected patients.

**9. What signs and symptoms suggest that a work-up for secondary hypertension is needed?**

A work-up for secondary hypertension is indicated in the following circumstances:

- Patients whose blood pressure responds poorly to adequate drug therapy (three antihypertensive drugs at maximal dosage, including a diuretic)
- Patients who were well-controlled in the past and now have difficult-to-control hypertension
- Sudden onset of hypertension
- Onset of hypertension at a younger or older than usual age
- Signs and symptoms of known secondary causes of hypertension (see Chapter 62, Other Causes of Secondary Hypertension, and Chapter 63, Hypertensive Emergencies)

**10. How is cardiovascular risk assessed in patients with hypertension? How does cardiovascular risk influence management of hypertension?**

The presence of target organ damage and other concomitant risk factors influences the overall cardiovascular risk of hypertensive patients and, therefore, is used to stratify the risk in each individual and guide management of hypertension. Refer to the table below for the stratification scheme proposed in the Sixth Joint National Committee on Hypertension.

*Risk Stratification and Treatment of Hypertension*

| BLOOD PRESSURE STAGES | RISK GROUP A (NO RISK FACTORS, NO TOD/CCD) | RISK GROUP B (AT LEAST 1 RISK FACTOR, NOT DIABETES; NO TOD/CCD) | RISK GROUP C (TOD/CCD AND/OR DIABETES WITH OR WITHOUT OTHER RISK FACTORS) |
|---|---|---|---|
| High normal | Lifestyle modification | Lifestyle modification | Drug therapy |
| Stage 1 | Lifestyle modification | Lifestyle modification | Drug therapy |
| Stages 2 and 3 | Drug therapy | Drug therapy | Drug therapy |

TOD = target organ damage; CCD = clinical cardiovascular disease
Data from National Institutes of Health: Sixth Report of the Joint National Committee on Prevention, Detection, Evaluation, and Treatment of High Blood Pressure. Bethesda, MD, NIH, 1997, NIH publication 98-4080.

The major risk factors to consider are smoking, dyslipidemia, diabetes, age older than 60 years, sex (men and postmenopausal females), and family history of cardiovascular disease. The presence of heart disease (left ventricular hypertrophy, angina or myocardial infarction, coronary revascularization, and heart failure), stroke or transient ischemic attack, nephropathy, peripheral arterial disease, and retinopathy is evidence of target organ damage, and prompt institution of drug therapy is indicated.

**11. What lifestyle modifications are recommended for patients with essential hypertension?**

Lifestyle modification is an important part of management of patients with hypertension. All patients should be counseled to maintain desirable body weight, limit alcohol intake to less than 1 oz/day, and increase aerobic physical activity. In addition, sodium intake should be restricted to less than 100 mmol/day, and adequate dietary intake of potassium, calcium, and magnesium should be maintained. Smoking cessation and reduced dietary intake of saturated fat should be encouraged in all patients to improve overall cardiovascular health.

**12. What are the general principles of antihypertensive drug therapy?**

In patients with stage 1 or 2 hypertension, drug therapy should be initiated with a low dose of a single agent, preferably once a day. The dose should be titrated upward as needed for blood pressure control. If the blood pressure remains greater than 140/90 after 1–2 months despite monotherapy, a second agent from a different class (particularly a diuretic if not already being used) should be added. If blood pressure is not controlled with adequate doses of three antihypertensive medications, a work-up for resistant hypertension should be started in consultation with a hypertension specialist. Once-daily dosing is generally preferred due to better adherence, smooth and persistent control of hypertension, and lower cost.

**13. What are the main classes of antihypertensive drugs?**

**Diuretics**
Beta blockers
Alpha blockers
Angiotensin-converting enzyme
  (ACE) inhibitors

**Angiotensin receptor antagonists**
Calcium channel antagonists
Centrally acting agents
Direct vasodilators

**14. In patients with uncomplicated essential hypertension, which drugs are recommended for initial use?**

Diuretics and beta blockers are the preferred drugs for initial therapy in patients with uncomplicated essential hypertension. These drugs are effective in lowering blood pressure, are generally well tolerated, and have been shown in several prospective trials to lower morbidity and mortality. Diuretics are particularly effective in African-American and elderly patients. They may cause some metabolic side effects including short-term increases in glucose and cholesterol levels, hypokalemia, and hyperuricemia. Therefore, these biochemical parameters should be monitored on a periodic basis in patients on diuretic therapy. There are several different types of beta blockers depending on their cardioselectivity, lipid solubility, and intrinsic sympathomimetic activity. This class of drugs is a good choice in patients with coexisting coronary artery disease because of its antianginal properties. Beta blockers are contraindicated in patients with bronchospasm or advanced heart block and may mask insulin-induced hypoglycemia in diabetic patients.

**15. How do ACE inhibitors act? When should they be used and what are their side effects?**

The renin angiotensin system is an important homeostatic mechanism involved in maintaining blood pressure and salt and water balance. ACE inhibitors act by inhibiting the enzyme that converts angiotensin I to angiotensin II, which is a potent vasoconstrictor that also promotes renal retention of sodium. Captopril, lisinopril, enalapril, ramipril, and quinapril are some of the commonly used ACE inhibitors.

Due to their unique effects on lowering intraglomerular pressure, ACE inhibitors are particularly useful in diabetics and those with mild to moderate chronic renal insufficiency. In addition, this class of drugs has been shown to reduce morbidity and mortality in patients with congestive heart failure. The side effect profile is attributed to reduced degradation of bradykinin and similar vasodilator metabolites. Angioedema and agranulocytosis are rare but serious side effects of ACE inhibitor therapy. A dry cough is the most common side effect, occurring in 10–15% of patients.

**16. What is the mechanism of action of the angiotensin II receptor blockers? How do they differ from ACE inhibitors?**

Recently, a new class of drugs has been introduced that acts by blocking the angiotensin II receptors (losartan, candesartan, valsartan, irbesartan). These products do not interfere with the production of angiotensin II but bind to the angiotensin I receptor preventing the actions of angiotensin II in the target tissues. In theory, these drugs should have all the beneficial effects of ACE inhibition; in addition, because they do not interfere with bradykinin metabolism, the incidence of cough is much lower than ACE inhibitors. Long-term studies with angiotensin II receptor antagonists are currently under way.

**17. What are the commonly used calcium channel blockers and what are their common side effects?**

The dihydropyridine calcium channel blockers, including amlodipine, nifedipine, and felodipine, act primarily as vasodilators and are effective antihypertensive agents. The short-acting formulations of nifedipine may be associated with excessive and rapid lowering of blood pressure and are not recommended for routine use. The long-acting formulations are well-tolerated and are among the most frequently prescribed antihypertensive medications in the United States currently. Ankle edema, flushing, and headache are the common side effects of these agents. The nondihydropyridine calcium channel blockers are diltiazem and verapamil. In addition to their antihypertensive efficacy, they also can depress cardiac contractility and inhibit atrioventricular node conduction. These are generally well tolerated but should be used with caution in patients with impaired systolic function or bradyarrhythmias.

**18. What are some reasons for resistance to antihypertensive therapy?**

Patients may not respond adequately to antihypertensive therapy for several reasons. Nonadherence to therapy is always a consideration in a chronic and asymptomatic condition such as hypertension. Educating patients about the disease and using simple, once-a-day, and affordable drug regimens can help to improve patient compliance. Volume overload and excessive salt intake, particularly in patients with impaired renal function, are common causes of poor blood pressure control and require appropriate diuretic therapy. Use of inadequate doses of antihypertensive drugs, ingestion of other medications such as nonsteroidal anti-inflammatory drugs (NSAIDs) and sympathomimetic agents, and associated conditions such as obesity, sleep apnea, and excessive ethanol intake can also contribute to poor blood pressure control.

**19. What are the features of hypertension in African Americans?**

The prevalence of hypertension in African Americans is among the highest in the world. Compared with whites, hypertension develops earlier in life, and average blood pressures and risk of target organ damage are much higher in African Americans. Diuretics are the agents of choice in hypertensive African Americans and should be used unless there are compelling indications for alternative drugs. ACE inhibitors may be less potent in this population but, at higher doses and in combination with diuretics, are still effective antihypertensive agents.

**20. What are the clinical features of hypertension in elderly patients?**

Hypertension is very common in patients older than 60 years with prevalence of 60–70%. These patients frequently have predominantly systolic hypertension, and systolic blood pressure has been shown to be a better predictor of cardiovascular events than diastolic blood pressure. Blood pressure can sometimes be falsely high due to arterial stiffness and should be evaluated using Osler's maneuver. In addition, older patients are more likely to have an orthostatic fall in blood pressure; therefore, blood pressure should always be measured in the standing and supine positions.

Diuretics have been shown to lower morbidity and mortality from hypertension in older patients and are, therefore, recommended as initial therapy. Calcium channel blockers can also be used as alternative therapy. The goal of treatment is the same as in younger persons (less than 140/90 mmHg), though an interim goal of systolic blood pressure less than 160 mmHg may be necessary in patients with marked systolic hypertension.

**21. What are the treatment considerations in hypertensive patients who have coexistent cardiovascular disease?**

Patients with coronary heart disease are at high risk for cardiovascular morbidity and mortality and will benefit from good control of blood pressure. Excessively rapid lowering of blood pressure, particularly associated with reflex tachycardia, should be avoided in these patients. In patients who have had a myocardial infarction (MI), beta blockers without sympathomimetic activity are the drugs of choice. If there is evidence of left ventricular systolic dysfunction following an MI, then ACE inhibitors are especially beneficial.

Left ventricular hypertrophy (LVH) is an independent risk factor for cardiovascular events. Most antihypertensive agents (except direct vasodilators such as hydralazine and minoxidil) are capable of reducing left ventricular mass and wall thickness. In some studies, ACE inhibitors, perhaps due to their actions on the local renin angiotensin systems, have been shown to be more effective in inducing regression of LVH. Whether regression of LVH reduces morbidity and mortality independent of blood pressure reduction has not been shown.

Hypertension is a leading factor in the development of congestive heart failure. ACE inhibitors, when used alone or in conjunction with diuretics or digoxin, are effective in lowering morbidity and mortality in patients with congestive heart failure. When ACE inhibitors are not tolerated, a combination of hydralazine and isosorbide dinitrate can be used. Angiotensin receptor antagonists have recently been shown to be beneficial in the treatment of congestive heart failure.

### 22. What is salt-sensitive hypertension?

Salt-sensitive hypertension is a form of essential hypertension defined by an increment in mean arterial blood pressure > 10 mmHg with a salt challenge. Salt-resistant individuals have a negligible changes in blood pressure after a salt challenge. About two-thirds of hypertensive African Americans are salt-sensitive compared to one-third of non-African Americans.

### 23. What populations are more susceptible to salt sensitivity of blood pressure regulation?

African Americans
Elderly
Diabetics
Individuals with insulin resistance

BIBLIOGRAPHY

1. Brown NJ, Vaughan DE: Angiotensin-converting enzyme inhibitors. Circulation 97:1411–1420, 1998.
2. Cutler JA, Follman D, Allender PS: Randomized trials of sodium reduction: An overview. Am J Clin Nutr 65(suppl):643S–651S, 1997.
3. Douglas JG, Onwuzulike KC: Pathophysiology of primary (essential) hypertension. In Hricik DE, Wright JT, Smith MC (eds): Hypertension Secrets. Philadelphia, Hanley & Belfus, 2002, pp 21–28.
4. Freis ED: Current status of diuretics, beta-blockers, alpha-blockers, and alpha-beta-blockers in the treatment of hypertension. Med Clin North Am 81:1305–1317, 1997.
5. Kaplan NM: Resistant hypertension: What to do after trying "the usual." Geriatrics 50:24–38, 1995.
6. Lever A, Ramsay LE: Treatment of hypertension in the elderly. J Hypertens 13:571–579, 1995.
7. National Institutes of Health: Sixth Report of the Joint National Committee on Prevention, Detection, Evaluation, and Treatment of High Blood Pressure. Bethesda, MD, NIH, 1997, NIH publication 98-4080.
8. Rahman M, Douglas JG, Wright JT Jr: Pathophysiology and treatment implications of hypertension in the African American population. Endocrinol Metab Clin North Am 26:125–144, 1997.

# 59. RENAL PARENCHYMAL HYPERTENSION

*Michael C. Smith, M.D.*

### 1. Why is hypertension important in patients with renal disease?

1. Hypertension associated with renal parenchymal disease is the most common form of secondary hypertension; 5% of all hypertensive patients have underlying renal disease.

2. Hypertension is prevalent in renal disease. Of patients with pre-end-stage renal disease (ESRD), > 80% are hypertensive, and hypertension is present in 90% by the time ESRD ensues.

3. In addition to increasing cardiovascular morbidity and mortality, hypertension in patients with renal disease accelerates the loss of renal function. Glomerular filtration rate (GFR) declines more rapidly in hypertensive patients with renal disease compared with their normotensive counterparts.

### 2. Does hypertension occur in patients with acute renal disease? What are its causes?

Hypertension can complicate acute poststreptococcal glomerulonephritis, acute tubular necrosis, and minimal change disease. Twenty percent to 30% of adults with minimal change disease are hypertensive at initial presentation, whereas 40% of patients with acute tubular necrosis and 80% of those with acute poststreptococcal glomerulonephritis exhibit hypertension at some time during their clinical course. Evidence to date suggests that the majority of hypertensive patients with acute renal disease demonstrate volume-dependent hypertension that improves with resolution of the underlying disease or with salt removal during dialysis. In some, however, vasoconstrictor mechanisms (i.e., angiotensin II, activation of the sympathetic nervous system) contribute to the increase in blood pressure (BP).

### 3. What is the prevalence of hypertension in chronic renal parenchymal disease?

Estimates of hypertension in various chronic renal diseases range from 35% to 80% (see table).

| RENAL DISEASE | PERCENT OF PATIENTS WITH HYPERTENSION |
|---|---|
| Chronic glomerular disease | |
|     Focal glomerulosclerosis | 75–80 |
|     Membranoproliferative glomerulonephritis | 65–70 |
|     Diabetic nephropathy | 65–70 |
|     Membranous nephropathy | 40–50 |
|     Mesangioproliferative glomerulonephritis | 35–40 |
|     IgA nephropathy | 30–35 |
| Polycystic kidney disease | 60 |
| Chronic interstitial nephritis | 35 |

Hypertension is less prevalent early in the course of most renal diseases but is present in 80–90% of patients with end-stage renal disease.

### 4. What factors are causally related to the development of hypertension in patients with chronic renal disease?

Renal parenchymal hypertension results from the integrated interaction of multiple factors that affect cardiac output, peripheral resistance, or both. Although alterations in the production of natriuretic peptides, prostaglandins (PGs), and endothelin have been implicated in the genesis of experimental renal hypertension, their relevance to renal hypertension in humans is unclear. On the other hand, a positive salt balance, increased activity of the renin-angiotensin-aldosterone system (RAAS), and stimulation of the sympathetic nervous system (SNS) are important contributors to human renal parenchymal hypertension.

## 5. What evidence supports a crucial role for salt in the initiation and maintenance of renal parenchymal hypertension?

1. Many studies have shown that hypertensive subjects with mild-to-moderate renal impairment have increased total body sodium. Small changes in total body sodium often precede frank elevations of BP or increments in serum creatinine.

2. Increases in dietary salt expand extracellular fluid volume and augment arterial pressure in most patients with renal dysfunction. This hypertensive effect of dietary salt loading is inversely related to GFR and most evident in patients with ESRD.

3. Dietary salt restriction or diuretic administration in patients with pre-ESRD or salt removal during dialysis in patients with ESRD decreases total body sodium, extracellular fluid volume, and BP in renal parenchymal hypertension.

## 6. What data indicate an important role for the RAAS in renal parenchymal hypertension?

Activation of the RAAS increases BP not only through the vasoconstrictor action of angiotensin II (AII), but also because of augmented renal sodium reabsorption mediated by AII and aldosterone. In many, but not all, patients with pre-ESRD, plasma renin activity (PRA) and AII concentration are increased and correlate with BP. AII receptor blockade in some hypertensive patients with renal parenchymal disease results in a decrement in BP that is inversely proportional to baseline PRA. In 10% to 20% of patients with ESRD, BP is clearly renin dependent. In these patients, PRA often is increased, and BP does not normalize with salt removal during dialysis. Before the advent of minoxidil and angiotensin-converting enzyme (ACE) inhibitors, bilateral nephrectomy often was required to control BP in ESRD patients with resistant hypertension and elevated PRA.

## 7. How does increased SNS activity contribute to hypertension in renal disease?

Many studies have shown increased plasma norepinephrine concentrations in hypertensive patients with pre-ESRD. This enhanced SNS activity not only directly increases BP by increasing cardiac output and total peripheral resistance, but also indirectly augments BP by stimulation of the RAAS. Activation of renal sympathetic nerves increases sodium reabsorption, contributing to volume expansion and further increments in BP. The reason that patients with renal disease exhibited enhanced SNS activity had been unclear. Emerging experimental and clinical data support the concept that in diseased kidneys there is increased renal afferent sympathetic nerve traffic, which signals the anterior hypothalamus to increase central sympathetic outflow.

## 8. How are PGs involved in renal parenchymal hypertension?

Renal and extrarenal PGs play important roles in regulating vascular tone and salt excretion. Some PGs ($PGF_{2\alpha}$ and thromboxane $A_2$) are vasoconstrictor and antinatriuretic, whereas others ($PGE_2$ and $PGI_2$) are vasodilator and natriuretic. On balance, however, stimulation of endogenous PG synthesis tends to decrease BP. A decrease in renal PG production theoretically could contribute to renal parenchymal hypertension. PG production tends to be normal or increased in hypertensive patients with renal disease, however. This is due to the fact that AII and enhanced SNS activity directly stimulate renal synthesis of $PGE_2$ and $PGI_2$, and they modulate the direct intrarenal vasoconstrictor and antinatriuretic effects of AII and the SNS.

This has important therapeutic implications. Inhibition of renal PG production by administration of nonsteroidal anti-inflammatory drugs (NSAIDs) to hypertensive patients with renal disease can decrease salt excretion and exacerbate hypertension as well as causing acute-on-chronic renal failure. Sulindac and piroxicam may be more renal sparing than other nonselective cyclooxygenase (COX) inhibitors. Selective COX-2 inhibitors have the same adverse intrarenal hemodynamic profile as their nonselective counterparts. All NSAIDs should be used cautiously, if at all, in hypertensive patients with renal disease and only with careful monitoring of renal function and serum potassium.

**9. Describe the effect hypertension has on renal function in patients with renal disease.**
Hypertension accelerates the decline of renal function. This effect is mediated largely by hemodynamic mechanisms. The figure shows a schematic representation of glomeruli from a normal individual and a patient with hypertension and renal disease.

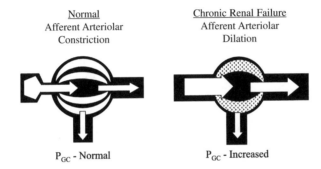

Normal
Afferent Arteriolar
Constriction

Chronic Renal Failure
Afferent Arteriolar
Dilation

$P_{GC}$ - Normal

$P_{GC}$ - Increased

Intrarenal response to systemic hypertension. (From Smith MC: Renal parenchymal hypertension. In Hricik DE, Wright JT, Smith MC (eds): Hypertension Secrets. Philadelphia, Hanley & Belfus, 2002, pp 31–36, with permission.)

Under normal circumstances (*left panel*), renal blood flow (RBF) and GFR are held constant over a wide range of mean arterial pressures (MAP) by constriction or dilation of the afferent arteriole. If systemic BP increases, the afferent arteriole constricts and intraglomerular capillary pressure ($P_{GC}$) remains normal. In renal disease (*right panel*), enhanced PG synthesis dilates the afferent arteriole and results in transmission of systemic BP to the glomerulus with a consequent increase in $P_{GC}$. This elevated glomerular pressure results in further hydraulically mediated damage, proteinuria, glomerulosclerosis, and a more rapid decrease in GFR.

**10. Does control of blood pressure retard the rate of decline in glomerular filtration rate?**
Reduction of systemic blood pressure limits glomerular damage and slows the rate of loss of kidney function in animal models of renal disease. Further, numerous prospective clinical trials have shown that excellent blood pressure control slows the progression of human renal parenchymal disease. Current recommendations suggest that reduction of blood pressure to a level of 130/80 mmHg should be a minimum goal in patients with chronic renal disease. Patients with diabetic nephropathy and nondiabetic patients with urine protein excretion greater than 1 gm/day, and especially those with greater than 3 gm/day, have a slower progression of renal disease with even lower blood pressure (i.e., 125/75 mmHg).

**11. Describe the initial therapeutic strategy in treating renal parenchymal hypertension.**
Because salt retention is central to the pathogenesis of hypertension in renal disease, a logical initial therapeutic approach requires dietary sodium restriction to 80 to 100 mmol/d.

When dietary salt restriction is in place, most patients still require diuretic therapy to achieve desired salt balance. Thiazide diuretics are generally ineffective with creatinine clearances < 30 ml/min. Hypertensive patients with this degree of renal insufficiency require loop-blocking diuretics, generally in a twice-a-day dosing regimen to achieve the requisite natriuresis. Diuretic therapy should be increased until the patient is free of edema. This approach can normalize BP in 25% to 30% of patients; the remainder require additional drug therapy to achieve goal BP.

## 12. If diuretic therapy does not control BP, what drug classes should be added next?

In patients with pre-ESRD, an antihypertensive drug should be logical from a pathophysiologic perspective, have a favorable side effect profile, exert a beneficial effect on cardiovascular morbidity and mortality, and retard the progression of renal disease.

- ACE inhibitors and angiotensin receptor blockers (ARBs) exert a unique renoprotective effect independent of their ability to lower BP. These drugs should be added to dietary salt restriction and diuretic therapy if BP is not at goal, provided that no contraindication (i.e., hyperkalemia, angioedema) exists.
- Calcium channel antagonists reduce BP despite extremes of dietary salt intake and are a logical next step if further reduction of BP is required.
- Centrally acting sympatholytics are excellent drugs from a pathophysiologic and practical perspective and often control BP in patients who have been resistant to the first three drug classes.

## 13. Is it the norm to require three or more drug classes in patients with renal parenchymal hypertension to achieve goal BP?

Yes, especially if the goal is ≤ 125/75 mmHg.

## 14. Are there risks to the use of ACE inhibitors or ARBs in hypertensive patients with renal insufficiency?

Yes. Two are most important.

1. Hyperkalemia can occur and is more likely with more severe renal dysfunction and in the face of additional constraints on potassium homeostasis (e.g., diabetes, nonselective β-blockade, digitalis). Serum potassium should be monitored frequently.

2. ACE inhibition or AII blockade can result in acute-on-chronic renal failure. These drugs dilate the efferent arteriole and in the face of a dilated afferent arteriole make GFR exquisitely dependent on systemic BP. If BP decreases excessively, filtration is compromised, and acute-on-chronic renal failure ensues (i.e., *no BP, no pee pee*).

## 15. What is the approach to the treatment of hypertension in patients with end-stage renal disease?

Eighty percent to 90% of hypertensive dialysis patients become normotensive if sufficient salt and water are removed by dialysis to achieve a true dry weight. The remaining patients require nondiuretic antihypertensive therapy. Because the pathogenesis of hypertension in dialysis patients is similar to that in patients with advanced chronic renal failure, selection of pharmacologic agents should be comparable. In this regard, ACE inhibitors, ARBs, centrally acting sympatholytics, and calcium channel antagonists are logical and effective selections.

### BIBLIOGRAPHY

1. Agodoa LY, Appel L, Bakris GL, et al: Effect of ramipril vs amlodipine on renal outcomes in hypertensive nephrosclerosis. JAMA 285:2719–2728, 2001.
2. Converse RL, Jacobsen TN, Toto RP, et al: Sympathetic overactivity in patients with chronic renal failure. N Engl J Med 327:1912–1918, 1992.

3. GISEN Group: Randomized placebo-controlled trial of effect of ramipril on decline in glomerular filtration rate and risk of terminal renal failure in proteinuric nondiabetic nephropathy. Lancet 349:1857–1863, 1997.
4. Ihle BU, Whitworth JA, Shahinfar S, et al: Angiotensin-converting enzyme inhibition in nondiabetic renal insufficiency: A controlled double-blind trial. Am J Kidney Dis 27:489–495, 1996.
5. Klahr S, Levey AS, Beck GJ, et al: The effects of dietary protein restriction and blood pressure control on the progression of chronic renal disease. N Engl J Med 330:877–894, 1994.
6. Kshirsagar AV, Joy MS, Hogan SL, et al: Effect of ACE inhibitors in diabetic and nondiabetic chronic renal disease: A systematic overview of randomized placebo-controlled trials. Am J Kidney Dis 35:695–707, 2000.
7. Lewis EJ, Hunsicker LG, Bain RP, Rohde KD: The effect of angiotensin-converting enzyme inhibition on progression of diabetic nephropathy. N Engl J Med 329:1456–1462, 1993.
8. Ligtenberg G, Blankestijn PJ, Oey PL, et al: Reduction of sympathetic hyperactivity by enalapril in patients with chronic renal failure. N Engl J Med 340:1321–1328, 1999.
9. Maschio G, Alberti D, Janin G, et al: Effect of the angiotensin-converting inhibitor benazepril on the progression of chronic renal insufficiency. N Engl J Med 334:939–945, 1996.
10. Peterson JC, Adler S, Burkhart JM, et al: Blood pressure control, proteinuria, and the progression of renal disease. The modification of diet in renal disease study. Ann Intern Med 123:754–762, 1995.
11. Rahman M, Smith MC: Chronic renal insufficiency. Arch Intern Med 158:1743–1752, 1998.
12. Schlondorff D: Renal complications of nonsteroidal anti-inflammatory drugs. Kidney Int 44:643–653, 1993.
13. Smith MC, Rahman M, Dunn MJ: Hypertension associated with renal parenchymal disease. In Schrier RW (ed): Diseases of the Kidney and Urinary Tract, 7th ed. Vol. 2. Philadelphia, Lippincott Williams & Wilkins, 2001, pp 1363–1397.

# 60. RENOVASCULAR HYPERTENSION

*Michael C. Smith, M.D., and Donald E. Hricik, M.D.*

### 1. What is renovascular hypertension?

The term *renovascular hypertension* refers to high blood pressure caused by occlusive disease of one or both main renal arteries or their branches. A diagnosis of renovascular hypertension can be made with certainty only by showing that high blood pressure is improved or cured after correction of the occlusion. However, decisions to proceed with interventions to correct occlusive renal arterial disease are based on a tentative diagnosis that requires anatomic or functional tests.

### 2. What is the pathophysiology of renovascular hypertension?

Renovascular hypertension results from activation of the renin-angiotensin-aldosterone system (RAAS) mediated by ischemia (see figure). Decreased perfusion to the affected kidney results in the release of renin, which, in turn, accelerates the conversion of angiotensinogen to angiotensin I. Angiotensin-converting enzyme (ACE) converts angiotensin I to angiotensin II, a peptide with potent vasoconstrictor properties. Angiotensin II also increases renal sodium absorption both directly and indirectly by stimulating the adrenal gland to release aldosterone. Hence, activation of the RAAS increases blood pressure through vasoconstrictor and volume-mediated mechanisms.

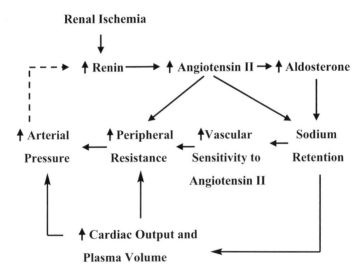

Pathophysiologic mechanism responsible for the development of renovascular hypertension. The solid line (—) indicates stimulation or augmentation; the dashed line (- - -) indicates inhibition.

The pathophysiology of renovascular hypertension varies depending on whether renal occlusive disease occurs in one kidney in a patient with two kidneys and a normal contralateral kidney ("two-kidney, one-clip model") or in a solitary kidney in a patient with no contralateral kidney ("one-kidney, one-clip model"). In the two-kidney model, the ischemic kidney secretes renin and retains salt and water, but the normal contralateral kidney exhibits a pressure natriuresis that actually leads to negative sodium balance, further exacerbating the release of renin. The clinical analogy is unilateral renal artery stenosis in a patient with two kidneys. In the one-kidney model, absence of a contralateral kidney prevents sodium loss. Extracellular volume expansion ensues, plasma renin activity is suppressed, and hypertension persists largely because of volume overload. Clinical analogies include renal artery stenosis in a patient with a solitary kidney and bilateral renal artery stenoses in a patient with two kidneys.

**3. What are the causes of renovascular hypertension?**
**Common causes of renovascular hypertension** (~ 95% of all cases):
- Atherosclerosis (75%)
- Fibromuscular dysplasia (20%)

**Rare causes of renovascular hypertension** (~ 5% of cases):
- Neurofibromatosis
- Extrinsic compression
- Congenital anomalies
- Radiation fibrosis
- Arterial thromboembolism
- Vasculitis
- Aortic dissection

**4. How common is renovascular hypertension?**
The reported prevalence of renovascular hypertension varies widely depending on the population studied and the type of tests performed to make the diagnosis. Autopsy studies suggest that as many as 40% of adults have at least mild narrowing of the renal arteries, but many cases may be clinically insignificant. Among severely hypertensive patients referred to tertiary care centers, the prevalence of renovascular hypertension may exceed 20% in patients studied with angiography. Most authorities agree, however, that renovascular disease probably accounts for high blood pressure in no more than 2–3% of the general population of patients with hypertension.

**5. What is fibromuscular dysplasia?**
Fibromuscular dysplasia is a nonarteriosclerotic occlusive vascular disease of unknown etiology. The disorder occurs most commonly in young or middle-aged adult women and is uncommon in African Americans. The dysplastic process primarily involves the renal arteries, but other vascular beds (e.g., cerebral vessels) can be involved. Four pathologic variants have been described. **Medial fibroplasia** is the most common (accounting for 70% of all cases) and is recognized angiographically by the classic "string of beads" appearance (see figure at top of next page). The less common variants are **intimal, perimedial,** and **adventitial fibrous dysplasia.**

**6. What clinical characteristics are typical of patients with renovascular hypertension?**
In most cases, renovascular hypertension cannot be differentiated clinically from essential hypertension. However, the following clinical features should increase suspicion and prompt diagnostic evaluation for possible renovascular disease:
- Progression in the severity of chronic hypertension
- Recent onset of hypertension in a patient without a family history of increased blood pressure
- Grade III or IV hypertensive retinopathy
- Moderate hypertension in a patient with diffuse vascular disease (especially if the patient is a smoker)

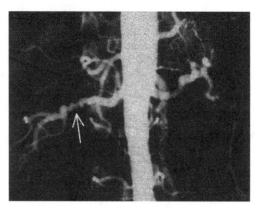

Renal angiogram demonstrating medial fibrous dysplasia in a main renal artery.

- Early (age < 25 years) or late (age > 60 years) onset
- Renal failure during treatment with an ACE inhibitor or angiotensin receptor blocker
- Abdominal or flank bruit
- Recurrent episodes of "flash" pulmonary edema
- Refractory hypertension (≥ 3 drugs)
- Unilateral small kidney

**7. What tests are used to make a diagnosis of renovascular hypertension?**

Angiography remains the gold standard for determining whether a patient has occlusive disease of the renal arteries. Digital subtraction angiography is preferred in some centers in an effort to minimize the amount of administered contrast dye. However, digital studies may not provide adequate images of the peripheral branches of the arterial tree. Angiographic techniques can detect anatomic abnormalities, but they do not provide information about the functional significance of a renal artery stenosis. Most clinicians would agree, however, that luminal narrowing of 70% or greater is usually clinically significant.

Because of the potential morbidity of angiography, numerous less-invasive tests have been developed to confirm the diagnosis of renovascular disease. Although many have been abandoned because of lack of sensitivity and specificity, some have proven valuable, and new tests have been developed that promise greater utility (see table). Recent experience suggests that computed tomography (CT) angiography, magnetic resonance angiography (MRA), and duplex ultrasonography are preferred tests to diagnose renovascular disease. However, selection among these tests should be based on local expertise.

*Diagnostic Tests for Renal Artery Stenosis*

| TEST | SENSITIVITY | SPECIFICITY |
| --- | --- | --- |
| CT angiography | 95% | 95% |
| MRA | 95% | 90% |
| Duplex ultrasonography | 85% | 90% |
| Captopril scintigraphy | 85% | 85% |
| Captopril test | 50% | 85% |

**8. How can you estimate the functional significant of RAAS in a hypertensive patient?**

Identification of a critical renal artery stenosis in a hypertensive patient does not necessarily indicate a causal relation. Moderate to severe renal artery stenoses have been found in a large proportion of normotensive patients at autopsy. Consequently, tests have been developed to predict the functional significance of renal artery stenosis in a hypertensive patient. Renal venous renin ratios ≥ 1.5 that lateralize to the ipsilateral side have a sensitivity of 70% and a specificity of 85% in predicting the response to percutaneous transluminal angioplasty (PTA), PTA plus stenting, or surgical revascularization. On the other hand, captopril renography utilizing hippuran has a sensitivity and specificity of 75% and 80%, respectively. Nevertheless, because the operating characteristics of these tests are suboptimal, most clinicians consider intervention on clinical grounds alone.

**9. How do angiotensin inhibitors cause renal failure in patients with renovascular disease?**

ACE inhibitor–induced renal failure was first described in patients with bilateral renal artery stenosis or renal artery stenosis involving a solitary kidney. Under circumstances in which the entire renal mass is hypoperfused as a consequence of arterial occlusion, intrarenal hemodynamics are altered such that autoregulation of glomerular filtration rate becomes critically dependent on the effects of angiotensin II on the efferent (postglomerular) capillaries. When angiotensin II is inhibited by an ACE inhibitor (or by an angiotensin receptor blocker), postglomerular resistance decreases. In theory, renal blood flow is maintained or increased, but glomerular filtration rate may fall dramatically. The hemodynamic pattern is best described as a dissociation in the autoregulation of renal blood flow and glomerular filtration rate.

The same phenomenon forms the basis for ACE inhibitor renography. In this diagnostic test, glomerular filtration rate is estimated by the clearance of a radioisotope under baseline conditions and again after administration of an ACE inhibitor. A decrease in the glomerular filtration rate suggests the presence of a functionally significant occlusion.

**10. What are the objectives of therapy in patients with renovascular disease?**
1. Control systemic blood pressure
2. Preserve or improve renal function

**11. What treatments are available for patients with renovascular hypertension?**
1. Medical therapy (i.e., antihypertensive drugs)
2. PTA
3. PTA with stenting
4. Surgical revascularization

**12. What are the management principles underlying the choice of therapy for patients with renovascular hypertension?**

The choice of therapy depends on the severity of hypertension, the pathologic process (i.e., atherosclerosis vs. fibromuscular dysplasia), the presence or absence of renal impairment, location of the lesion (see question 17), and the presence of comorbid conditions (e.g., coronary or cerebrovascular disease) that may affect life expectancy. In addition, selection of therapy will depend on whether the goal is control of blood pressure, improvement or preservation of renal function, or both. With the wide array of antihypertensive agents currently available, indications for radiologic or surgical intervention have shifted over the past decade from simply control of blood pressure to preservation or improvement of renal function.

Medical therapy can adequately control blood pressure but, in patients with renal insufficiency, will not likely decrease the risk of progressive renal impairment resulting from renal ischemia. In fact, medical therapy can *contribute* to progressive ischemic injury by reducing systemic pressure and further decreasing perfusion to the affected kidney(s). For patients who are candidates for invasive therapy, PTA alone or PTA with stenting is preferred because either procedure can be performed without general anesthesia or prolonged hospitalization. The main limitations of angioplasty are technical failures, vascular accidents (e.g., dissection or rupture), and recurrence of stenosis. The latter, however, is substantially reduced with stenting. In patients with fibromuscular dysplasia, PTA alone has a high success rate. On the other hand, in patients with atherosclerotic renal artery disease, PTA with stent deployment provides superior results.

### 13. What are the results of medical therapy in hypertensive patients with renal artery stenosis?

Recently, several prospective, randomized, controlled trials have clarified the role of medical therapy in renovascular hypertension. These trials compared PTA to medical treatment in hypertensive patients with atherosclerotic renal artery stenosis. Overall, although there was no difference in blood pressure between the treatment groups, PTA resulted in a significantly decreased requirement for antihypertensive therapy. In the largest trial, however, 44% of patients assigned to the medical treatment group required PTA because of resistant hypertension or deterioration in renal function.

### 14. What are the indications for medical therapy in patients with renovascular hypertension?

Medical therapy is reasonable:
• In most hypertensive patients with renovascular disease unless they demonstrate resistant hypertension or deteriorating renal function
• In patients with bilateral or segmental lesions deemed to be nondilatable and inoperable
• In patients with high operative risks (e.g., elderly patients with prohibitive coronary or cerebrovascular disease)
• In patients who refuse invasive therapy

### 15. Are certain classes of antihypertensive agents preferable in patients with renovascular hypertension?

From a pathophysiologic perspective, patients with renovascular hypertension due to unilateral renal artery stenosis respond well to drugs that inhibit the RAAS. In this regard, ACE inhibitors, angiotensin II receptor blockers (ARBs), and β-blockers are effective antihypertensive agents. However, because of the risk of precipitating acute renal failure, ACE inhibitors and ARBs should be avoided in patients with bilateral renal artery stenosis and in those with stenosis in a solitary kidney (see question 9). In azotemic patients with unilateral renal artery stenosis, there is a volume-dependent component of the hypertension. Under these circumstances, dietary salt restriction and diuretic therapy are key components of the antihypertensive regimen. Calcium channel blockers and centrally acting sympatholytics are useful adjunctive classes in patients with unilateral renovascular disease who do not normalize their blood pressure with ACE inhibition or angiotensin II antagonism and diuretic administration.

### 16. What are the results, with respect to control of blood pressure and preservation of renal function of PTA, PTA plus stenting, and surgery for atherosclerotic renovascular disease?

Overall, the results are comparable among the three treatment modalities with respect to change in blood pressure and preservation of renal function (see table). Ten percent to 20% of patients will be cured of their hypertension, 50% will require fewer antihypertensive medications, and 30–40% will derive no benefit from revascularization. Renal function will improve in approximately one-third of patients, stabilize in about 40%, and continue to decline in the remainder.

*Comparative Effects of PTA, PTA Plus Stenting, and Surgery on Blood Pressure and Renal Function in Patients with Atherosclerotic Renovascular Disease*

|  | PTA | PTA + STENT | SURGERY |
|---|---|---|---|
| **Blood Pressure** | | | |
| Cure (%) | 10 | 20 | 15 |
| Improved (%) | 50 | 50 | 50 |
| No Change (%) | 40 | 30 | 35 |
| **Renal Function** | | | |
| Improved (%) | 40 | 30 | 30 |
| No Change (%) | 40 | 40 | 45 |
| Worse (%) | 20 | 30 | 25 |

## 17. How does the location of an atherosclerotic renal artery stenosis influence therapy?

Angioplasty alone is often successful in correcting lesions of fibromuscular dysplasia involving the distal two-thirds of the main renal artery. On the other hand, PTA plus stenting is preferable in atherosclerotic lesions involving the renal ostia. Surgical intervention is required in fibromuscular disease involving branches of the main renal artery and in lesions that fail to respond to PTA plus stenting.

### BIBLIOGRAPHY

1. Conlon PJ, O'Riordan E, Kalra PA: New insights into the epidemiologic and clinical manifestations of atherosclerotic renovascular disease. Am J Kidney Dis 35:573–587, 2000.
2. Hricik DE, Dunn MJ: Angiotensin-converting enzyme inhibitor–induced renal failure: Causes, consequences, and diagnostic uses. J Am Soc Nephrol 1:845–858, 1990.
3. Leertouwer TC, Gussenhoven EJ, Bosch JL, et al: Stent placement for renal arterial stenosis: Where do we stand? A meta-analysis. Radiology 216:78–85, 2000.
4. Martinez-Maldonado M: Pathophysiology of renovascular hypertension. Hypertension 17:707–719, 1991.
5. National High Blood Pressure Education Program Working Group: 1995 Update of the working group reports on chronic renal failure and renovascular hypertension. Arch Intern Med 156:1938–1947, 1996.
6. Plouin P-F, Rossignol P, Bobrie G: Atherosclerotic renal artery stenosis: To treat conservatively, to dilate, to stent, or to operate? J Am Soc Nephrol 12:2190–2196, 2001.
7. Safian RD, Textor SC: Renal-artery stenosis. N Engl J Med 344:431–442, 2001.
8. van de Ven PJG, Kaatee R, Beutler JJ, et al: Arterial stenting and balloon angioplasty in ostial atherosclerotic renovascular disease: A randomised trial. Lancet 353:282–286, 1999.
9. van Jaarsveld BC, Krijnen P, Pieterman H, et al: The effect of balloon angioplasty on hypertension in atherosclerotic renal-artery stenosis. N Engl J Med 342:1007–1014, 2000.
10. Vasbinder GBC, Nelemans PJ, Kessels AGH, et al: Diagnostic tests for renal artery stenosis in patients suspected of having renovascular hypertension: A meta-analysis. Ann Intern Med 135:401–411, 2001.

# 61. PHEOCHROMOCYTOMA

## Donald E. Hricik, M.D.

### 1. What is pheochromocytoma?

The term *pheochromocytoma* is derived from the Greek words *phios* ("dusky") and *chroma* ("color"). Pheochromocytoma is a catecholamine-producing tumor arising from the chromaffin cells of the sympathetic nervous system that are distinguished by their embryonic derivation from the primitive neural crest cells and their uptake of chromium salts. Most pheochromocytomas arise from the adrenal gland. About 10% arise from extra-adrenal sites such as the carotid body and abdominal sympathetic ganglia—including the organ of Zuckerkandl, which consists of ganglia at the bifurcation of the aorta.

### 2. What is the incidence of pheochromocytoma?

Pheochromocytoma is responsible for less than 0.1% of all patients with hypertension.

### 3. What catecholamines are produced by pheochromocytoma?

Norepinephrine is the catecholamine secreted predominantly by most pheochromocytomas. Tumors that predominantly secrete epinephrine are less common and more often are malignant or extra-adrenal in location. Synthesis of catecholamines begins with the amino acid tyrosine, derived either from the diet or from hydroxylation of phenylalanine. The metabolism of tyrosine within the sympathetic nervous system is shown in the figure below.

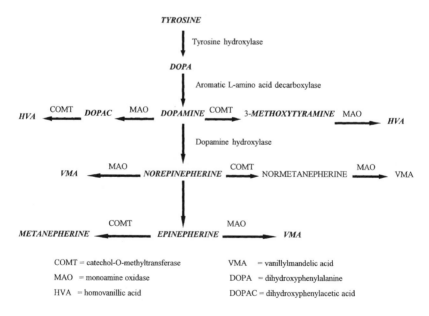

Norepinephrine is the catecholamine secreted predominantly by most pheochromocytomas. Tumors that predominantly secrete epinephrine or dopamine are less common and more often are malignant or extra-adrenal in location.

Pheochromocytomas also store and secrete a variety of peptides: endogenous opioids, endothelin, erythropoietin, parathyroid hormone–related protein, neuropeptide-y, and chromogranin-A. Little is known about the mechanism of hormone release from pheochromocytomas, but changes in blood flow and necrosis within the tumor may be the cause in some cases.

### 4. What are the clinical manifestations of pheochromocytoma?

The most common finding is hypertension, which occurs in more than 90% of patients and which is paroxysmal in character in 20–25% of cases. Paroxysmal episodes of hypertension are typically associated with other signs and symptoms of catecholamine excess: tremor, tachycardia, hyperhydrosis, headache, and pupillary dilatation. Orthostatic hypotension may occur as a result of decreased sympathetic reflexes reflecting downregulation of adrenergic receptors. Weight loss may result from chronic hypermetabolism. Hyperglycemia may occur and reflects the inhibitory effects of catecholamines on pancreatic beta cells.

### 5. What are the five H's associated with pheochromocytoma?

This mnemonic derives from the clinical manifestations defined in the question above:
Hypertension
Headache
Hypermetabolism
Hyperhydrosis
Hyperglycemia

### 6. What is the "rule of ten percent"?

Each of the following accounts for 10% of all pheochromocytomas:
- Bilateral (in adrenal gland)
- Extra adrenal
- Malignant
- Familial (associated with multiple endocrine neoplasia [MEN] syndromes)
- Pediatric

### 7. What conditions are associated with pheochromocytoma?

von Recklinghausen's disease (neurofibromatosis)
Tuberous sclerosis
Sturge-Weber syndrome
von Hippel-Lindau disease
Ataxia telangiectasia
MEN syndrome
- MEN Type 2: Pheochromocytoma, parathyroid adenoma, medullary carcinoma of thyroid
- MEN Type 3: Pheochromocytoma, medullary carcinoma of thyroid, mucosal neuromas, abdominal gangliomas, marfanoid body habitus

### 8. What are some clinical clues to the diagnosis of pheochromocytoma?

1. Sustained or paroxysmal hypertension associated with triad of headache palpitations and diaphoresis
2. Hypertension and family history of pheochromocytoma.
3. Refractory hypertension especially if associated with weight loss.
4. Sinus tachycardia
5. Orthostatic hypotension
6. Recurrent arrhythmias
7. Features of MEN type 2 or 3

8. Hypertensive crises during surgery or anesthesia
9. Pressor response to beta-blocker.
10. Incidentally discovered adrenal mass

**9. What are the causes of death of patients with pheochromocytoma?**
Myocardial infarction
Arrhythmias
Cerebrovascular accident
Renal failure
Dissecting aortic aneurysm.

**10. Elaborate on the biochemical screening for pheochromocytoma.**
Measurement of catecholamines and their metabolites in the plasma and urine are recommended for screening. Small tumors may exhibit rapid turnover rates and release mainly unmetabolized catecholamines. Larger tumors often exhibit slower turnover rates associated with higher concentrations of catecholamine metabolites in plasma and urine. Resting plasma catecholamine concentrations greater than 2000 pg/ml suggest a pheochromocytoma while values less than 500 pg/ml are normal. Intermediate values (500–2000 pg/ml) are equivocal and mandate additional testing if clinical suspicion is high. Urine screening consists of measuring metanephrines, vanillylmandelic acid, and free catecholamines in a 24-hour urine collection.

An algorithm for diagnosis and treatment of pheochromocytoma is shown in the figure.

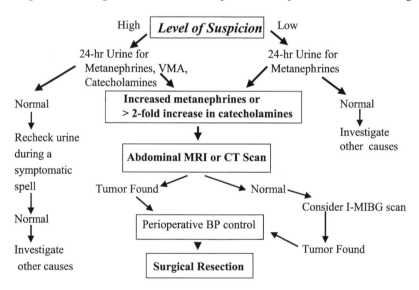

Diagnosis and treatment of pheochromocytoma. (From Desai UA: Pheochromocytoma. In Hricik DE, Wright JT, Smith MC (eds): Hypertension Secrets. Philadelphia, Hanley & Belfus, 2002, pp 49–54, with permission.)

**11. What are the potential sources of error in chemical screening tests?**
Plasma catecholamines levels may be elevated falsely with any kind of stress. In patients with paroxysmal hypertension, urinary concentration of catecholamines and their metabolites may be normal if the 24-hour urine is collected when the patient is normotensive and asymptomatic. Drugs that alter the measured levels of catecholamines and its metabolites are listed in the table.

| INCREASE | DECREASE |
|---|---|
| Tricyclic antidepressants | Metyrosine |
| Amphetamine | Methylglucamine |
| Beta blocker (labetalol, sotalol) | |
| Benzodiazepines | |
| L-dopa, methyldopa | |
| Ethanol | |
| Withdrawal from clonidine | |

## 12. What tests should be performed in equivocal cases?

A number of provocative pharmacologic tests can be performed:

| TEST | RATIONALE |
|---|---|
| Regitine (phentolamine) test | Phentolamine is an alpha blocker, and a reduction in blood pressure suggests catecholamine excess. Not very sensitive or specific. |
| Glucagon stimulation test | Glucagon stimulates catecholamine release. Associated with a risk of precipitating a hypertensive crisis. |
| Clonidine suppression test | Clonidine decreases central sympathetic outflow but does not suppress autonomous production by a tumor. Failure to suppress plasma norepinephrine by more than 50% after administration of clonidine suggests a pheochromocytoma. |

## 13. What studies are used to localize a pheochromocytoma?

Computed tomography (CT) scan or magnetic resonance imaging (MRI) of the abdomen are imaging studies of choice. I-metaiodobenzylguanidine (MIBG) scintigraphy employs an isotope with affinity for chromaffin tissue and can be used to detect extra-adrenal tumors or to confirm that an adrenal mass is a pheochromocytoma. When imaging studies are equivocal, selective venous sampling of the vena cava at various levels can help to locate the tumor. In general, imaging studies are used to confirm and localize a pheochromocytoma only after biochemical screening has suggested the presence of the tumor. Screening a hypertensive patient with a CT scan or MRI prior to biochemical screening may lead to identification of "incidentalomas" (i.e., nonfunctioning tumors incidentally present in a hypertensive patient without catecholamine excess).

## 14. What is the treatment of choice for pheochromocytoma?

Surgical removal of the tumor is the treatment of choice and is curative in 90% of cases. Medical therapy is used mainly for perioperative management. Chronic medical therapy in form of alpha and beta blockade or inhibition of catecholamine synthesis with alpha-methyl-paratyrosine can be used in patients with inoperable, recurrent, multicentric or malignant pheochromocytoma.

## 15. Describe perioperative management.

The goal of preoperative medical therapy is to control blood pressure (for 1–4 weeks prior to surgery) and to block the consequences of increased circulatory catecholamines. Alpha-blockers are the agents of choice and phenoxybenzamine, a long-acting, noncompetitive alpha-blocker, is preferred. The newer competitive, postsynaptic alpha-blockers (prazosin, terazosin) have a shorter action and provide incomplete alpha-blockade so are used less commonly. When tachycardia or arrhythmias persist, beta-adrenergic blockade is indicated, but only after achieving alpha-blockade in order to avoid unopposed alpha-receptor stimulation.

## 16. What clinical parameters should monitored in the postoperative period?
1. Persistent hypertension reflects:
   - Fluid overload
   - Return of autonomic reflexes
   - Inadvertent ligation of renal artery
   - Presence of residual tumor
2. Persistent hypotension reflects:
   - Blood loss
   - Altered vascular compliance
   - Residual effect of preoperative alpha-blockade
3. Hypoglycemia
   - Removal of inhibitory effect of catecholamines on pancreatic islet cells
   - Increased sensitivity of the beta cells to glucose level after tumor removal
   - Cessation of enflurane anesthesia–reactive increase in insulin

## 17. What about treatment for malignant pheochromocytoma?
Malignant pheochromocytoma accounts for less than 10% of all pheochromocytomas. These are slow growing and poorly responsive to radio- or chemotherapy. Surgical debulking may be necessary to decrease catecholamine synthesis. Radioactive MIBG has been used with some success to ablate primary and metastatic sites. Alpha-methyl-tyrosine has been tried in inoperable cases.

## 18. What is the prognosis of pheochromocytoma?
- 5-year survival:  > 95% in nonmalignant pheochromocytoma
                     < 50% in malignant pheochromocytoma
- Recurrence rate after surgery is < 10% in nonmalignant pheochromocytoma.
- Complete resection cures hypertension in approximately 75% of patients. In the remaining 25%, hypertension persists but is usually mild and well controlled with standard antihypertensive agents.

### BIBLIOGRAPHY

1. Bravo EL: Pheochromocytoma: New concepts and future trends: Kidney Int 40:544–556, 1991.
2. Kebew E, Duh QY: Benign and malignant pheochromocytoma: Diagnosis, treatment and follow up. Surg Oncol Clin North Am 7:765–789, 1998.
3. Russel WJ, Metcalf IR, Tonkin AL, Frewin DB: The preoperative management of pheochromocytoma. Anesth Intens Care 26:196–200, 1998.
4. Venkata C, Ram S, Fierro-Carrion G: Pheochromocytoma. Semin Nephrol 15:126–137, 1995.
5. Young WF: Pheochromocytoma and primary aldosteronism: Diagnostic approaches. Endocrinol Metab Clin North Am 26:801–827, 1997.

# 62. OTHER CAUSES OF SECONDARY HYPERTENSION

*Mahboob Rahman*, M.D., M.S.

**1. What are some of the relatively uncommon causes of secondary hypertension?**

Primary aldosteronism
Cushing's syndrome
Coarctation of the aorta
Hypothyroidism
Acromegaly
Sleep apnea
Drugs

Cyclosporine
Erythropoietin
Estrogens
Cocaine
Anabolic steroids
Glucocorticoids
Monoamine oxidase (MAO) inhibitors
Bromocriptine

**2. What are the clinical features of primary aldosteronism?**

Primary aldosteronism is a rare cause of secondary hypertension. It is usually seen in patients between the ages of 30 and 50 years and in women more frequently than in men. The typical clinical features of this syndrome are hypertension associated with hypokalemia, excessive urinary potassium excretion, and metabolic alkalosis. This clinical picture may be due to an aldosterone-producing adenoma or, less commonly, due to bilateral adrenal hyperplasia or adrenal carcinoma.

**3. What laboratory tests are helpful in diagnosis of primary aldosteronism?**

Unexplained hypokalemia is usually the first marker suggesting the possibility of underlying primary aldosteronism. The excretion of greater than 30 mEq/day of potassium in the presence of hypokalemia confirms urinary potassium wasting and supports a diagnosis of primary aldosteronism.

The plasma aldosterone (PA) and plasma renin activity (PRA) are important biochemical markers in the diagnosis of primary aldosteronism. The PA/PRA ratio is normally 10; patients with primary aldosteronism frequently have a ratio of greater than 20. Ideally, this test should be done in the absence of drug therapy such as diuretics, beta blockers, or angiotensin-converting enzyme (ACE) inhibitors, which can affect these measurements.

Once an abnormal PA/PRA ratio is seen, it is important to document whether the excessive aldosterone production is autonomous or responsive to normal homeostatic mechanisms. This can be accomplished either by saline infusion or by the captopril suppression test. If the elevated aldosterone levels are not suppressed by these maneuvers, it is likely that an aldosterone production is autonomous.

**4. What radiologic tests are helpful in the diagnosis of this condition?**

Both computed tomography (CT) and magnetic resonance imaging (MRI) are effective in visualizing aldosterone-producing adenomas greater than 1 cm in diameter. Adrenal scintigraphy and adrenal venous sampling are useful in special circumstances.

**5. What are the therapeutic options in patients with primary aldosteronism?**

The treatment depends on the type of adrenal pathology. Surgical removal is the treatment of choice for patients with adrenal adenomas or carcinomas, and medical therapy with spironolactone is recommended for those with bilateral adrenal hyperplasia. Spironolactone is an aldosterone antagonist and is used in doses ranging between 50 and 200 mg/day. Impotence and gynecomastia are common side effects of long-term therapy with aldosterone.

**6. What are some causes of mineralocorticoid excess–like states other than primary hyperaldosteronism?**

When patients exhibit the manifestation of mineralocorticoid excess in the presence of low serum or urinary aldosterone levels, it is likely that a nonaldosterone mineralocorticoid is responsible. This can occur in patients taking fludrocortisone. Increased levels of deoxycorticosterone can occur in rare patients with adenomas producing this hormone and with some types of congenital adrenal hyperplasia. Black licorice contains glycyrrhetinic acid, a steroid that inhibits 11-beta-hydroxysteroid dehydrogenase. The latter enzyme usually converts cortisol (with mineralocorticoid activity) to cortisone (with little mineralocorticoid activity). By effectively increasing levels of cortisol, ingestion of licorice can be associated with signs and symptoms of mineralocorticoid excess. In patients with ectopic adrenocorticotropic hormone (ACTH) production, extremely high levels of cortisol overwhelm the capacity for conversion to cortisone, also leading to mineralocorticoid excess. Liddle's syndrome is a rare autosomal-dominant condition involving mutation in the gene for the sodium channel of the collecting duct. This results in excessive sodium reabsorption and, in most cases, augmented potassium excretion, resulting in a syndrome sometimes referred to as *pseudohyperaldosteronism*.

**7. What is glucocorticoid-remediable aldosteronism?**

Glucocorticoid-remediable aldosteronism is a genetic disorder in which there is excess secretion of aldosterone due to ectopic production in the zona fasciculata of the adrenal gland resulting in all the clinical manifestations described above. This secretion is regulated by ACTH; therefore, suppression of ACTH by administration of exogenous steroids results in complete resolution of the symptoms. The diagnosis can be confirmed by genetic analysis.

**8. What clinical signs and symptoms suggest a diagnosis of Cushing's syndrome?**

Cushing's syndrome is another relatively rare cause of secondary hypertension. The typical clinical features include truncal obesity, facial plethora ("cushingoid facies"), hirsutism, striae, easy bruising, neuropsychiatric disturbances, osteopenia, and glucose intolerance. Hypertension is present in 80% of patients with Cushing's syndrome.

**9. What are the common screening tests used in the diagnosis of Cushing's syndrome?**

An overnight dexamethasone suppression test is a good screening test in patients with suspected Cushing's syndrome. After a bedtime dose of 1 mg of dexamethasone is given, the plasma cortisol is measured at 8:00 the next morning. A level of less than 5 µg/dl indicates normal suppression. If the screening test is abnormal, further testing is needed to establish the cause of the syndrome (i.e., adrenal hyperplasia, ectopic ACTH production, or pituitary disease).

**10. What are the treatment options in Cushing's syndrome?**

Hypertension can be difficult to treat in patients with Cushing's syndrome. A diuretic, in combination with spironolactone, is usually the first choice with additional antihypertensive therapy as needed. After definitive therapy of the underlying cause of Cushing's syndrome, the hypertension usually resolves. The definitive therapy depends on the underlying disease. Surgical removal is the treatment of choice for benign adrenal tumors. For adrenal cancers and ectopic ACTH production, adjuvant chemotherapy may be required. Transsphenoidal removal is the treatment of choice for pituitary tumors.

**11. What signs suggest coarctation of the aorta?**

Hypertension in the arms with weak femoral pulses in a young person is suggestive of coarctation of the aorta. The chest x-ray will typically show the "3 sign" from the dilatation of the aorta above and below the constriction and notching of the ribs by enlarged collateral vessels. The diagnosis is usually made by echocardiography and by color-flow Doppler imaging.

**12. Why should thyroid function tests be considered in hypertensive patients?**

Hypothyroidism is associated with elevated diastolic pressure due to increased peripheral vascular resistance. Blood pressure can improve when patients are treated with thyroid hormone replacement therapy.

**13. What are the symptoms of sleep apnea? What is its association with hypertension?**

Patients with obstructive sleep apnea present with excessive snoring, daytime somnolence, and nocturia. The diagnosis is confirmed by an overnight sleep study. It is important to keep this diagnosis in mind, particularly in obese hypertensive patients. The pathogenesis of hypertension in sleep apnea is not clear; however, correction of the defect by surgery or by continuous positive airway pressure (CPAP) is associated with improvement in blood pressure.

**14. What are some of the neurologic disorders associated with hypertension?**

Patients with intracranial brain tumors, quadriplegia, or severe head injury may have hypertension due to excessive sympathetic nervous system activity.

**15. What is the relationship among oral contraceptives, estrogen replacement therapy, and hypertension?**

Hypertension is reported to be two to three times more common in women taking oral contraceptives, especially in obese and older women, than in those not taking oral contraceptives. Blood pressure should be monitored every 6 months in patients taking oral contraceptives. If hypertension develops, oral contraceptives should be stopped, and blood pressure will normalize in most cases in a few months. Hypertension is not a contraindication for postmenopausal hormone replacement therapy. However, a few women may experience a rise in blood pressure attributable to hormone replacement therapy. Therefore, all women treated with hormone replacement therapy should have their blood pressure monitored periodically.

**16. Does cocaine use cause hypertension?**

There is no evidence that ongoing cocaine use causes chronic hypertension. However, it can cause an acute rise in blood pressure and can be associated with ischemia from coronary and cerebral vasoconstriction or acute renal failure from rhabdomyolysis.

### BIBLIOGRAPHY

1. Bravo EL: Primary aldosteronism. Issues in diagnosis and management. Endocrinol Metab Clin North Am 23:271–283, 1994.
2. Dluhy RG, Lifton RP: Glucocorticoid remediable aldosteronism (GRA): Diagnosis, variability of phenotype, and regulation of potassium homeostasis. Steroids 60:48–51, 1995.
3. Danese RD, Aron DC: Cushing's syndrome and hypertension. Endocrinol Metab Clin North Am 23:299–324, 1994.
4. Kaplan NM: Other forms of secondary hypertension. In Kaplan NM (ed): Clinical Hypertension. Baltimore, Williams & Wilkins, 1988, pp 395–406.
5. Madhun ZT, Aron DC: Hyperaldosteronism. In Hricik DE, Wright JT, Smith MC (eds): Hypertension Secrets. Philadelphia, Hanley & Belfus, 2002, pp 43–47.

# 63. HYPERTENSIVE EMERGENCIES

*Mahboob Rahman, M.D., M.S.*

### 1. What constitutes a hypertensive emergency?

A hypertensive emergency is a clinical situation characterized by marked elevation of blood pressure associated with progressive target organ damage that requires immediate reduction of blood pressure. Situations include:

- Hypertensive encephalopathy
- Hypertension associated with acute left ventricular failure
- Subarachnoid or intracerebral bleed
- Aortic dissection
- Acute myocardial infarction or unstable angina
- Adrenergic crises
- Malignant hypertension
- Eclampsia

It is important to emphasize that evidence of new or progressive target organ damage and not the absolute levels of blood pressure determine the urgency of treatment. For example, relatively modest acute increases in blood pressure may lead to target organ damage in previously normotensive patients (as in eclampsia) and in those with accompanying medical conditions (aortic dissection or myocardial infarction). Elevated blood pressure alone, in the absence of symptoms or new or progressive target organ damage, rarely requires emergency therapy.

### 2. What is malignant hypertension?

**Malignant hypertension** is a syndrome of severe elevation of arterial pressure (usually, but not always, the diastolic pressure exceeds 140 mmHg) associated with vascular damage manifested by retinal hemorrhages, exudates, and papilledema. **Accelerated hypertension** is the term used for a similar syndrome without papilledema.

### 3. What are the clinical circumstances associated with malignant hypertension?

Patients presenting with malignant hypertension may have a history of severe and inadequately treated essential hypertension and frequently are smokers. It is important to evaluate these patients for secondary hypertension because renovascular and renal parenchymal disease can be present in many patients presenting with malignant hypertension.

### 4. What is the pathophysiology leading to development of malignant hypertension?

A rapid and progressive rise in blood pressure causes endothelial damage in the blood vessels, leading to platelet and fibrin deposition and fibrinoid necrosis. In addition, due to tissue ischemia, there is increased production of angiotensin II, which is a potent vasoconstrictor. Due to the higher blood pressure, a pressure natriuresis promotes volume depletion and further activation of the renin angiotensin axis. These events form a positive feedback loop and result in progressive elevation of blood pressure and the vascular sequelae seen in malignant hypertension.

### 5. What are the typical pathologic lesions seen in malignant hypertension?

The vascular lesions consist predominantly of myointimal proliferation and fibrinoid necrosis. Vascular smooth muscle hypertrophy and collagen deposition contribute to medial thickening, which, accompanied by cellular intimal proliferation, results in the onion skin appearance of the small vessels.

## 6. What are the clinical features of malignant hypertension?

The blood pressure is usually, but not always, markedly elevated (diastolic > 140 mmHg). The presence of hemorrhages, exudates, and papilledema on funduscopic exam is typical in patients with malignant hypertension. Neurologic symptoms may include headache, confusion, somnolence, visual loss, seizures, or coma. Renal involvement is common, and patients may have oliguria or azotemia. Generalized weakness, nausea, vomiting, and malaise may be present. Microangiopathic hemolytic anemia with red cell fragmentation can be seen in association with fibrinoid necrosis. The urine may contain protein and red cells.

## 7. What are the principles of antihypertensive therapy in patients with hypertensive emergencies?

Patients with hypertensive emergencies should be admitted to intensive care settings. An intra-arterial line should be placed to monitor the response to therapy. Parenteral antihypertensive therapy should be initiated as early as possible. It is important to avoid abrupt falls and excessive lowering of blood pressure to minimize precipitating cardiac or cerebral ischemia. Patients with chronic hypertension and elderly patients have impaired ability to autoregulate blood flow and are at greater risk for hypoperfusion. The initial goal of therapy in hypertensive emergencies is to reduce mean arterial pressure by no more than 25% in the first minutes to 2 hours, then reducing it toward 160/100 mmHg within 2–6 hours. Once blood pressure is controlled, oral antihypertensive drugs should be introduced and intravenous therapy weaned.

## 8. What drugs are available for treatment of hypertensive emergencies?

Sodium nitroprusside is the drug of choice in many hypertensive emergencies because of its rapid onset and efficacy in lowering blood pressure. In addition, the antihypertensive effect disappears within minutes of the drug being stopped, making it easier to titrate therapy. It is an arterial and venous dilator, reducing cardiac preload and afterload and myocardial oxygen consumption. Nitroprusside is metabolized to thiocyanate and excreted in the urine. Prolonged administration of nitroprusside can result in thiocyanate toxicity, which manifests as blurred vision, confusion, tinnitus, and hyperreflexia. Therefore, use of nitroprusside should be limited to a rate of less than 3 μg per minute for less than 72 hours.

Labetalol is a combined alpha and beta blocker and reduces peripheral resistance without increasing cardiac output. It can be used as repeated IV boluses or as a continuous infusion and is contraindicated in bradycardia, heart block, bronchospasm, or congestive heart failure. IV nitroglycerin, because of its properties of afterload reduction and improved myocardial perfusion, is the treatment of choice in patients with myocardial ischemia. Esmolol is a short-acting beta blocker that is particularly useful in the treatment of hypertension associated with aortic dissection to reduce the shear stress in the vessel wall. Details of these and other agents are listed in the table at the top of the next page.

## 9. What is the long-term prognosis and outcome of patients with malignant hypertension?

Patients with untreated malignant hypertension have a high mortality rate with a 1-year survival rate as low as 10–20% reported in a series in 1958. However, with improved antihypertensive therapy, survival has improved considerably in the last few years. The presence of renal failure at the time of initial presentation is associated with a poorer prognosis. After the initiation of vigorous antihypertensive therapy, renal function may deteriorate transiently but usually improves with good blood pressure control. In fact, several studies show that some patients recover enough renal function to allow withdrawal of dialysis.

*Parenteral Therapy for Hypertensive Emergencies*

| DRUG | ONSET OF ACTION | DOSE | COMMENTS |
|------|------|------|------|
| Sodium nitroprusside | Immediate | 0.25–10 µg/kg/min as IV infusion | Effective in most hypertensive emergencies; caution with high intracranial pressure or azotemia |
| Nitroglycerin | 2–5 minutes | 5–100 µg/min IV | Particularly useful in hypertension associated with coronary ischemia |
| Nicardipine | 5–10 minutes | 5–15 mg/hr IV | Avoid in acute heart failure and coronary ischemia |
| Enalaprilat | 15–30 minutes | 1.25–5 mg every 6 hr IV | Useful in acute left ventricular failure; avoid in acute myocardial infarction |
| Labetalol | 5–10 minutes | 20–80 mg IV bolus every 10 minutes; 0.5–2.0 mg/min IV infusion | Avoid in acute heart failure |
| Esmolol | 10–20 minutes | 250–500 µg/kg/min for 1 min, then 50–100 µg/kg/min for 4 min; may repeat sequence | Particularly useful in aortic dissection and perioperative hypertension |

### 10. What are the clinical features of hypertensive encephalopathy?

Patients with hypertensive encephalopathy can present with headache, somnolence, seizures, or focal neurologic abnormalities. Funduscopic exam usually shows stage 3 or 4 hypertensive retinopathy, and there is frequently evidence of prior target organ damage in the kidneys or the heart. Definitive diagnosis of hypertensive encephalopathy requires exclusion of other neurologic processes, usually by computed tomography (CT) scan and other diagnostic work-up.

### 11. How do patients with aortic dissection present? How is hypertension treated in the presence of aortic dissection?

A history of severe hypertension and inherited disorders of connective tissue, such as Marfan syndrome or Ehlers-Danlos syndrome, increases the risk for developing an aortic dissection. Patients usually present with severe chest or upper back pain, which may radiate into the arms or upper abdomen and is associated with difference in blood pressure between the two arms. In addition, a murmur of aortic regurgitation, a pericardial rub, or evidence of a pleural effusion may be present. The diagnosis is confirmed by computed tomography (CT) scan or transesophageal echocardiography.

The goal of treatment of hypertension in the setting of an aortic dissection is to reduce the shear force of the pressure upstroke. The combination of intravenous beta blockade and sodium nitroprusside is the treatment of choice, and blood pressure should be maintained as low as possible. Definitive treatment depends on the location of the dissection. Lesions before the aortic arch (type A) require immediate surgery, whereas those distal to the arch (type B) can have a trial of medical therapy.

**12. What are the clinical features of hypertension associated with acute left ventricular failure and pulmonary edema? How is this condition treated?**

Patients present with severe shortness of breath associated with a cough producing a frothy, pink-tinged sputum. The blood pressure is markedly elevated, neck veins are distended, and crackles or wheezes are present in both lung fields. An S3 or S4 gallop may be heard. The chest x-ray shows bilateral cephalization, hilar congestion, and pulmonary edema. Treatment should be initiated immediately with oxygen, intubation, or, if necessary, intravenous furosemide. IV nitroglycerin is very effective because it lowers preload and afterload, improves coronary perfusion, and, therefore, is the treatment of choice in this setting. IV morphine is also helpful as an adjunctive measure.

**13. What is an adrenergic crisis? How is it treated?**

Adrenergic crises are clinical situations characterized by abrupt increases in alpha-adrenergic tone and plasma catecholamine levels. These can occur because of withdrawal of clonidine, cocaine and amphetamine overdose, and monoamine oxidase–tyramine syndrome. Alpha blockers such as phentolamine, phenoxybenzamine, and combined alpha and beta blockers such as labetalol are effective antihypertensive agents in this scenario. Sodium nitroprusside can be used if necessary.

### BIBLIOGRAPHY

1. Berger BE: Hypertensive crises. In Hricik DE, Wright JT, Smith MC (eds): Hypertension Secrets. Philadelphia, Hanley & Belfus, 2002, pp 13–16.
2. Gifford RW: Management of hypertensive crises. JAMA 266:829–835, 1991.
3. Kitiyakara C, Guzman NJ: Malignant hypertension and hypertensive emergencies. J Am Soc Nephrol 9:133–142, 1998.
4. National Institutes of Health: Sixth Report of the Joint National Committee on Prevention, Detection, Evaluation, and Treatment of High Blood Pressure, Bethesda, MD, NIH, 1997, NIH publication 98-4080.
5. Phillips RA, Krakoff LR: Hypertensive Emergencies. True and False. New York, American Society of Hypertension, 1997.

# 64. CHILDHOOD HYPERTENSION

*Ira D. Davis, M.D.*

## 1. What is the definition of hypertension in children?

Hypertension is based on the normal distribution of systolic and diastolic blood pressure in the general population for children of comparable age, weight, and height. High normal blood pressure is defined as pressures between the 90th and 95th percentile; significant hypertension is defined as pressures greater than the 95th–99th percentile; severe hypertension is defined as pressures greater than the 99th percentile (see tables).

*90th and 95th Percentiles of Blood Pressure (BP) for Girls*

| AGE (YRS) | BP PERCENTILE | SYSTOLIC BP (mmHg) BY PERCENTILE OF HEIGHT | | | DIASTOLIC BP (mmHg) BY PERCENTILE OF HEIGHT | | |
|---|---|---|---|---|---|---|---|
| | | 25% | 75% | 95% | 25% | 75% | 95% |
| 2 | 90th | 100 | 103 | 105 | 58 | 59 | 61 |
| | 95th | 104 | 107 | 109 | 62 | 63 | 65 |
| 4 | 90th | 103 | 106 | 108 | 64 | 65 | 67 |
| | 95th | 107 | 109 | 111 | 68 | 69 | 71 |
| 8 | 90th | 110 | 112 | 114 | 71 | 72 | 74 |
| | 95th | 113 | 116 | 118 | 75 | 76 | 78 |
| 10 | 90th | 114 | 116 | 118 | 73 | 75 | 76 |
| | 95th | 117 | 120 | 122 | 77 | 79 | 80 |
| 14 | 90th | 121 | 124 | 126 | 78 | 79 | 81 |
| | 95th | 125 | 128 | 130 | 82 | 83 | 85 |

*90th and 95th Percentiles of Blood Pressure (BP) for Boys*

| AGE (YRS) | BP PERCENTILE | SYSTOLIC BP (mmHg) BY PERCENTILE OF HEIGHT | | | DIASTOLIC BP (mmHg) BY PERCENTILE OF HEIGHT | | |
|---|---|---|---|---|---|---|---|
| | | 25% | 75% | 95% | 25% | 75% | 95% |
| 2 | 90th | 100 | 104 | 106 | 56 | 58 | 59 |
| | 95th | 104 | 108 | 110 | 60 | 62 | 63 |
| 4 | 90th | 105 | 109 | 111 | 63 | 65 | 66 |
| | 95th | 109 | 113 | 115 | 67 | 69 | 71 |
| 8 | 90th | 110 | 114 | 116 | 72 | 74 | 75 |
| | 95th | 114 | 118 | 120 | 76 | 78 | 80 |
| 10 | 90th | 113 | 117 | 119 | 74 | 76 | 78 |
| | 95th | 117 | 121 | 123 | 79 | 80 | 82 |
| 14 | 90th | 123 | 126 | 128 | 77 | 79 | 80 |
| | 95th | 127 | 130 | 132 | 81 | 83 | 85 |

Adapted from National High Blood Pressure Education Program Working Group on Hypertension Control in Children and Adolescents: Update on the 1987 task force report on high blood pressure in children and adolescents: A working group report from the National Blood Pressure Education Program. Pediatrics 98:649–658, 1996.

**2. When should the blood pressure be checked in the pediatric patient?**

The American Academy of Pediatrics recommends that annual blood pressure screening should begin at 3 years of age.

**3. Does essential hypertension occur in children?**

Essential hypertension accounts for only 10–20% of the cases of hypertension in children younger than 10 years. On the other hand, essential hypertension accounts for about 35% of cases of hypertension in the adolescent population. The majority of hypertension in the pediatric population is due to secondary or identifiable causes.

**4. What is the primary cause of hypertension in newborn infants?**

The most frequent cause of hypertension in this population is renovascular disease associated with renal arterial thromboemboli or renal artery stenosis. Other causes include coarctation of the aorta, congenital renal malformations such as obstructive uropathy or polycystic kidney disease, and bronchopulmonary dysplasia.

**5. What are the most common causes of hypertension in infants through preschool-age children?**

Hypertension secondary to renal parenchymal disease, renal artery stenosis, or coarctation of the aorta occurs most frequently in this age group.

**6. What are the most common causes of hypertension in children aged 6–10 years?**

Hypertension secondary to either renal parenchymal disease or renal artery stenosis occurs most frequently in this age group.

**7. What are the most common causes of secondary hypertension in the adolescent population?**

The primary cause of secondary hypertension in adolescence is renal parenchymal disease. Etiologies include acute or chronic forms of glomerulonephritis and renal scarring associated with a remote history of pyelonephritis.

**8. Which clinical characteristics are commonly associated with essential hypertension?**

Typical characteristics include mild blood pressure elevations to the 95th percentile with significant variability in measurements, a strong family history, and obesity.

**9. What important features of the patient history need to be assessed when evaluating a child with hypertension?**

A careful family history including the age of onset of hypertension and the presence of complications such as myocardial infarction, kidney failure, heart failure, stroke, and peripheral vascular disease in first- and second-degree relatives is essential. The patient's growth pattern and neonatal history also should be assessed. Patients also should be questioned regarding the intake of foods and medications (including over-the-counter and illicit drugs including caffeine, nicotine, sodium, sympathomimetics, steroids, cocaine, and amphetamines) that cause elevations in blood pressure. The patient should be questioned regarding the presence of symptoms suggestive of hypertension, renal disease, or other acute or chronic illnesses.

**10. What are the symptoms of hypertension in children?**

Children with essential hypertension or mildly elevated blood pressure due to secondary causes are usually asymptomatic. Severe hypertension may be associated with headaches, epistaxis, dizziness, blurred vision, nausea, changes in mental status, or seizures.

Neonates with hypertension may present with poor feeding, irritability, lethargy, respiratory distress, seizures, or apnea.

## 11. What are the important features of the physical exam when evaluating a child with hypertension?
These include:
- Growth assessment
- Four extremity blood pressure measurements for evidence of coarctation of the aorta
- Funduscopic exam and a careful neurologic exam
- Neck exam for evidence of thyromegaly
- Cardiopulmonary exam for evidence of congestive heart failure or murmurs
- Abdominal exam for masses or bruits
- Skin exam looking for manifestations of rheumatologic diseases (such as systemic lupus erythematosus) or neurocutaneous syndromes (such as neurofibromatosis or tuberous sclerosis)
- Genitalia

## 12. What is the initial approach to the laboratory evaluation of hypertension in children?
All patients with hypertension require a urinalysis, serum chemistries, blood urea nitrogen (BUN), and creatinine determination. Patients with suspected essential hypertension should have a fasting lipid profile checked. Those with suspected secondary hypertension due to urologic abnormalities or pyelonephritis should have a urine culture. Children with severe hypertension and all children younger than 13 years should undergo a renal ultrasound. Patients with tachycardia or thyromegaly should have thyroid function studies. Echocardiography should be performed in patients with blood pressure above the 95th percentile and when pharmacotherapy is being considered.

## 13. What are the nonpharmacologic approaches to the treatment of hypertension in children?
Weight reduction, aerobic exercise, and dietary modifications (low salt and low fat) are standard approaches for the treatment of essential hypertension in the adolescent with high-normal blood pressure or significant hypertension.

## 14. When are the pharmacologic approaches necessary in treating childhood hypertension?
The indications for pharmacologic therapy include:
- Presence of significant hypertension unresponsive to nonpharmacologic approaches
- Presence of symptoms
- Presence of end-organ injury evidenced by increased left ventricular mass or left ventricular dysfunction on echocardiogram
- Presence of severe hypertension
The goal of treatment is to reduce the blood pressure below the 95th percentile.

## 15. What are the current recommendations regarding children's participation in competitive contact sports if they have hypertension?
According to the Academy of Pediatrics, no limitations exist for children with blood pressure in the 95th–99th percentile who have no evidence of target organ injury (e.g., retinopathy, congestive heart failure, or left ventricular hypertrophy). Children with blood pressure readings above the 99th percentile must restrict participation in competitive contact sports and highly static activities (e.g., weight lifting) until their blood pressure is below the 99th percentile.

BIBLIOGRAPHY

1. Bartosh S, Aronson A: Childhood hypertension, diagnosis, and treatment. Pediatr Clin North Am 46:235–251, 1999.
2. Coody DK, Yetman RJ, Portman RJ: Hypertension in children. J Pediatr Health Care 9:3–11, 1995.
3. Flynn J: Neonatal hypertension: Diagnosis and management. Pediatr Nephrol 14:332, 2000.
4. National High Blood Pressure Education Program Working Group on Hypertension Control in Children and Adolescents: Update on the 1987 task force report on high blood pressure in children and adolescents: A working group report from the National High Blood Pressure Education Program. Pediatrics 98:649–658, 1996.

# IX. Acid-Base and Electrolyte Disorders

## 65. METABOLIC ACIDOSIS

*Bruce E. Berger, M.D.*

### 1. What is pH and how can I translate pH to free H⁺?

pH is the negative logarithm of the hydrogen ion concentration of a solution, expressed in equivalents per liter. The concentration of free hydrogen ion in body fluids is approximately $40 \times 10^{-9}$ Eq/L, or 40 nanoequivalents per liter (nEq/L). This corresponds to a pH of approximately 7.40. The number of free hydrogen ions per liter of body fluid can be calculated using the following approximation: A pH of 7.00 equals 100 nEq/L. For every 0.10 increase in pH, the corresponding $H^+$ number is 80% of the preceding value. For example, at a pH of 7.10, $H^+$ = 80 nEq/L; at a pH of 7.20, $H^+$ = 64 nEq/L).

### 2. How can I adapt the Henderson-Hasselbach equation for clinical practice?

Use this equation:

$$H^+ = 24 \times pCO_2/HCO_3^-$$

If one knows two of the three variables in the equation, the third can be calculated, allowing quick bedside assessment of acid-base disorders.

### 3. What are the major sources and disposition of metabolic acids?

The body produces both organic and mineral acids as a product of normal metabolic processes. The oxidation of carbohydrates, amino acids, and fatty acids results in the formation of approximately 15,000 mmoles of carbon dioxide per day, which are rapidly excreted by the lungs. The typical Western diet is an acid-ash diet because its metabolism results in the generation of approximately 1 mEq/kg body weight of fixed, nonvolatile acids. These mineral acids consist of sulfates, which are derived from sulfur-containing amino acids in the diet, and phosphates, which are abundant in most foodstuffs. Because the concentration of free hydrogen ion in the body is approximately $40 \times 10^{-9}$ Eq/L, it is obvious that even a slight accumulation of the $60-70 \times 10^{-3}$ equivalents of hydrogen ion produced daily would be rapidly fatal. Therefore, endogenously produced mineral acids must be immediately buffered so that free hydrogen ion does not accumulate in body fluids. The body defends pH by recruiting a number of extracellular and intracellular buffers, including bicarbonate, proteins, and bone. The most important buffer system is the bicarbonate–carbonic acid buffer pair in the extracellular fluid. The kidney's role in acid-base balance is to excrete the mineral ion associated with the endogenously produced mineral acids and to regenerate the 60–70 mEq of bicarbonate consumed daily in buffering the endogenous acid load.

### 4. Distinguish the roles of the proximal and distal renal tubules in maintaining acid-base balance.

The proximal tubule reabsorbs the majority of filtered bicarbonate (approximately 85%), thereby conserving the extracellular bicarbonate buffer pool. The proximal tubule also defends extracellular bicarbonate concentration by rejecting filtered bicarbonate in excess of the normal extracellular fluid bicarbonate concentration of 25–28 mEq/L, so that bicarbonate cannot accumulate to abnormally high levels in the plasma. Under normal circumstances, by the time the glomerular filtrate has reached the end of the distal tubule, most if not all of the filtered bicarbonate has been reabsorbed. In the cortical collecting duct, hydrogen ion is secreted against a gradient into the tubular lumen, acidifying the urine to a pH of around 5.0. This process of urinary acidification does not increase the amount of free hydrogen ions enough to maintain hydrogen ion balance (at a pH of 5, there are only $10 \times 10^{-6}$ Eq/L of hydrogen ion compared to the $60–70 \times 10^{-3}$ equivalents of hydrogen ion that must be excreted to maintain acid balance). Rather, the purpose of acidifying the urine is to promote the proteination of buffers (primarily phosphate) that are present in the glomerular filtrate. These "titratable acids" constitute approximately one third of net acid excretion under normal circumstances. Urinary ammonium, which is produced by both proximal and distal tubular cells, comprises the remaining two thirds of net acid excretion. By metabolizing one molecule of glutamine, renal tubular cells produce two molecules of ammonium and one molecule of alpha-ketoglutarate. As the alpha-ketoglutarate (a divalent anion) is further metabolized to $CO_2$ and water through the Krebs cycle or to glucose through gluconeogenesis, it takes on two hydrogen ions from intracellular carbonic acid, leaving two bicarbonate molecules behind. These two bicarbonates are then returned to the extracellular fluid, regenerating the bicarbonate that was consumed in the initial process of buffering the mineral acids. As every milliequivalent of ammonium excreted represents a milliequivalent of bicarbonate regenerated by the kidney to replenish the bicarbonate buffer pool, every milliequivalent of titratable acid excreted also represents a milliequivalent of bicarbonate regenerated by the kidneys. Net acid excretion equals the total of ammonium and titratable acid excreted minus any bicarbonate present in the urine. In order to maintain acid-base homeostasis, daily net acid excretion must equal daily mineral acid production. In states of sustained metabolic acidosis, the kidneys must increase net acid excretion and do so almost entirely by increasing ammonium excretion.

**5. What is the difference between metabolic acidosis and metabolic acidemia?**

Metabolic acidosis describes a process that may or may not lead to a state of metabolic acidemia (a decrease in arterial pH). By definition, in order to have metabolic acidemia, a state of metabolic acidosis must exist. The corollary, however, is not necessarily correct. Metabolic acidosis need not result in metabolic acidemia if there is a concomitant state of metabolic or respiratory alkalosis.

**6. What are the three major processes that can result in a metabolic acidosis?**

1. Acid production in excess of the kidneys' ability to excrete the acid and regenerate bicarbonate

2. Decreased ability of a diseased kidney to excrete acid and regenerate bicarbonate

3. Loss of bicarbonate from the extracellular fluid through either the kidneys or the gastrointestinal tract

**7. What is the anion gap and how does it help to distinguish the causes of metabolic acidosis?**

The anion gap is the difference between the sum of the serum chloride and bicarbonate concentrations and the serum sodium concentration (see figure).

A normal anion gap is 10–14 mEq/L. An elevated anion gap generally indicates the presence of a metabolic acidosis, but an anion gap up to 16–18 mEq/L may sometimes be found in patients with metabolic alkalemia (pH > 7.50). A metabolic acidosis with an elevated anion gap generally results from the overproduction of endogenously produced organic acids, such as lactic acid and ketoacids, or the generation of acid metabolites from the ingestion of certain toxins, such as salicylates, methanol, and ethylene glycol. Advanced renal failure can

$$\text{Anion gap} = Na^+ - (Cl^- + HCO_3^-)$$

Constituents of normal extracellular fluid used in calculating the anion gap. Note that the gap actually reflects the difference between "unmeasured" anions and cations although it is calculated based on commonly measured electrolytes (i.e., $Na^+$, $Cl^-$, and $HCO_3^-$).

also lead to a metabolic acidosis with an elevated anion gap because of the decreased ability of the kidneys to keep up with the normal production of endogenously produced acids. A metabolic acidosis with a normal anion gap is generally due to bicarbonate loss from the extracellular fluid (through the kidneys or gastrointestinal tract) or the administration of a chloride-containing acid. This is referred to as a **hyperchloremic metabolic acidosis**.

**8. What is the urinary anion gap? How is it used in the differential diagnosis of metabolic acidosis? What are it's clinical limitations?**

The normal renal response to sustained states of metabolic acidosis is to increase net acid excretion. The resulting increase in bicarbonate regeneration is reflected by a commensurate increase in urine ammonium excretion. Each ammonium ion must be excreted with an anion. The urinary anion gap is the difference between the urine chloride concentration and the sum of the urine sodium and potassium concentrations. The urinary anion gap can be used to estimate ammonium excretion in states of hyperchloremic non–anion gap metabolic acidosis. A urine anion gap that is more negative than −30 reflects an appropriate renal acidification as seen, for example, with diarrhea. A positive urinary anion gap in this setting suggests impaired urinary acidification as in type I (distal) renal tubular acidosis. The urine anion gap is useful in estimating ammonium excretion only when $Cl^-$ is the predominant urine anion, when bicarbonaturia and organic anion (e.g., ketonuria) are absent, and when urine $NH_4^+$ excretion is expected to be high (i.e., > 100 mM).

**9. If the normal response to sustained metabolic acidosis is an increase in urine ammonium excretion, how can I estimate its production?**

Clinical studies have shown that the urine osmolality is approximately equal to twice the positively charged urine solutes and the sum of the major uncharged solutes, glucose and urea (all expressed in millimoles per liter).

$$\text{Urine osmolality} = [2 \times (NH_4^+ + Na^+ + K^+)] + \text{urea} + \text{glucose}$$

$$\text{Urine } NH_4^+ = \frac{\text{Osmolality} - [2(Na^+ + K^+) + \text{urea} + \text{glucose}]}{2}$$

The determination of urine $NH_4^+$ concentration by this equation will be overestimated, however, when there is a significant amount of nonionic urine solute (e.g., alcohol).

**10. What is the osmolal gap, and what is its role in the differential diagnosis of metabolic acidosis?**

The osmolal gap is the difference between the measured serum osmolality and the calculated serum osmolality, which is determined by the following formula:

$$\text{Serum osmolality} = 2 \times [\text{Na}^+ \text{ (mEq/L)}] + \frac{[\text{glucose (mg/dl)}]}{18}$$

$$+ \frac{[\text{blood urea nitrogen (mg/dl)}]}{2.8}$$

The osmolality as determined by the laboratory should not exceed the calculated osmolarity by greater than 10 mOsm/kg. An elevated osmolal gap in the setting of a metabolic acidosis with an increased anion gap suggests intoxication with a low–molecular-weight substance such as methanol or ethylene glycol.

**11. What are the four major factors that affect renal tubular bicarbonate reabsorption?**

Renal tubular bicarbonate reabsorption ($T_m$ bicarbonate) is increased in the setting of decreased extracellular fluid volume, hypokalemia, increased $\text{Paco}_2$, and increased mineralocorticoid activity. Conversely, renal tubular bicarbonate reabsorption is suppressed by expanded extracellular fluid volume, hyperkalemia, decreased $\text{Paco}_2$, and decreased mineralocorticoid activity.

**12. Compare and contrast type I (distal) renal tubular acidosis (RTA) and type II (proximal) RTA.**

By definition, type I and type II RTA are metabolic acidoses that are a result of a renal tubular disorder. The glomerular filtration rate is classically normal. In **type I RTA**, a defect in urinary acidification and renal ammoniagenesis results in a failure of net acid excretion to keep pace with mineral acid production. Consequently, there is an ongoing and daily accumulation of acids within body fluids, a downward titration of extracellular bicarbonate, and recruitment of nonbicarbonate buffers such as bone. It is important to appreciate that patients with type I RTA never achieve a state of acid-base balance. Buffering of hydrogen ions by bone buffers results in the release of calcium, which is filtered through the kidneys and easily precipitated in the tubules because of impaired urine citrate excretion and the failure of urinary acidification to keep it in solution. As a result, patients with type I RTA often develop chronic progressive renal failure as a result of nephrocalcinosis. Finally, in type I RTA, there is an augmentation of renal potassium secretion in exchange for sodium in the distal nephron. This can lead to profound hypokalemia. Muscle weakness due to hypokalemia is a common presenting symptom in type I RTA. Once the diagnosis is made, type I RTA is not difficult to treat. Because many of these patients present with both profound hypokalemia and metabolic acidosis, it is important to replace the potassium first, because alkalization of the plasma will lead to a shift of potassium into cells, which may aggravate the hypokalemia to a life-threatening degree. Once serum potassium levels are stabilized, alkali can be administered to restore plasma pH and serum bicarbonate levels to normal. Once the serum bicarbonate has been normalized, the maintenance bicarbonate dose is merely that required to buffer the daily excess of mineral acid production over net urinary acid excretion. Even if a patient with type I RTA had zero net acid excretion, which would be most unusual, his or her daily bicarbonate requirement would only be required to neutralize the 1 mEq/kg body weight (60–70 mEq) of mineral acid produced daily.

In **type II RTA**, a major defect is in the proximal tubular reabsorption of filtered bicarbonate. As a result, bicarbonate is lost in the urine, the extracellular bicarbonate buffer pool is reduced, and plasma bicarbonate concentration decreases. However, as the filtered load of bicarbonate decreases to a point that matches the degree of reduction in proximal bicarbonate absorption, a new steady state of bicarbonate filtration and reabsorption is achieved, bicarbonate disappears from the urine, and plasma bicarbonate remains stable at a reduced level. Unlike patients with type I RTA, patients with type II RTA are not in a continuous state of net acid accumulation, and long-term metabolic consequences from type II RTA are minimal. However, correcting the reduced plasma bicarbonate level in patients with type I RTA is very difficult, because the administration of exogenous bicarbonate will again cause the filtered load of bicarbonate to exceed the proximal tubular capacity to reabsorb bicarbonate. Administered bicarbonate is promptly excreted in the urine along with potassium, which may induce hypokalemia.

**13. What are the indications for bicarbonate therapy in patients with acute metabolic acidosis?**

Bicarbonate therapy should be reserved for patients with severe metabolic acidosis, characterized by hemodynamic instability, blood pH less than 7.15, or serum bicarbonate less than 12 mEq/L. Bicarbonate therapy is most beneficial in patients with metabolic acidosis that is due to bicarbonate loss from the body (such as severe diarrhea). It is generally not indicated if accumulated bicarbonate precursors (such as lactic acid or ketoacids) can be metabolized to generate bicarbonate once the underlying metabolic abnormality is corrected. The greatest degree of bicarbonate precursor accumulation occurs in patients with azotemia because there will be less filtration and secretion of these sodium salts. The goal of bicarbonate therapy is not to normalize serum bicarbonate but to improve hemodynamic and central nervous system function and severe acidemia. Bicarbonate dose should be calculated to increase the serum bicarbonate to 15 mEq/L or blood pH to 7.15, but no higher. In more severe and chronic metabolic acidosis, as nonbicarbonate buffers are recruited, the volume of distribution for administered bicarbonate increases and may approximate total body weight. Therefore, it is important to realize that these calculations are only estimates. If the serum bicarbonate is greater than 10 mEq/L, the volume of distribution in liters for administered bicarbonate is 0.5 times the body weight in kilograms. If the serum bicarbonate is 5–10 mEq/L, then the volume of distribution of administered bicarbonate is 0.75 times the body weight in kilograms. If the serum bicarbonate is less than 5 mEq/L, then the volume of distribution of administered bicarbonate is 1.0 times the body weight in kilograms. Bicarbonate dose should be equal to the body weight × the volume distribution × (15 – the initial bicarbonate concentration). Fifty percent of the calculated bicarbonate dose should be administered immediately by intravenous bolus, with the remainder administered over 6–12 hours by intravenous infusion. Ongoing generation of acid may require frequent monitoring of the response to bicarbonate administration and adjustment of the dosage accordingly.

**14. What are the causes of lactic acidosis and their implications regarding management and prognosis?**

**Type A lactic acidosis** is associated with decreased delivery of oxygen to the tissues, as a result of either hypoxemia or hypotension. Patients with ongoing sepsis may have shunting of blood flow away from capillaries, leading to tissue hypoxia in the absence of overt hypotension, and also fall into the type A lactic acidosis group. **Type B lactic acidosis** is due to abnormalities of cellular metabolism, frequently associated with an uncoupling of oxidative phosphorylation, as may be seen in the setting of disseminated malignancy or certain toxins, including cyanide, phenformin, metformin, and salicylates. Prognosis of lactic acidosis depends on reversal of the underlying illness. If the underlying illness cannot be identified or corrected, as is more often the case in type B lactic acidosis, then the prognosis for survival tends to be very poor.

### 15. Should bicarbonate be administered to patients with lactic acidosis?

The role of bicarbonate therapy in patients with lactic acidosis is controversial. No study has demonstrated a relationship between the amount of bicarbonate administered to patients with lactic acidosis and the eventual outcome. Some experimental studies have demonstrated that bicarbonate administration results in the paradoxic acidification of the cerebrospinal fluid (because the $CO_2$ generated from some of the administered bicarbonate diffuses into the cerebrospinal fluid faster than the bicarbonate itself), results in the generation of more carbon dioxide and a higher $Paco_2$, and actually increases lactic acid production by the cells—all resulting in a potential exacerbation rather than amelioration of the acidosis. However, because the goal of alkali administration in the setting of metabolic acidosis is stabilization of the cardiovascular system, raising the pH to greater than 7.15 may improve cardiac performance and enhance tissue oxygen delivery, thus decreasing lactate production.

### 16. What is the expected respiratory compensation in metabolic acidosis?

Compensatory hyperventilation is expected. The expected $Paco_2$ should be 1.5 times the serum bicarbonate + 8 ± 2.

### 17. What is the pathophysiology and treatment of the metabolic acidosis in patients with chronic renal failure?

A major defect in acid-base homeostasis in patients with chronic renal failure is decreased renal ammoniagenesis resulting from the decrease in functioning nephron mass. As a result of decreased net acid excretion, the rate of renal bicarbonate regeneration falls short of the rate of mineral acid production, and the patient goes into a state of positive acid balance, leading to titration of bicarbonate and nonbicarbonate buffers and a metabolic acidosis. Therefore, the initial acid-base disorder in progressive chronic renal insufficiency is a hyperchloremic metabolic acidosis. This is typically seen when the glomerular filtration rate declines to approximately 25 ml/minute. An anion gap metabolic acidosis develops when the glomerular filtration rate falls to approximately 15 ml/minute because the kidneys are no longer able to excrete endogenously produced mineral acid salts (e.g., sulfates and phosphates). Dietary protein restriction has been advocated to decrease the imbalance between acid production and excretion, which thereby ameliorates the acidosis of chronic renal failure. As is the case in patients with type I RTA, a shortfall between real bicarbonate regeneration and acid production can be made up with exogenous alkali administration.

### 18. What is type IV RTA?

A subset of patients with chronic renal failure who have hyperkalemia and metabolic acidosis out of proportion to their degree of renal function impairment carry a diagnosis of type IV RTA. This condition appears to be more common in patients whose renal disease is due to diabetic nephropathy, chronic interstitial nephritis, obstructive uropathy, sickle cell nephropathy, and chronic transplant rejection. Many of these patients will prove to have a subnormal plasma renin and aldosterone response to diuretic-induced volume depletion and upright posture, a condition known as *hyporeninemic hypoaldosteronism*. Because the hyperkalemia in this condition tends to be more problematic than the metabolic acidosis, therapy is primarily directed at augmenting renal potassium excretion with loop diuretics and exogenous mineralocorticoid. These therapies tend to have a modest effect on correcting the metabolic acidosis.

BIBLIOGRAPHY

1. Arieff A: Indications for use of bicarbonate in patients with metabolic acidosis. Br J Anaesth 67:165–177, 1991.

2. Battle DC, Hizon M, Cohen E, et al: The use of the urinary anion gap in the diagnosis of hyper-chloremic metabolic acidosis. N Engl J Med 318:594–599, 1988.
 3. Dyck RF, Asthana S, Kalra J, et al: A modification of the urine osmolal gap: An improved method for estimating urine ammonium. Am J Nephrol 10:359–362, 1990.
 4. Gabow PA: Disorders associated with an altered anion gap. Kidney Int 27:472–483, 1985.
 5. Garella S, Dana C, Chazan J: Severity of metabolic acidosis is a determinant of bicarbonate requirements. N Engl J Med 289:121–126, 1973.
 6. Halperin ML, Vasuvattakul S, Bayoumi A: A modified classification of metabolic acidosis: A pathophysiologic approach. Nephron 60:129–133, 1992.
 7. Madias NE: Lactic acidosis. Kidney Int 29:752–774, 1986.
 8. Narins RG, Emmett M: Simple and mixed acid-base disorders: A practical approach. Medicine 59:161–187, 1980.
 9. Schelling JR, Howard RL, Winter SD, Linas SL: Increased osmolal gap in alcoholic ketoacidosis and lactic acidosis. Ann Intern Med 113:580–582, 1990.
10. Stacpoole PW: Lactic acidosis: The case against bicarbonate therapy. Ann Intern Med 105:276–279, 1986

# 66. METABOLIC ALKALOSIS

*Bruce E. Berger, M.D.*

### 1. What is metabolic alkalosis?
Metabolic alkalosis is an acid-base disturbance characterized by an increased blood pH due to a primary increase in plasma bicarbonate concentration.

### 2. What is the difference between metabolic alkalosis and metabolic alkalemia?
**Metabolic alkalosis** describes a process that may or may not lead to a state of metabolic alkalemia. By definition, a state of metabolic alkalosis must exist in order to have metabolic alkalemia. The converse is not necessarily true. Metabolic alkalosis need not result in alkalemia if there is a concomitant state of metabolic or respiratory acidosis.

### 3. What mechanisms account for the increase in the anion gap occasionally observed in patients with metabolic alkalemia?
1. Independent of hypoxemia, lactate dehydrogenase is stimulated by alkalemia. However, this generally increases lactate levels by no more than 4 mmol/L.

2. Volume depletion, common in many clinical states associated with metabolic alkalosis, results in an increase in plasma albumin concentration. Because each gram per deciliter of albumin contributes about 2.0–2.5 mEq/L to the anion gap, an increase in albumin concentration increases the anion gap.

3. Because albumin is a buffer, as arterial pH increases, $H^+$ ions dissipate from albumin exposing more anionic sites. Thus, the net charge of albumin molecules increases and each gram per deciliter of albumin possesses a greater anionic charge.

### 4. What factors influence renal handling of bicarbonate?
Under normal circumstances, absorption of filtered bicarbonate plateaus at the normal serum bicarbonate concentration of 25–28 mEq/L. At higher levels of serum bicarbonate, the incremental bicarbonate present in the glomerular filtrate is rejected by the renal tubules and appears in the urine. This phenomenon is known as the tubular transport maximum ($T_m$) for bicarbonate. Four factors may increase the $T_m$ for bicarbonate, allowing for tubular reabsorption of increased amounts of filtered bicarbonate and the maintenance of elevated serum bicarbonate concentrations:
1. Extracellular volume depletion (resulting in a decrease glomerular filtration rate and, therefore, filtered load of bicarbonate)
2. Hypokalemia
3. Hypercapnia
4. Increased mineralocorticoid activity

### 5. Distinguish between the generation stage and maintenance stage of metabolic alkalosis.
The generation of metabolic alkalosis refers to the condition that results in the initial elevation in serum bicarbonate concentration. This is due either to a net loss of hydrogen ions from the body (as occurs in vomiting or with loop diuretics) or from addition of bicarbonate in excess of that required by net acid excretion. However, the accumulation of bicarbonate in the extracellular fluid is not sufficient to sustain a meta-

bolic alkalosis, because a normal $T_m$ for bicarbonate would cause the additional bicarbonate to be excreted rapidly in the urine. In order for a metabolic alkalosis to be maintained, one or more of the factors described in question 4 must be present to raise the $T_m$ of bicarbonate above normal, maintaining a higher-than-normal serum bicarbonate concentration. The factor or factors that raise the $T_m$ for bicarbonate and perpetuate the elevated serum bicarbonate concentration maintain the metabolic alkalosis. In the most common type of metabolic alkalosis (i.e., chloride responsive), approximately two thirds of the maintenance of the alkalosis is due to an increase in net acid excretion (resulting from increased bicarbonate reabsorption) and one third is due to a decrease in the filtered load of bicarbonate.

### 6. What conditions may lead to the generation of a metabolic alkalosis?

The etiologies of metabolic alkalosis fall into three major categories:

1. Extracellular volume depletion caused by the loss of chloride-rich fluid from the body, resulting in a secondary increase in aldosterone

2. A primary increase in mineralocorticoid or mineralocorticoid-like activity

3. Administration of alkali in a patient with renal insufficiency.

Extracellular volume depletion is a chloride-deficient state. This is seen in vomiting (where hydrochloric acid is lost), with the use of diuretics (which inhibit chloride reabsorption in the loop of Henle and early distal nephron), and with a villous adenoma of the colon (which secretes a chloride-rich diarrheal fluid). These conditions result in a state of secondary hyperreninemic hyperaldosteronism. As such, there will be an increase in proximal tubule fractional reabsorption of sodium and bicarbonate (due to increased levels of angiotensin II) and an increase in collecting duct secretion of $H^+$ (due to increased levels of aldosterone). The kidney's response to volume depletion takes precedence over maintaining acid-base balance. However, the amount of sodium bicarbonate the tubules can reabsorb will be limited by those factors described in question 4. In addition, at times when bicarbonate generation is occurring and the plasma bicarbonate is rising, the filtered load of bicarbonate transiently increases. As this happens, there will be even less tubular reabsorption, and bicarbonaturia ensues. Because sodium is the major urine cation, it will be excreted even in the setting of volume depletion. Chloride reabsorption, however, remains intact, and the urine chloride concentration will be low (typically less than 20 mEq/L). It is important to note that the metabolic alkalosis will be maintained through this mechanism long after the initial loss of chloride-rich fluid has ceased, as long as exogenous chloride is not provided to replace the deficit.

The second major mechanism by which metabolic alkalosis can be generated is through a primary or autonomous increase in mineralocorticoid activity. The increase in hydrogen ion secretion by distal tubular cells is accompanied by the production of additional bicarbonate, which accumulates in the extracellular fluid. At the same time, sodium reabsorption and potassium secretion in the distal nephron also are accelerated, leading to potassium losses in the urine and hypokalemia. The metabolic alkalosis is maintained both by hypokalemia and by the effect of the mineralocorticoid on the renal tubule. The primary increase in sodium reabsorption by the distal nephron usually leads to expansion of extracellular intravascular fluid volume and hypertension.

Metabolic alkalosis due to excessive alkali administration in the setting of renal insufficiency is much less common than the etiologies described above. It may occur in patients with renal insufficiency who are given alkali-rich intravenous fluid such as Ringer's lactate or intravenous hyperalimentation. It also may occur in a condition known as the **milk-alkali syndrome**, in which excessive consumption of milk and calcium-containing antacids for treatment of dyspepsia leads to renal insufficiency due to nephrocalcinosis and impaired alkali excretion.

## 7. How is metabolic alkalosis classified?

Metabolic alkalosis can be classified based on the urine chloride concentration. A **chloride responsive** or **sensitive** metabolic alkalosis is present when urine chloride concentration is less 20 mEq/L. Volume depletion stimulates both extrarenal and renal baroreceptor activation that results in avid sodium and chloride reabsorption in the proximal tubule and collecting tubule nephron segments.

A **chloride unresponsive** or **resistant** metabolic alkalosis is present when the urine chloride is greater than 20 mEq/L. This condition is a reflection of a *primary* increase in mineralocorticoid activity and, as such, is associated with extracellular volume expansion. This leads to suppression of sodium and chloride reabsorption out of the proximal tubule and from the nonmineralocorticoid sensitive regions of the collecting tubules (the latter in part is due to atrial natriuretic factor). The table lists common causes for metabolic alkalosis.

*Diagnosis of Metabolic Alkalosis*

| CHLORIDE RESPONSIVE (URINE CHLORIDE < 20 mEq/L) | CHLORIDE UNRESPONSIVE (URINE CHLORIDE > 20 mEq/L) |
|---|---|
| **Normotensive or hypotensive** | **Hypertensive** |
| Vomiting | Primary mineralocorticoid excess |
| Nasogastric suction |   Adrenal adenoma/hyperplasia |
| Diuretics |   Cushing's disease/syndrome |
| Posthypercapnic |   Natural licorice ingestion |
| Bicarbonate administration | Adrenal enzymatic defects |
| Potassium deficiency | Renal artery stenosis |
| | **Normotensive** |
| | $Mg^{++}$ deficiency |
| | Severe $K^+$ deficiency |
| | Bartter's syndrome |
| | Gitelman's syndrome |

## 8. What is "paradoxical aciduria"?

It is a common misconception that urine pH must always reflect the arterial pH. The urine pH is a reflection of urinary buffers (primarily titratable acids), ammonium, bicarbonate, and free $H^+$ and need not reflect what is happening to plasma pH. Metabolic alkalosis is an example. Paradoxical aciduria occurs when three conditions coexist:

1. There is a chloride responsive metabolic alkalosis.
2. Volume contraction is severe.
3. The generation stage has ceased.

As described in question 6, bicarbonaturia only occurs during the generation stage of metabolic alkalosis. During the maintenance stage, bicarbonaturia ceases (1) because the increased filtered load of sodium bicarbonate that was present during the generation stage decreases due to reduction in glomerular filtration rate, which occurs consequent to worsening volume depletion, and (2) because of the ongoing enhanced fractional reabsorption of bicarbonate in the proximal tubule occurring from increased angiotensin II production. A state of marked secondary hyperaldosteronism is reflected both by the low urine chloride and by the enhanced distal secretion of $H^+$. The secretion of $H^+$ is in excess of urinary buffers and, therefore, results in a urine pH that is not alkalotic (pH ~ 6.8).

## 9. What is post-hypercapnic metabolic alkalosis?

This condition is found most often in patients with cor pulmonale and chronic respiratory acidosis. The metabolic response to chronic respiratory acidosis is an increased net acid excretion and, therefore, bicarbonate regeneration and production. The classic clinical scenario begins with an event that results in intubation and mechanical ventilation. The patient is ventilated down to a $Paco_2$ that is less than his or her baseline level (e.g., $Paco_2$ of 40 mmHg versus 60 mmHg). This results in the "unmasking" of the initial compensatory state of metabolic alkalosis to that of a "primary" state. Because the renal response of bicarbonaturia requires at least many hours to unfold, therapy is directed at allowing for hypoventilation to recur.

**10. What are Bartter's and Gitelman's syndromes?**

Both are disorders characterized by a chloride-resistant hypokalemic metabolic alkalosis, normal blood pressure, hyperreninemic hyperaldosteronism, and juxtaglomerular cell hyperplasia. Bartter's syndrome most commonly occurs in children. These individuals have findings akin to a nephrogenic diabetes insipidus, and they have hypercalciuria. Gitelman's syndrome is more common in adults and is associated with hypocalciuria and hypomagnesemia. Bartter's syndrome is now known to be the result of mutational defects in the thick ascending limb of the loop of Henle. These defects involve the apical NaK2Cl transporter, the apical membrane $K^+$ conductance channel, or the basolateral chloride channel. These patients behave as though they are receiving chronic treatment with furosemide. Gitelman's syndrome results from mutational defects in the thiazide-sensitive NaCl transporter. These patients behave as though they are receiving chronic treatment with thiazides.

Treatment strategies for these disorders have generally been of limited efficacy but have included the use of nonsteroidal anti-inflammatory drugs (NSAIDs), aldosterone antagonists, angiotensin-converting enzyme inhibitors, potassium supplementation, magnesium supplementation, and propranolol. Because these are very uncommon disorders, it is important, especially in adults, to exclude surreptitious vomiting and diuretic usage.

**11. What is the treatment for metabolic alkalosis?**

Treatment for metabolic alkalosis depends on the mechanism by which the alkalosis was generated and maintained. In patients with metabolic alkalosis associated with extracellular volume depletion and excessive loss of chloride-containing fluids, the therapy is directed at restoring effective extracellular fluid volume through the administration of chloride-containing solutions. These patients have a secondary increase in mineralocorticoid activity due to the volume depletion. Consequently, potassium secretion in the distal nephron is accelerated, leading to urinary potassium losses and hypokalemia. Treatment includes administration of potassium chloride to correct the hypokalemia and sodium chloride to correct the hypovolemia. In patients in whom there is a contraindication to the administration of sodium chloride (e.g., congestive heart failure or cor pulmonale), the metabolic alkalemia can be treated by the use of either a potassium-sparing diuretic (e.g., amiloride) or a carbonic anhydrase inhibitor (e.g., acetazolamide). Amiloride may be preferable for the following reasons: (1) it corrects the metabolic alkalemia by inhibiting $H^+$ secretion, (2) it minimizes ongoing kaliuresis present with this state of secondary hyperaldosteronism, and (3) it decreases the magnesuria induced by loop diuretics. Acetazolamide will be of limited efficacy if there is significant volume depletion and pre-renal azotemia. Should a bicarbonaturia ensue, there will be an enhanced kaliuresis. This will require additional potassium supplementation to avoid potentially serious hypokalemic associated arrhythmias. Bicarbonaturia also results in phosphaturia and the possible need for phosphorus supplementation. Intravenous 0.1N hydrochloric acid is reserved for the truly rare patient with severe metabolic alkalemia in whom no other therapy is possible (e.g., the renal failure patient in whom the gastrointestinal tract cannot be used).

The treatment for metabolic alkalosis due to a primary increase in mineralocorticoid or mineralocorticoid-like activity is to eliminate or antagonize the mineralocorticoid activity.

If it is due to a surgically resectable adenoma, efforts should be made to excise the adenoma. In the case of adrenal hyperplasia, spironolactone, a direct antagonist of the action of aldosterone, is the treatment of choice. These patients are often profoundly hypokalemic because of the increased urinary potassium excretion. Large doses of oral potassium supplements may be required to correct the hypokalemia.

The treatment of metabolic alkalosis due to excessive alkali administration in the setting of renal insufficiency is obviously to decrease the alkali administration. In most of these situations, the kidney will eventually excrete the excessive bicarbonate, returning plasma bicarbonate pH to normal.

### BIBLIOGRAPHY

1. Berger BE, Cogan MG, Sebastian A: Reduced glomerular filtration rate and enhanced bicarbonate reabsorption metabolic alkalosis in humans. Kidney Int 26:205–208, 1984.
2. Harrington JT: Metabolic alkalosis. Kidney Int 26:88–97, 1984.
3. Knutsen OH: New method for administration of hydrochloric acid in metabolic alkalosis. Lancet 1:53–55, 1983.
4. Koch SM, Taylor RW: Chloride ion in intensive care medicine. Crit Care Med 20:227–240, 1992.
5. Rimmer JM, Gennari FJ: Metabolic alkalosis. J Intens Care Med 78:482–485, 1985.
6. Simon DB, Lifton RP: Ion transporter mutations in Gitelman's and Bartter's syndromes. Curr Opin Nephrol Hypertens 7:43–47,1998.
7. Vaziri ND, Byrne C, Barton CH, et al: Prevention of metabolic alkalosis induced by gastric fluid loss using H2 receptor antagonists. Gen Pharmacol 16:141–144, 1985.

# 67. RESPIRATORY ACIDOSIS

*Andrew S. O'Connor, D.O.*

**1. What is respiratory acidosis? What are some clinical characteristics of respiratory acidosis?**

Acidosis is a metabolic disturbance characterized by a fall in arterial pH (i.e., an increase in $[H^+]$). Acidosis can be separated into **metabolic** causes, those associated with a "primary" disturbance in $[HCO_3]$, and **respiratory** causes, those associated with a "primary" disturbance in the elimination of $CO_2$. Therefore, respiratory acidosis is characterized clinically by a decreased pH (acidemia), an elevated $pCO_2$ (hypercapnia), and a variable change in $HCO_3^-$.

**2. How is $CO_2$ produced by the body? What are some conditions that can alter the production of $CO_2$ by the body? How is $CO_2$ eliminated by the body?**

$CO_2$ is produced as a byproduct of endogenous metabolism, especially of carbohydrates. These processes lead to the production of approximately 15,000 mmol of $CO_2$ per day. Any condition that affects the basal metabolic rate can alter the production of $CO_2$. Examples of such conditions include increased activity (exercise) and febrile states (fevers). $CO_2$ production rises approximately 13% for every 1°C rise above normal. The major route of elimination of $CO_2$ from the body is via the lungs in a process termed *ventilation*. The relationship between the production and elimination of $CO_2$ can be expressed as:

$$Paco_2 = K (V_{CO_2}/V_A)$$

K is a constant with a value of 0.863 under standard conditions.
$V_{CO_2}$ = carbon dioxide production
$V_A$ = alveolar ventilation

**3. How is arterial $Paco_2$ regulated?**

The arterial $Paco_2$ (normally 40 ± 4 mmHg) and $PaO_2$ are closely linked and determined by alveolar ventilation. An acute increase in $Paco_2$ stimulates chemosensitive areas in the carotid sinus and in the aortic arch. These chemoreceptors are also especially sensitive to changes in arterial oxygen content ($PaO_2$). Over time, the increase in $Paco_2$ leads to a decrease in central nervous system pH and direct stimulation of respiratory centers located within the ventrolateral medullary surface. The latter response is much more pronounced than the former, and in normal subjects, alveolar ventilation rises by 1–4 L/min for every 1 mmHg increase in $Paco_2$.

**4. What is the relationship between $CO_2$ and pH?**

$CO_2$ is not an acid in itself. Rather, it is closely related to $[H^+]$ as demonstrated by the following relationship:

$$CO_2 + H_2O \Leftrightarrow H_2CO_3 \Leftrightarrow H^+ + HCO_3^-$$

$[H^+]$ (nanomoles/L) can be predicted by:

$$[H^+] = 24 \times (Pco_2 / [HCO_3^-])$$

or, in logarithmic terms:

$$pH = 6.10 + \log ([HCO_3^-] / 0.03\ Pco_2)$$

which, you will notice, is the Henderson-Hasselbach equation.

## 5. What is the pathophysiology of respiratory acidosis?
Under steady-state conditions, the rate of elimination of $Paco_2$ matches the rate of $Paco_2$ production. Thus:

$$Paco_2 = K\ (V_{CO_2}/V_A)$$

where $Vco_2 = CO_2$ production, $V_A$ = alveolar ventilation, and $K = 0.863$ (a constant).

Hypercapnia can result either from increased $CO_2$ production or from decreased alveolar ventilation. Increased $CO_2$ production is an uncommon cause of respiratory acidosis because the body normally can raise its ventilatory rate to match almost any increase in $CO_2$ production. Thus, hypercapnia and respiratory acidosis are usually the results of decreased alveolar ventilation.

## 6. What is the pathophysiology of decreased alveolar ventilation?
Alveolar ventilation is expressed as:

Alveolar ventilation = minute ventilation – dead space ventilation

Decreased alveolar ventilation results from decreased minute ventilation in states of central nervous system depression, advanced neuromuscular disease, and respiratory muscle fatigue. Increased dead space ventilation mainly results from disorders associated with ventilation-perfusion mismatching.

## 7. How does the body respond to an acute increase in $Paco_2$?
An acute increase in $Paco_2$ results in an immediate small increase in plasma $HCO_3^-$, averaging 1 mEq/L for every 10 mmHg rise in $PCO_2$. This minimal elevation in $HCO_3^-$ is a consequence of the inability of $HCO_3^-$ to buffer $H_2CO_3$. Therefore, the acute rise in $[H^+]$ related to the elevation of $PCO_2$ must be buffered by cellular protein buffers such as hemoglobin. The maximum concentration of $HCO_3^-$ reached during compensation for acute hypercapnia is about 30 mEq/L. This chemical adaptation is complete in 5–10 minutes. For instance, if $PCO_2$ acutely rises from 40 mmHg to 80 mmHg, the expected rise in $HCO_3$ would be 4 mEq/L to roughly 28. Using the relationship between $[HCO_3^-]$, $PCO_2$, and pH:

$$pH = 6.10 + \log[28 / (0.03 \times 80)]$$
$$pH = 7.17$$

## 8. What is the adaptive response seen in chronic respiratory acidosis?
The adaptive response to chronic respiratory acidosis is an increase in plasma $HCO_3^-$ generated mainly by the kidney. This response is accomplished by a net increase in the secretion of $H^+$ and reabsorption of filtered $HCO_3^-$.

## 9. How do the kidneys generate bicarbonate in chronic respiratory acidosis?
The kidneys generate bicarbonate by the following mechanisms:
• Increased net urinary acid excretion (as ammonium and titratable acids)
• Increased renal bicarbonate reabsorption

## 10. In chronic respiratory acidosis, how does serum $HCO_3^-$ change in response to an increase in $Paco_2$?
The serum $HCO_3^-$ increases by about 3.5 mEq/L for every 10-mmHg rise in $Paco_2$. This physiologic adaptation usually requires 3–5 days.

**11. What are the causes of acute respiratory acidosis?**

| CAUSE | EXAMPLE |
|---|---|
| Central nervous system disorders | Head trauma<br>Drugs (e.g., opiates, sedatives, anesthetics)<br>Cerebrovascular accident<br>Central sleep apnea |
| Neuromuscular disorders | High spinal cord injury<br>Guillain-Barré syndrome<br>Myasthenic crisis<br>Drugs (e.g., aminoglycosides, succinylcholine)<br>Hypokalemic or hyperkalemic paralysis |
| Restriction to ventilation | Flail chest<br>Pneumothorax, hemothorax |
| Upper airway dysfunction | Aspiration of foreign body, food<br>Laryngospasm<br>Obstructive sleep apnea |
| Alveolar causes | Severe pneumonia<br>Adult respiratory distress syndrome |
| Impaired pulmonary perfusion | Massive pulmonary embolism<br>Cardiac arrest |
| Iatrogenic | Complications of mechanical ventilation |

**12. What are the causes of chronic respiratory acidosis?**

| CAUSE | EXAMPLE |
|---|---|
| Central nervous system disorders | Pickwickian syndrome (obesity-hypoventilation syndrome)<br>Brain tumor<br>Chronic use of sedatives, opiates |
| Neuromuscular disorders | Poliomyelitis<br>Multiple sclerosis<br>Myxedema<br>Amyotrophic lateral sclerosis |
| Restrictive to ventilation | Kyphoscoliosis<br>Extreme obesity<br>Fibrothorax<br>Hydrothorax |
| Upper airway obstruction | Vocal cord paralysis<br>Tracheal stenosis after prolonged intubation |
| Lower airway obstruction | Chronic obstructive pulmonary disease (COPD) |

**13. What are the neurologic manifestations of respiratory acidosis?**

The neurologic manifestations depend on the magnitude and rapidity with which respiratory acidosis develops and on the degree of accompanying hypoxemia. Patients may present with irritability, confusion, headaches, agitation, delirium, or hallucinations. Extreme elevations of $Paco_2$ are associated with myoclonic jerks, tremors, and even coma. Deep tendon reflexes are increased with lesser degrees of hypercapnia and are depressed in patients with severe hypercapnia. Pupillary constriction also may be observed.

## 14. What are cardiovascular manifestations of respiratory acidosis?

Mild to moderate respiratory acidosis is associated with an increase in cardiac output and blood pressure. Myocardial contractility may be impaired in patients with severe hypercapnia with a resulting decrease in cardiac output and blood pressure. Cardiac arrhythmias, mainly supraventricular arrhythmias, may be observed, but probably reflect not just the elevated $Paco_2$ but a combination of factors such as hypoxemia, electrolyte imbalance, sympathetic overactivity, and concomitant drug use.

## 15. What is the treatment for acute respiratory acidosis?

The mainstays of treatment of acute respiratory acidosis are to identify and treat the underlying cause with emphasis on maintaining airway patency and to use bronchodilators, corticosteroids, and antibiotics when clinically indicated. Alkali therapy is generally not used because it can be associated with the risk of volume overload and depression of ventilation mediated by an increase in pH. Alkali therapy may have a useful role in severe asthma in order to prevent barotrauma, which may result from attempts to improve pH by mechanical ventilation.

### BIBLIOGRAPHY

1. Adrogue HJ, Madias NE: Management of life-threatening acid-base disorders. N Engl J Med 378:107–111, 1998.
2. Berger AJ, Mitchell RA, Serveringhaus JW: Regulation of respiration. N Engl J Med 297:92, 138, 194, 1977.
3. Cohen JJ: Acid-base. In Kassirer JP, Hricik DE, Cohen JJ (eds): Repair of Body Fluids: Principles and Practices. Philadelphia, W.B. Saunders, 1989, pp 130–168.
4. Madias NE, Wolf CJ, Cohen JJ: Regulation of acid-base equilibrium in chronic hypercapnia. Kidney Int 27:538–543, 1985.
5. Rose BD (ed): Clinical Physiology of Acid-Base and Electrolyte Disorders, 4th ed. New York, McGraw-Hill, 1994.

# 68. RESPIRATORY ALKALOSIS

*Andrew S. O'Connor, D.O.*

### 1. What is respiratory alkalosis?

Respiratory alkalosis is an acid-base disturbance characterized by a primary decrease in $Paco_2$ leading to an elevated arterial pH. Respiratory alkalosis must be differentiated from other causes of a low $Paco_2$ such as metabolic acidosis. In metabolic acidosis, the primary disorder is one of an increase in $[H^+]$, or a decrease in $[HCO_3^-]$. This primary disturbance leads to a fall in arterial pH (i.e., acidosis). The clinically observed decrease in $Paco_2$ is secondary, reflecting compensation for the primary disturbance.

### 2. What is the pathophysiologic basis for respiratory alkalosis?

Under steady state conditions, $Paco_2$, is directly proportional to the rate of $CO_2$ production and inversely related to alveolar ventilation, as follows:

$$Paco_2 = K (V_{CO_2}/V_A)$$

K is a constant with a value of 0.863 under standard conditions.
$V_{CO_2}$ = carbon dioxide production
$V_A$ = alveolar ventilation
Respiratory alkalosis can result from increased alveolar ventilation (most common), decreased $CO_2$ production, or both. Hyperventilation, in turn, can result from hypoxemia that stimulates peripheral chemoreceptors mainly along the carotid bodies and the aortic arch, direct stimulation of the respiratory center, and/or secondary signals arising from the lungs.

### 3. How does the body respond to acute respiratory alkalosis?

The adaptation to acute respiratory alkalosis occurs within 5–10 minutes by a decrease in plasma $[HCO_3^-]$. When $Paco_2$ acutely decreases, hydrogen ions ($H^+$) are released from intracellular buffers and combine with extracellular $HCO_3^-$ in a chemical response to generate more $CO_2$, based on the following equilibrium:

$$H^+ + HCO_3^- \Leftrightarrow H_2CO_3 \Leftrightarrow CO_2 + H_2O$$

### 4. How much does the plasma $HCO_3^-$ decrease in response to an acute decrease in $Paco_2$?

The plasma $HCO_3^-$ decreases by approximately 2 mEq/L for every 10 mmHg decrease in $Paco_2$.

### 5. What other electrolyte abnormalities can be seen in acute respiratory alkalosis?

The small decrease in plasma bicarbonate is balanced by a small increase in plasma chloride, lactate, and other unmeasured ions. A decrease in $[K^+]$ also can be seen because of the movement of this ion from the extracellular to the intracellular space.

### 6. What is the physiologic response to chronic respiratory alkalosis?

The response to chronic respiratory alkalosis is mediated mainly by a decrease in $H^+$ secretion by the kidney as well as $HCO_3^-$ loss in the urine. The renal adaptation to respiratory alkalosis begins within 2 hours but requires 2–3 days to complete. As mentioned in other chapters, the secretion of $H^+$ by the kidney is accomplished mainly through the excretion of ammonium and titratable acids. $HCO_3^-$ is directly regulated by the proximal tubule.

**7. What is the magnitude of change in plasma $HCO_3^-$ in chronic respiratory alkalosis?**

The plasma $HCO_3^-$ decreases by approximately 4–5 mEq/L for every 10 mmHg decrease in $Paco_2$.

**8. What are the causes of respiratory alkalosis?**

1. Hypoxemia
   High altitude
   Ventilation-perfusion mismatch (e.g., pneumonia, pulmonary embolism)
   Cyanotic heart disease
2. Pulmonary disorders
   Pneumonia
   Obstructive airway disease (e.g., asthma, chronic obstructive pulmonary disease [COPD])
   Other parenchymal lung disease
3. Central nervous system stimulation
   Pain
   Anxiety
   Fever
   Structural brain lesions (e.g., stroke, tumors)
4. Drugs
   Salicylates
   Progesterone
5. Others
   Mechanical ventilation
   Gram-negative sepsis
   Pregnancy
   Liver failure

**9. What are the clinical manifestations of respiratory alkalosis?**

Acute respiratory alkalosis produces clinical manifestations more often than chronic respiratory alkalosis does. Hypocapnia-induced cerebral vasoconstriction has been implicated in the pathogenesis of the neurologic manifestations that include paresthesias, circumoral numbness, light-headedness, tetany, and seizures. A variety of supraventricular arrhythmias may occur, particularly in critically ill patients.

**10. What is the treatment for respiratory alkalosis?**

Treatment is directed at management of the underlying cause. In anxiety-induced hyperventilation, reassurance, sedatives, or rebreathing into a closed system (e.g., paper bag) may help increase the $Paco_2$. Patients on mechanical ventilation may require skeletal muscle paralysis if respiratory alkalosis is severe.

BIBLIOGRAPHY

1. Adrogue HJ, Madias NE: Management of life-threatening acid-base disorders. N Engl J Med 338:107–111, 1998.
2. Berger AJ, Mitchell RA, Serveringhaus JW: Regulation of respiration. N Engl J Med 297:92, 138, 194, 1977.
3. Gennari FJ, Kassirer JP: Respiratory alkalosis. In Cohen JJ, Kassirer JP (eds): Acid-Base. Boston, Little, Brown, 1982, pp 349–376.
4. Krapf R, Beeler I, Hertner D, Hutler HN: Chronic respiratory alkalosis: The effect of sustained hyperventilation on renal regulation of acid-base equilibrium. N Engl J Med 324:1394–1401, 1991.
5. Rose BD: Clinical Physiology of Acid-Base and Electrolyte Disorders. New York, McGraw-Hill, 1994.

# 69. HYPONATREMIA AND HYPERNATREMIA

*Bruce E. Berger, M.D.*

**1. What do serum sodium determinations of 130 mEq/L, 140 mEq/L, and 150 mEq/L have in common?**

They each represent a concentration of sodium present in a liter of plasma.

**2. What do serum sodium determinations of 130 mEq/L, 140 mEq/L, and 150 mEq/L tell you about total body sodium and water content?**

Absolutely nothing.

**3. So, how does one make sense of these different sodium concentrations?**

Because the serum sodium concentration tells you nothing about total body sodium content and total body water content, it is the task of the clinician to determine both. Sodium content can be determined by taking advantage of the fact that it is essentially restricted to the extracellular space and, therefore, determines volume status. The history and physical examination should enable you to assess whether there is a state of volume depletion or volume surfeit. Determining the fractional excretion of sodium and urea nitrogen further refines your evaluation of the source of total body sodium depletion or surfeit (i.e., is it renal or extrarenal). The fractional excretion of urea nitrogen is of special utility because, in states of volume depletion, its excretion is not affected by the use of diuretics (i.e., the $FE_{Urea\ nitrogen}$ remains $< 35\%$).

The determination of total body water content is more difficult but is generally made by the history more so than the physical exam and by interpreting the serum sodium concentration in light of your determinations of total body sodium stores. As an example, a patient who presents with vomiting and diarrhea, poor oral intake, orthostatic vital signs, and a serum sodium concentration of 130 mEq/L will be total body sodium depleted. It is more difficult to state whether total body water content compared to baseline is increased or decreased. What we can say is that, compared to the reduction in total body sodium content, the change in total body water content is less than that seen with sodium.

It is important to keep in mind that hyponatremia and hypernatremia can each exist in states of volume depletion, euvolemia, and hypervolemia.

**4. What does the term *dehydration* mean?**

For those of you who have a food dehydrator at home you know that the only thing it does is remove water. Clinical use of the term *dehydration* should refer to patients with pure water depletion resulting in *hyper*natremia. Having said that, the word *dehydration* has become (erroneously) synonymous with volume depletion. In fact, more often than not, the volume-depleted patient is *hypo*natremic.

**5. How is plasma osmolality determined?**

The lab will measure the plasma osmolality if you order it. You can calculate the plasma (and, therefore, extracellular fluid osmolality) by the use of the following formula:

$$\text{Plasma osmolality (mOsm/kg)} = \{2\ [Na^+]\ (mEq/L) + [K^+]\ (mEq/L)\} + [\text{urea (mg/dl)}/2.8] + [\text{glucose (mg/dl)}/18]$$

Normally, the measured plasma osmolality is no more than 10 mOsm/kg higher than the calculated plasma osmolality.

**6. Is every hypernatremic patient also hyperosmolar?**

Yes—and of equal importance is the appreciation that they are hypertonic.

**7. Is there a difference between hypertonicity and hyperosmolality?**

Yes. Hypertonicity occurs when there is an increase in an impermeable solute (e.g., sodium) in the extracellular space. As such, water will follow the osmotic gradient and leave the cellular space, causing intracellular dehydration. By definition, therefore, if you are hypertonic, you must be hyperosmolar. The corollary, however, is not necessarily true. If hyperosmolality is caused by an increase in a permeable solute (e.g., urea or alcohol), there will no difference in intracellular and extracellular osmolalities. Hypertonicity does not occur in this setting.

**8. Is every hyponatremic patient also hyposmolar?**

No. You can confirm hypo-osmolality (with one exception) in hyponatremic patients by measuring the plasma osmolality.

**9. In what instances does hyponatremia not reflect hypo-osmolality?**

**Pseudohyponatremia** is a laboratory phenomenon seen with flame photometry measurements and less so when ion-specific electrodes are used to measure sodium concentration. Sodium determination in plasma reflects its presence in the water component of plasma. Severe hypertriglyceridemia (generally > 2000 mg/dl) and hyperproteinemia (total proteins > 18 gm/dl) result in pseudohyponatremia (generally not less than 128–130 mEq/L) because the portion of water in plasma is reduced by the increase in the lipid or protein component. Sodium concentration is measured as milliequivalents per liter of *plasma* and not *water*. The plasma osmolality remains normal.

**Spurious hyponatremia** most frequently occurs in uncontrolled diabetes. The plasma osmolality is elevated because of hyperglycemia. The increase in the extracellular fluid (ECF) osmolality results in the movement of water out of cells, thus diluting the plasma sodium concentration. To correct for this effect, the plasma sodium concentration is increased by 1.6 mEq/L for every 100 mg/dl of glucose above normal.

**Renal failure with hyponatremia** is a clinical disorder where true hyponatremia exists with a *measured* plasma osmolality that is normal or increased depending on the severity of the azotemia. Urea nitrogen is an ineffective osmolyte (see question 7). As such, hyponatremia that occurs in the setting of renal failure reflects a reduction in the *effective* plasma osmolality ($2 \times$ plasma $[Na^+]$ + [glucose]/18) even though the plasma osmolality is normal or increased.

**10. What is the diagnostic approach to the patient with hyponatremia?**

After you have ascertained you are dealing with true hyponatremia, you may organize your approach by determining total body sodium content. Hyponatremia is a common medical problem in hospitalized patients. Approximately 20% of patients admitted to medical and surgical services will have serum sodium concentrations of less than 135 mEq/L. The table at the top of the next page lists common etiologies.

**11. What is the syndrome of inappropriate antidiuretic hormone secretion (SIADH)?**

SIADH is a disorder characterized by a pure and primary disturbance in water metabolism. As such it can only be diagnosed in the absence of renal, adrenal, cardiac, thyroid, or hepatic diseases and in the absence of disturbances in ECF volume. By definition, the release of ADH in this condition mandates that neither of the two usual stimuli for ADH release, hyperosmolality and hypovolemia, are present. Most patients with SIADH have an autonomous release of ADH (hypothalamic as seen with strokes, tumors, abscesses, or

*Diagnostic Approach to the Patient with Hyponatremia*

| HYPOVOLEMIC | | EUVOLEMIC | HYPERVOLEMIC | |
| --- | --- | --- | --- | --- |
| FENa < 1% | FENa > 1% | | FENa < 1% | FENa > 1% |
| Diarrhea | Adrenal | SIADH | Acute GN | CRF |
| Vomiting | insufficiency | Psychogenic | CHF | ATN |
| (maintenance) | Salt-losing | polydipsia | Cirrhosis | |
| Diuretics (chronic) | nephropathy | Pure cortisol | Nephrotic | |
| Blood loss | | deficiency | syndrome | |

FENa = fractional excretion of sodium; SIADH = syndrome of inappropriate secretion of antidiuretic hormone; GN = glomerulonephritis; CHF = congestive heart failure; CRF = chronic renal failure; ATN = acute tubular nephrosis.

ectopic, as seen with small-cell lung cancer, tuberculosis, pneumonia). This syndrome also can develop in settings in which renal responsiveness to ADH is potentiated (e.g., by drugs such as chlorpropamide or nonsteroidal anti-inflammatory agents) or in which ADH release is enhanced by drugs (e.g., carbamazepine, cyclophosphamide).

**12. How is SIADH diagnosed?**
As noted above, patients with SIADH have no osmotic or volume-mediated stimulus for ADH release. Thyroid and cortisol testing are also normal. They do not have chronic pain. Because of water expansion, the urine sodium concentration is generally > 40 mEq/L. However, it can be less than 20 mEq/L in patients with poor intake or vomiting or diarrhea. Because the normal response to hypo-osmolality is a maximally diluted urine, a urine osmolality > 75–100 mOsm/kg is abnormal and consistent with SIADH. Additional clues are serum uric acid levels < 4 mg/dl and blood urea nitrogen (BUN) levels < 10 mg/dl. In this disorder, the fractional excretion of uric acid will be > 10% and urea nitrogen > 60%. A plasma ADH level can be obtained but is rarely needed.

**13. What is psychogenic polydipsia?**
This is a disorder classically seen in the psychiatric patient (manic or schizophrenic) who ingests large volumes of water. The glomerular filtration rate (GFR) is normal and the urine osmolality is 50–75 mOsm/kg.

**14. If the urine osmolality is maximally diluted how do these patients become hyponatremic?**
The urine osmolality reflects the number of osmotically active solutes in a kilogram of urine. As such, like the serum sodium value, it is a concentration term. It tells nothing about the volume of urine or solute load being excreted. It is actually very difficult to induce hyponatremia from fluid ingestion. The kidneys are able to excrete 15–18% of our daily glomerular ultrafiltrate as free water (daily GFR is 180 L $\times$ 15% = 27 L). Therefore, a person would need to ingest *more than* 1 L an hour of water every hour of the day to first exceed the capacity of the kidneys to excrete free water. Thus, in addition to an increase in fluid intake, the reason patients with psychogenic polydipsia (or any patients, for that matter) become hyponatremic is because of a decrease in their solute intake or load.

**15. How does the solute load affect the abilities of the kidneys to excrete free water?**
In order for the kidneys to produce urine they must excrete solute (in humans the urine osmolality ranges between 50 and 1400 mOsm/kg). The average Western diet contains about

900 mOsm of solute. The solute is primarily composed of sodium and protein (excreted as urea nitrogen). In homeostasis, we must excrete what we ingest (or else hypovolemia or hypervolemia, or hyponatremia or hypernatremia develops). If a person's solute load has decreased to 300 mOsm per day because of illness or psychosis, at a urine of 50 mOsm/kg, he or she will be able to excrete 6 L of water a day. If he or she ingests more than 6 L, hyponatremia develops because he cannot further reduce the urine osmolality. If the patient ingests all of 100 mOsm of solute per day, then he or she is able to excrete 2 L of urine a day. If the person ingests more than 2 L of fluid, hyponatremia (often severe) develops. You can see how it now becomes much easier to develop hyponatremia when solute intake is low. The amount of fluid you need to ingest no longer seems Herculean.

## 16. How is the solute load determined?

A good dietary history is usually enough. If necessary you can obtain a timed (generally 24 hour) urine collection for creatinine, sodium, urea nitrogen, glucose, and osmolality. With the timed urine, you may also calculate the osmolar clearance to further confirm the solute intake.

## 17. What is the osmolar clearance and how is it calculated?

The osmolar clearance ($C_{osm}$) represents the excretion of the daily solute in a volume of urine that is isotonic to plasma. If we ingest and excrete 900 mOsm/kg of solute a day we would need 3 L of isotonic urine in order to excrete our solute load. We use the concept of urine that is isotonic to plasma because glomerular ultrafiltrate (the "forerunner" of urine) arises from plasma. The daily solute load is "dissolved" in plasma and is excreted as part of the glomerular ultrafiltrate. It is the task of the tubules to excrete that part of the filtered load of sodium and urea nitrogen in glomerular ultrafiltrate (i.e., tubular fluid) that is necessary to get rid of the daily solute load. As a result of this, the tubules normally reabsorb ~99% of the filtered load of sodium and 50% of the filtered load of urea nitrogen. Therefore, the normal $C_{osm}$ is about 2 ml/min. Individuals with a decrease solute load have a $C_{osm}$ < 2 ml/min.

$$C_{osm} = \frac{\text{Urine Osm (mOsm/kg)}}{P_{osm} \text{ (mOsm/kg)}} \times V \text{ (ml/min)}$$

## 18. What are the clinical manifestations of hyponatremia?

Symptoms include impaired concentration, anorexia, nausea and vomiting, seizures, coma, and death. The most important determinant of symptoms is the rate at which hyponatremia develops rather than the absolute concentration. Given time (several days to a week), the brain is able to reduce intracellular osmolytes and, therefore, decrease the degree of brain edema that arises from plasma hypo-osmolality. Thus, a serum sodium value of 125 mEq/L that develops within a few hours (as can be seen with psychogenic polydipsia or SIADH) will be associated with more symptoms (perhaps life threatening) than someone who has a serum sodium concentration of 110 mEq/L that developed gradually over 1–2 weeks (as can be seen with chronic volume depletion).

## 19. Who is most likely to develop hyponatremic-associated cerebral edema?

Women, especially premenopausal women, are at greater risk than men of developing severe irreversible neurologic damage. It is seen most often in the postoperative setting. Interestingly, there is no gender difference before puberty.

## 20. How is hyponatremia treated?

The treatment is based on the diagnosis of the etiology of the hyponatremia.

**Hypovolemic hyponatremia** is treated with volume repletion (isotonic saline, enteral salt). The onset of free water clearance, which corrects hyponatremia, follows repletion of salt.

**Hypervolemic hyponatremia** is treated (separate from the specific treatment for the underlying disorder) with water restriction (at times as limited as 250 ml/day) and a loop diuretic.

**Euvolemic hyponatremia secondary to psychogenic polydipsia** is treated by keeping the patient away from water and any therapy the physician might otherwise consider.

**Euvolemic hyponatremia secondary to SIADH** is treated (separate from treating the underlying disorder) with water restriction. If the patient is symptomatic or the hyponatremia is severe, then additional acute therapy with 3% saline and furosemide is required. The rationale behind this therapy is that when you induce a diuresis with furosemide, you produce urine that contains about 70 mEq/L of sodium. You will replace the sodium losses using a smaller volume of infused 3% saline. Three percent saline contains about 0.5 mEq of sodium per milliliter. Assume that, with the administration of 5 mg of intravenous furosemide over 1 hour, you will induce 1 L of urine that contains 70 mEq of sodium. Because the goal of therapy is to cause a loss of water and not sodium, you would administer about 150 ml of 3% saline over the hour. There would be a net loss of 850 ml of water.

Treatment of chronic **SIADH** (separate from treating the underlying disorder) can be done with a high-salt diet and a loop diuretic that renders the urine about isotonic to plasma over the entire day, or with demeclocycline.

### 21. What determines the speed with which I correct hyponatremia?

The three most important determinants are:
1. The etiology of the hyponatremia
2. The presence of symptoms
3. The rate with which hyponatremia developed

Issues regarding the speed of correction most often come up in patients with SIADH. In the asymptomatic patient with chronic hyponatremia (present > 3–5 days), look to correct the hyponatremia at a rate that mirrors the time it took to develop. However, even the chronic asymptomatic patient with a serum sodium of 110 mEq/L should receive treatment to get the sodium to a less dangerous level. Generally 115–120 mEq/L is the goal. A rate of correction of about 0.5–1 mEq/L/hour should be the goal unless you know the severe hyponatremia occurred over a time frame that would require more rapid correction over several hours. Even if this is the case (and it would be rare), you would not want to correct the serum sodium concentration above 125–130 mEq/L. Above all, common sense and prudence (and an experienced nephrologist) should guide you.

### 22. What happens if hyponatremia is corrected too rapidly?

Too rapid correction or correction to normal sodium concentrations has been associated with pontine and extrapontine myelinolysis. This can result in spastic quadraparesis, pseudobulbar palsies, coma, and death.

### 23. What is the diagnostic approach to the patient with hypernatremia?

As with the hyponatremic patient, your assessment is accomplished by your history and physical to ascertain whether the is hypovolemic, euvolemic, or hypervolemic. The table at the top of the next page lists some common etiologies.

### 24. What is the appropriate renal response to hypernatremia?

Oliguria. Therefore, you should always further evaluate the nonoliguric hypernatremic patient. The table lists the usual etiologies. The urine osmolality will be of limited utility because all of these conditions (except central diabetes insipidus) generally will present with urine osmolalities ranging from about 250 to 400 mOsm/kg. The patient with partial

*Diagnostic Approach to the Patient with Hypernatremia*

| HYPOVOLEMIC | | EUVOLEMIC | HYPERVOLEMIC | |
| --- | --- | --- | --- | --- |
| FENa < 1% | FENa > 1% | | FENa < 1% | FENa > 1% |
| Sweating | Osmotic diuresis | DI (central or | CHF | Hypertonic NaCl |
| Fever | (urea glucose, | nephrogenic) | | Hypertonic |
| Burns | mannitol) | Primary | | NaHCO₃ |
| Diarrhea | Salt-losing | hypodipsia | | Sea water |
| Vomiting | nephropathy | Essential | | Excess sodium |
| (maintenance) | | hypernatremia | | intake |
| Diuretics (chronic) | | | | ATN with sepsis |
| Blood loss | | | | |

FENa = fractional excretion of sodium; DI = diabetes insipidus; CHF = congestive heart failure; ATN = acute tubular nephrosis.

central or nephrogenic diabetes insipidus (DI) and the patient undergoing a solute diuresis will both have comparable urine osmolalities. Once more, it is experience and the $C_{osm}$ that will be of help.

*Classification of Hypernatremic Polyuria*

| OUTPATIENT SETTING | | INPATIENT SETTING | |
| --- | --- | --- | --- |
| PHYSIOLOGIC | PATHOPHYSIOLOGIC | PHYSIOLOGIC | PATHOPHYSIOLOGIC |
| None | Uncontrolled DM | Postobstructive | Postobstructive diuresis |
| | DI (central and | diuresis* | Uncontrolled DM |
| | nephrogenic) | Saline loading | High-protein diet |
| | Hypokalemia | | Recovery phase of ATN |
| | Hypercalcemia | | |
| | Salt-losing nephropathy | | |
| | (e.g., medullary cystic | | |
| | disease) | | |

*Postobstructive diuresis can be considered a physiologic response so long as the patient is volume overloaded *and* the hypernatremia improves as the volume overloaded state corrects.

DM = diabetes mellitus; DI = diabetes insipidus; ATN = acute tubular nephrosis.

## 25. What is diabetes insipidus?

Diabetes insipidus arises from the complete or partial deficiency of antidiuretic hormone (central or partial central) or because of an impaired renal response to ADH (nephrogenic). These patients generally maintain water balance because of an intake thirst mechanism. They complain of polyuria and polydipsia. Clinical clues can serve to distinguish between the two. Patients (other than infants or very young children) with central diabetes insipidus tend to present rather acutely (they can often times remember the date of onset) and they have a penchant for ice cold water. Patients (other than infants or very young children) with nephrogenic diabetes insipidus have a more gradual onset. The tables below list the etiologies of central diabetes insipidus and nephrogenic diabetes insipidus. Idiopathic DI accounts for about 30% of all cases. Nephrogenic DI is either acquired or congenital. Acquired nephrogenic DI most commonly arises from either a disturbance in the countercurrent multiplier system (which results in an impairment in the generation and maintenance of the hypertonic interstitium), or an impaired renal receptor response to ADH. ADH binds to the V2 receptor (V2R) present on the basolateral surface of collecting tubule cells. Following V2R binding by ADH, cyclic adenosine monophosphate (cAMP) is produced, which through a series of intracellular processes results in the formation and insertion of water channel proteins into the cell membrane. Congenital DI is an uncommon, X-linked recessive, familial disorder. There is variable penetrance in heterozygous females. In about 90% of patients, the defect is due to an impaired V2 receptor response to ADH. These gene coding mutations result in one of the following defects: a failure of the receptor to insert in the membrane, or normal insertion but failure to bind or respond to ADH, normal insertion and binding but subnormal response. The remaining 10% of patients appear to have defects in the metabolism of the water channel proteins (primarily aquaporin II that is present on the lumenal surface).

*Etiology of Central Diabetes Insipidus*

| | |
|---|---|
| Idiopathic | Neoplasm |
| Head trauma | Primary—craniopharyngioma, pinealoma |
| Hypoxic/ischemic | Metastatic—breast, lung |
|   Cardiopulmonary arrest | Other |
|   Sepsis/shock |   Histiocytosis X |
|   Sheehan's syndrome |   Sarcoidosis |
| Neurosurgical |   Meningoencephalitis |
|   Craniopharyngioma | |
|   Transsphenoidal surgery | |

*Etiology of Nephrogenic Diabetes Insipidus*

| V2 RECEPTOR/AQUAPORIN COMPLEX DEFECT | HYPERTONIC INTERSTITIUM DEFECT |
|---|---|
| Familial | Osmotic diuresis (glucose, urea, mannitol) |
| Hypokalemia | Loop diuretics |
| Hypercalcemia | Acute tubular necrosis |
| Lithium | Chronic renal failure, sickle cell disease, obstructive uropathy |
| Demeclocycline | Severe and chronic hypercalcemia |
| Amphotericin | Severe and chronic hypokalemia |

## 26. What is the primary defense against hypernatremia?

Thirst. The ability of the kidneys to concentrate our urine more than four times that of plasma (and, therefore, decrease our daily need of water to excrete our solute load from 3 L to as little as 500 ml) is a luxury.

## 27. What is the most common presentation for hypernatremia?

Hypovolemic dehydration in infants or in the elderly patient. A common thread among these patients is impaired thirst (e.g., from dementia, stroke, or illness) or inability to express one's thirst. The awake and alert patient must have a hypothalamic lesion to render them adipsic or hypodipsic. Symptoms are primarily neurologic and are similar to that seen in hyponatremia. They include impaired concentration, lethargy, irritability, seizures, coma, and death. The most important determinant of symptoms is the rate with which hypernatremia develops rather than the absolute concentration. Within hours of the onset of hypernatremia, the brain begins to increase brain intracellular osmolality. Within the first few hours, it does so by increasing $Na^+$, $K^+$, $Cl^-$ content. This is a limited response, because a significant increase in these cations can disrupt intracellular protein metabolism and cellular activity. Therefore, beginning by the end of the first day, the brain generates idiogenic osmolytes. These are organic solutes derived from glutamine and glutamate, and especially myoinositol (this is what enables cells within the medullary and papillary region of the kidney to function normally). This process requires the generation of new and increased number of transporters and thus takes days to reach maximum potential. This adaptive process preserves brain water content. Thus, patients with chronic severe hypernatremia (up to 180 or so mEq/L) may be only minimally symptomatic. Symptoms are primarily seen with acute hypernatremia (hours to a few days) and are related to brain cell dehydration.

### 28. How is hypernatremia treated?
The treatment is based on the diagnosis of the etiology of the hypernatremia.
- **Hypovolemic hypernatremia** is first treated with volume repletion (isotonic or hypo-tonic saline, enteral salt) as required to establish hemodynamic stability. After restora-tion of plasma volume, water or hypotonic fluids can be used as necessary.
- **Euvolemic hypernatremia** is treated with water. Antidiuretic hormone is used as well in central diabetes insipidus.
- **Hypervolemic hypernatremia** is treated with water and salt restriction. Because this disorder most commonly occurs in the critically ill patient with sepsis and central volume overload, a loop diuretic is necessary (often times the hypernatremia was generated by a loop diuretic, which produces hypotonic urine). In light of ongoing hypotonic renal losses and insensible losses, these patients will require large volumes of water.

### 29. How is the free water deficit calculated in a patient with hypernatremia?
Several important concepts should be kept in mind.
1. The volume of distribution of sodium is extracellular fluid space (20% of total body weight). Any equation that uses serum sodium concentration rather than osmolality assumes you know that you are using sodium as a marker for intracellular potassium. You are using this formula to determine water deficit and not sodium stores.
2. Unless you are treating diabetes insipidus, you will need to replenish sodium stores as well.
3. You will need to take into account ongoing losses of hypotonic fluid (e.g., from diar-rhea, burns).
4. Any equation you use is an estimate that will require frequent monitoring of labora-tory data to confirm that your rate of correction is on target.

With these caveats in mind, the goal is to determine the amount of water needed to cor-rect the hypernatremia to a desired goal. The following formula can be used:

$$\text{Water deficit} = (\text{observed } [Na^+]/140 \times \text{TBW}) - \text{TBW}$$

where TBW (total body water) is estimated to be ~50% total body weight.
As an example, a 70-kg patient with a serum sodium of 180 mEq/L has a water deficit of:

$$([180/140] \times 35) - 35 = 10 \text{ L}$$

Keep in mind the following points:
- There also will be a sodium deficit to correct. This will require additional water.
- This formula is an estimate. You will need to follow lab work appropriately.

### 30. What determines the speed with which hypernatremia is corrected?
The rate at which hypernatremia developed influences the rate at which it is corrected. If hypernatremia has been present within 24 hours, you can correct it within several hours. Once hypernatremia has been present for more than a day, it is best to aim for a reduction in serum sodium concentrations by 5–10 mEq/L daily. Above all, common sense and pru-dence (and an experienced nephrologist) should guide you.

## 31. What happens if hypernatremia is corrected too rapidly?

Cerebral edema and herniation can occur resulting in seizures, encephalopathy, coma, and death.

BIBLIOGRAPHY

1. Anderson RJ, Chung HM, Kluge R, et al: Hyponatremia: Prospective analysis of its epidemiology and the pathogenic role of vasopressin. Ann Intern Med 102:164–172, 1985.
2. Ayus JC, Arieff AI: Abnormalities of water metabolism in the elderly. Semin Nephrol 16:177–188, 1996.
3. Fried LF, Pavelsky PM: Hyponatremia and hypernatremia. Med Clin North Am 81:585–609, 1997.
4. Lauriat SM, Berl T: The hyponatremic patient: Practical focus on therapy. J Am Soc Nephrol 8:1599–1607, 1997.
5. Muloy AL, Carvana RJ: Hyponatremic emergencies. Med Clin North Am 79:155–168, 1995.
6. Pavelsky PM, Bhagrath R, Greenberg A: Hypernatremia in hospitalized patients. Ann Intern Med 124:197–203, 1996.

# 70. HYPOKALEMIA AND HYPERKALEMIA

*Thomas C. Knauss, M.D.*

**1. Describe normal potassium homeostasis.**

Total body potassium stores range between 3000 mmol and 4000 mmol. Approximately 98% of total body potassium is intracellular. Potassium absorption and excretion are regulated primarily by the gastrointestinal tract and the kidneys, respectively. Extracellular potassium concentration also depends critically on shifts of the cation between the intra- and extracellular pools. As a corollary, hypokalemia or hyperkalemia do not necessarily reflect total body potassium stores.

**2. What factors can cause hypokalemia by shifting potassium into cells?**

Increased insulin
Endogenous catecholamines
Beta-agonist drugs

**3. What factors can cause hyperkalemia by shifting potassium out of cells?**

Insulin deficiency (hyperglycemia)
Beta blockade
Metabolic acidosis
Hypertonicity
Muscle depolarizing agents such as succinylcholine
Exercise

**4. What electrocardiographic changes occur in patients with hypokalemia?**

Flattened T waves
Prominent U waves
ST segment depression

**5. What electrocardiographic changes occur in patients with hyperkalemia?**

- Initially, peaked, narrow T waves
- Subsequently, prolonged P waves, PR prolongation, QRS widening, and ST segment elevation or depression
- Eventually, cardiac standstill

**6. What are some of the signs and symptoms of hypokalemia?**

Paresthesias
Muscle weakness progressing to rhabdomyolysis
Paralytic ileus resulting in constipation

**7. What are some of the signs and symptoms of hyperkalemia?**

Paresthesias
Muscle weakness
Cardiac arrest

**8. What is pseudohyperkalemia and what are some of its causes?**

Pseudohyperkalemia is an elevated measured blood potassium level that does not reflect the true blood potassium value. It can be caused by release of potassium in the blood-drawing tube in patients with very high platelet counts. It also is seen when blood is drawn with prolonged tourniquet time or muscle clenching. If red blood cells hemolyze due to shaking of the blood-drawing tube, an artifactually elevated potassium level can result.

**9. How can one determine if an elevated serum potassium level is an artifact due to thrombocytosis?**
Blood can be drawn in a nonclotting tube using an anticoagulant such as heparin.

**10. Does pseudohypokalemia also exist?**
Yes. It can be seen in patients with leukemia and markedly elevated white blood cell counts. If blood drawn from such patients is not processed quickly, the white blood cells may reabsorb the potassium and artifactually lower the serum potassium concentration.

**11. What two physiologic factors are needed to facilitate renal potassium secretion?**
1. Adequate delivery of sodium to the distal nephron
2. Presence of aldosterone

**12. What conditions would decrease distal delivery of volume and sodium?**
1. Decreased glomerular filtration rate
2. Decreased distal tubular delivery of sodium

**13. What conditions stimulate release of aldosterone?**
Volume depletion or renal ischemia activate the renin-angiotensin system. Angiotensin II stimulates release of aldosterone from the zona fasciculata of the adrenal cortex. Hyperkalemia itself also directly stimulates aldosterone release from the adrenal gland.

**14. How do diuretics cause renal potassium loss?**
All diuretics cause sodium and volume loss leading to activation of the renin-angiotensin-aldosterone axis. They also increase distal delivery of volume and sodium to the distal portion of the nephron in which potassium is secreted.

**15. What is the mechanism for hyperkalemia in patients with hyporeninemic hypoaldosteronism (type IV renal tubular acidosis)?**
Decreased production of renin leads to decreased generation of angiotensin I and thus less angiotensin II. Less angiotensin II results in impaired stimulation of aldosterone synthesis and release and thus a defect in secretion of potassium. In addition, most of these patients have at least mild intrinsic renal scarring and end-organ resistance to aldosterone, further limiting potassium excretion.

**16. What are some other causes of hypoaldosteronism?**
Low aldosterone levels and hyperkalemia also can occur in the case of congenital adrenal aldosterone synthetic enzyme deficiencies, diffuse medical disease of the adrenals (Addison's disease), surgical removal of the adrenals, or acquired blockade of aldosterone synthesis.

**17. What medication commonly used in hospitalized patients to prevent or treat clotting disorders partially blocks aldosterone synthesis?**
Heparin. Even the low-dose heparin used for deep venous thrombosis prophylaxis can cause hyperkalemia, probably by impairing tubular responsiveness to aldosterone.

**18. Which class of diuretics can result in hyperkalemia?**
Potassium-sparing diuretics either competitively inhibit aldosterone (e.g., spironolactone) or block the sodium channel (e.g., amiloride or triamterene) and can result in hyperkalemia.

**19. What is the treatment of choice for life-threatening hyperkalemia?**
Intravenous calcium gluconate or calcium chloride will antagonize the cardiac effects of hyperkalemia. It works within 5 minutes with a duration of 30–60 minutes. This drug does not correct the hyperkalemia but stabilizes the cell membrane and provides time for more definitive therapy.

**20. What other acute treatments can be used for management of severe hyperkalemia?**
Administration of insulin causes potassium to shift into cells from the extracellular compartment. Glucose is given simultaneously to prevent hypoglycemia. These drugs can be given either by intravenous bolus or by constant infusion to achieve a more sustained effect. An alternative approach is to use beta-agonist drugs (inhaled or intravenous). This requires doses higher than those typically used for bronchodilator therapy and may cause cardiac irritability. If the patient is acidotic, infusion of sodium bicarbonate may have some beneficial effect. Potassium can be removed from the body with cation exchange resins (e.g., Kayexalate) given orally with a cathartic such as sorbitol. Ischemic lesions in the colon may complicate rectal use of this drug. If some renal function remains, loop diuretics and saline infusion may help. If renal function is minimal, dialysis may be required.

**21. What is the value in measuring a urine potassium level?**
Hypokalemia can develop with excessive losses in the urine or through extrarenal losses. In hypokalemic patients ingesting a "normal sodium" diet (> 100 mEq/day), the urine potassium should be less than 20 mEq/day with extrarenal potassium losses. In contrast, hypokalemic patients with active renal losses of potassium generally excrete more than 20 mEq of potassium daily.

**22. What are common causes of extrarenal potassium loss?**
The extrarenal conditions are categorized by those that cause:
• Acidosis (e.g., diarrhea, lower gastrointestinal fistulas)
• Alkalosis (diuretics, vomiting, nasogastric suction)
• Normal acid-base status (e.g., profuse sweating, cathartics)

BIBLIOGRAPHY

1. De Fronzo RA: Hyperkalemia and hyporeninemic hypoaldosteronism. Kidney Int 17:118–134, 1980.
2. Kassirer JP: Potassium. In Kassirer JP, Hricik DE, Cohen JJ (eds): Repairing Body Fluids: Principles and Practices. Philadelphia, W.B. Saunders, 1989, pp 46–72.
3. Rabelink TJ, Koomans HA, Hene RJ, Dourhout Mees EJ: Early and late adjustment to potassium loading in humans. Kidney Int 38:942–949, 1990.
4. Sterns RH, Cox M, Feig PU, Singer I: Internal potassium balance and the control of the plasma potassium concentration. Medicine 60:339–351, 1981.

# 71. HYPOCALCEMIA AND HYPERCALCEMIA

*Lavinia A. Negrea, M.D.*

### 1. What are the most common causes of hypocalcemia?

Chronic renal failure
Vitamin D deficiency
Hyperphosphatemia
Hypoalbuminemia (artifactual)

Hypomagnesemia
Hypoparathyroidism
Pseudohypoparathyroidism

### 2. What are the clinical manifestations of hypocalcemia?

The symptoms of hypocalcemia depend as much on the rate of its occurrence as on the degree of the reduction in plasma calcium. Symptoms include neuromuscular manifestations such as tetany, muscle spasm, cramps, carpopedal spasm, irritability, and seizures. Cardiovascular manifestations include arrhythmias, hypotension, and congestive heart failure .

### 3. How does hypoalbuminemia cause hypocalcemia?

A reduction in serum albumin will result in a reduction in the total serum calcium, whereas the ionized portion (the physiologically important one) remains normal. A reduction in albumin concentration of 1 gm/dl is associated with a fall in total serum calcium concentration of approximately 0.8 mg/dl.

### 4. Describe the vitamin D–related causes of hypocalcemia.

- Vitamin D **deficiency** associated with inadequate exposure to ultraviolet light, poor dietary intake, or malabsorption
- Abnormalities of vitamin D **metabolism**: either reduced hydroxylation of vitamin D to 25-hydroxyvitamin D in chronic liver diseases or reduced hydroxylation of 25-hydroxyvitamin D to 1,25-dihydroxyvitamin D in renal failure
- **Resistance** to the actions of vitamin D (e.g., vitamin D–dependent rickets type I [deficiency of renal 1α-hydroxylase], and type II [molecular defects in the vitamin D receptor])

Anticonvulsant use is associated with decreased levels of 25-hydroxyvitamin D through an uncertain mechanism.

### 5. How does hypomagnesemia cause hypocalcemia?

Hypomagnesemia is a common cause of functional hypoparathyroidism, resulting from impaired secretion of parathyroid hormone (PTH) and from resistance to the action of PTH on the end organs.

### 6. Explain how hypocalcemia can result from hyperphosphatemia.

Hyperphosphatemia can abruptly induce hypocalcemia through an increase in calcium × phosphorus product with subsequent spontaneous precipitation of calcium phosphate salts in soft tissues. This commonly occurs with excessive enteral or parenteral phosphate administration (during treatment of hypophosphatemia) or with massive release of intracellular phosphate in patients with tumor lysis syndrome or acute rhabdomyolysis.

### 7. What factors contribute to hypocalcemia in chronic renal failure?

The factors responsible for hypocalcemia in chronic renal failure are hyperphosphatemia, decreased levels of 1,25-dihydroxyvitamin D, and skeletal resistance to the calcemic action of PTH.

## 8. What are some causes of hypoparathyroidism?

Idiopathic hypoparathyroidism may be due to absence of the parathyroid glands, branchial dysembryogenesis (DiGeorge syndrome), or a polyglandular autoimmune disorder. Acquired hypoparathyroidism can result from surgery, neck irradiation, or infiltrative disease (hemochromatosis, amyloidosis, thalassemia).

## 9. What is pseudohypoparathyroidism?

In contrast to hypoparathyroidism, in which the synthesis or secretion of hormone (PTH) is impaired, in pseudohypoparathyroidism, target tissues are unresponsive to the actions of PTH. Chronic hypocalcemia in this disorder leads to hyperplastic parathyroid glands and increased levels of PTH.

## 10. Can hypocalcemia be associated with malignant disease?

Yes. Osteoblastic metastases, most commonly associated with cancer of the prostate or breast, can cause hypocalcemia as a consequence of accelerated bone formation. The osteoblastic lesions are usually evident on plain radiography, and the serum alkaline phosphatase is generally elevated.

## 11. What laboratory tests are helpful in the evaluation of hypocalcemia?

Once true hypocalcemia is confirmed, serum magnesium should be measured to exclude hypomagnesemia. If this is not present, measurement of intact PTH should help differentiate between hypoparathyroidism (low PTH) and conditions associated with elevated PTH levels, such as pseudohypoparathyroidism and vitamin D deficiency. Serum phosphorus is elevated in pseudohypoparathyroidism and decreased in vitamin D deficiency.

## 12. What is the treatment for acute symptomatic hypocalcemia?

Acute symptomatic hypocalcemia requires therapy with intravenous calcium. This can be given as 10–20 ml of calcium gluconate (90 mg of $Ca^{++}$ per 10-ml ampule), infused at no more than 2 ml/min. This should be repeated as needed to keep the patient free of symptoms.

## 13. What are the most common causes of hypercalcemia?

Hyperparathyroidism
Malignancy
Granulomatous diseases (e.g., sarcoidosis, tuberculosis)
Thyrotoxicosis
Immobilization
Vitamin D intoxication

## 14. What are the clinical manifestations of hypercalcemia?

Common clinical manifestations of hypercalcemia include lethargy, confusion, irritability, stupor, coma, anorexia, nausea, vomiting, constipation, polyuria, and hypertension.

## 15. Describe the mechanisms leading to hypercalcemia in primary hyperparathyroidism.

Primary hyperparathyroidism is the most common cause of hypercalcemia, accounting for over 50% of all cases. PTH causes hypercalcemia by stimulating osteoclastic bone resorption and by decreasing renal calcium excretion. PTH also increases 1,25-dihydroxyvitamin D synthesis, which leads to increased calcium absorption from the gut.

**16. What is the association between hypercalcemia and malignancy?**

Malignancy is the second most common cause of hypercalcemia. *Humoral hypercalcemia of malignancy* refers to hypercalcemia that results from secretion of PTH-related peptide (PTH-rP) by tumors including squamous cell carcinomas of the lung, head, or neck and renal cell carcinoma. PTH-rP mimics the actions of PTH by binding to the same receptor. Other tumors secrete either bone-resorbing cytokines (such as lymphotoxin, interleukin-1, and interleukin-6 in some patients with multiple myeloma) or 1,25-hydroxyvitamin D (certain lymphomas), with resultant hypercalcemia. In addition to these mechanisms, local osteolytic hypercalcemia is believed to result from resorption by cancer cells, either directly or by secreting osteoclast-activating factors such as prostaglandins.

**17. What are the mechanisms responsible for hypercalcemia in granulomatous disorders?**

Hypercalcemia in sarcoidosis, tuberculosis, and other granulomatous diseases results from increased production of 1,25-hydroxyvitamin D by the macrophage, a prominent constituent of the sarcoid granuloma.

**18. How does thyrotoxicosis lead to hypercalcemia?**

The thyroid hormones thyroxine and triiodothyronine stimulate osteoclastic bone resorption.

**19. How does hypercalcemia occur during immobilization?**

Immobilization regularly leads to accelerated bone resorption and hypercalcemia in individuals with high rates of bone turnover (e.g., adolescents, patients with Paget's disease). Hypercalcemia is preceded by hypercalciuria, which may lead to renal stones. Hypercalcemia promptly reverses with the resumption of normal weight bearing.

**20. What medications have been associated with hypercalcemia?**

The hypercalcemia of vitamin D intoxication usually develops in vitamin faddists and has gastrointestinal, renal, and skeletal components. Vitamin A intoxication, more commonly seen today with dermatologic or oncologic use of vitamin A analogues, causes hypercalcemia mediated by osteoclast-mediated bone resorption. Excessive oral ingestion of calcium-containing compounds can occasionally result in hypercalcemia. Thiazide diuretics can cause mild and usually transient hypercalcemia by increased renal calcium reabsorption.

**21. What is the milk-alkali syndrome?**

This syndrome consists of hypercalcemia, hyperphosphatemia, metabolic alkalosis, and renal failure. It was most commonly observed years ago in patients who were treated for peptic ulcer disease with large doses of calcium carbonate and milk. Renal failure was mediated by metastatic calcification of the kidney resulting from excessive calcium and phosphorus absorption. Renal failure accounted for impairment of bicarbonate excretion.

**22. Which laboratory tests are helpful in the evaluation of hypercalcemia?**

In patients with normal renal function, an elevated serum intact-PTH level will diagnose primary hyperparathyroidism in over 90% of cases. Serum phosphorus is usually decreased in PTH or PTH-rP–mediated hypercalcemias and elevated in 1,25-dihydroxyvitamin D–mediated hypercalcemias. Elevated serum levels of PTH-rP can be helpful in diagnosing hypercalcemia of malignancy. Elevated levels of 1,25-dihydroxyvitamin D are detected in patients with certain lymphomas and granulomatous diseases. Elevated serum levels of 25-hydroxyvitamin D suggest vitamin D intoxication.

**23. What are the general therapeutic interventions in the management of hypercalcemia?**

In symptomatic patients, general measures that facilitate urinary calcium excretion include administration of intravenous saline, followed by furosemide. The latter is calciuric and helps prevent pulmonary congestion. Patients with impaired renal function who are unable to excrete the sodium load may require hemodialysis against a low calcium bath.

**24. What specific treatment should be employed in hypercalcemia associated with granulomatous disease?**

Glucocorticoids are the mainstay of therapy. These agents inhibit the macrophage hydroxylation reaction and prompt a decrease in the circulating levels of 1,25-dihydroxy-vitamin D.

**25. What specific treatment should be employed in hypercalcemia of malignancy?**

Hypercalcemia of malignancy almost always is associated with increased osteoclastic bone resorption. Osteoclast activity is best inhibited by drugs such as calcitonin (effect often transient) or biphosphonates (etidronate, pamidronate).

BIBLIOGRAPHY

1. Marx SJ: Hyperparathyroid and hypoparathyroid disorders. N Engl J Med 343:1863–1875, 2000.
2. Mundy GR, Reasner CA: Hypercalcemia. In Jacobson HR, Striker GE, Klahr S (eds): The Principles and Practice of Nephrology, 2nd ed. St. Louis, Mosby, 1995, pp 977–986.
3. Mundy GR, Reasner CA: Hypocalcemia. In Jacobson HR, Striker GE, Klahr S (eds): The Principles and Practice of Nephrology, 2nd ed. St. Louis, Mosby, 1995, pp 971–977.
4. Shane E: Hypercalcemia: Pathogenesis, clinical manifestations, differential diagnosis, and management. In Favus MJ (ed): Primer on the Metabolic Bone Diseases and Disorders of the Mineral Metabolism, 3rd ed. Philadelphia, Lippincott-Raven, 1996, pp 177–181.
5. Shane E: Hypocalcemia: Pathogenesis, differential diagnosis, and management. In Favus MJ(ed): Primer on the Metabolic Bone Diseases and Disorders of Mineral Metabolism, 3rd ed. Philadelphia, Lippincott-Raven, 1996, pp 217–219.
6. Thomas MK, Demay MB: Vitamin D deficiency and disorders of vitamin D metabolism. Endocrinol Metab Clin North Am 29:611–627, 2000.
7. Ziegler R: Hypercalcemic crisis. J Am Soc Nephrol 12:S3–S9, 2001.

# 72. PHOSPHORUS

*Donald E. Hricik, M.D.*

**1. What is the chemical relationship between phosphorus and phosphate?**

Phosphorus circulates in serum as a constituent of both organic (i.e., phospholipids) and inorganic molecular species. The term *inorganic phosphate* refers to ionic species derived either from pyrophosphoric acid (a component of bone) or orthophosphoric acid ($H_3PO_4$). The equilibrium shown in the equation below is governed by pH. Within the pH range of blood, the concentrations of undissociated phosphoric acid and trivalent phosphate are extremely small.

$$H_3PO_4 \rightleftharpoons H^+ + H_2PO_4^- \rightleftharpoons H^+ + HPO_4^{2-} \rightleftharpoons H^+ + PO_4^{3-}$$

At the normal plasma pH of 7.4, the molar ratio of $H_2PO_4^-$ to $HPO_4^{2-}$ is 1.4, and the average valence of the mixture is 1.8. Because variations in plasma pH alter the molar ratio and average valence, the milliequivalent is not a convenient term for expressing phosphate concentration. Instead, concentrations of inorganic phosphate are conventionally expressed in terms of elemental phosphorus. Each millimole of phosphate contains 31 mg of elemental phosphorus.

**2. Describe normal phosphate homeostasis.**

The average adult consumes 800–1200 mg of phosphate per day, largely in the form of meats, cereals, and dairy products. Approximately 80% of ingested phosphate is absorbed in the small bowel under the influence of vitamin D. About 40% of the dietary intake is excreted in the stool, suggesting that intestinal phosphate excretion contributes to phosphate balance. However, the kidney is primarily responsible for regulating serum phosphorus levels. Normally, 80–90% of the inorganic phosphate filtered through glomeruli is reabsorbed by the renal tubules. Tubular transport of phosphates is influenced by a number of hormones; parathyroid hormone and 1,25-dihydroxyvitamin $D_3$ decrease phosphate reabsorption, whereas growth hormone and thyroxine increase reabsorption.

Impairment of renal function per se is by far the most common underlying cause of phosphate retention. The distribution of phosphate within body compartments also is influenced by acid-base balance. Respiratory and metabolic alkalosis are accompanied by a fall in serum phosphorus that results from the intracellular migration of phosphate in exchange for organic acids destined to buffer the alkalosis. Considering the large number of factors that influence the internal distribution of phosphorus, it is clear that serum phosphorus levels, like serum levels of any predominantly intracellular ion, may not reflect total body stores.

**3. What are the causes of phosphate depletion?**

Three categories of disturbances may cause hypophosphatemia, phosphate depletion, or both:

1. Decreased intestinal absorption
   - Prolonged, inadequate dietary intake
   - Vitamin D deficiency
   - Malabsorption
   - Chronic administration of magnesium- or aluminum-containing antacids

2. Increased urinary losses
    Diuretic therapy
    Hyperparathyroidism
    Fanconi syndrome
    Vitamin D deficiency
    Diabetic ketoacidosis
    Volume expansion
        Saline infusion
        Aldosteronism
3. Transcellular redistribution
    Chronic alkalosis
    Increased insulin levels
        Exogenous administration
        After glucose loads
        Following refeeding after prolonged starvation
        Hyperalimentation

In many cases, some combination of the above factors can be implicated in patients with hypophosphatemia. For example, in diabetic ketoacidosis, phosphate depletion can occur in part because of urinary losses related to osmotic diuresis and also because of transcellular shifts that occur after administration of insulin. In patients with severe burns, hypophosphatemia can result from excessive urinary losses during the diuresis that follows an initial period of fluid retention and from incorporation of phosphorus into new tissues during the healing phase.

## 4. What mechanisms account for hypophosphatemia in alcoholic patients?

Hypophosphatemia occurs in up to 50% of hospitalized patients with chronic alcoholism. A number of factors may play a role: poor dietary intake, diarrhea, vomiting, use of antacids, and the effects of refeeding. In addition, it has been speculated that alcoholic ketoacidosis may serve to decompose organic phosphates within cells and lead to urinary loss of phosphate analogous to that observed in diabetic ketoacidosis.

## 5. Grade the severity of hypophosphatemia.

In adults, normal serum concentration of phosphorus ranges from 2.5 to 4.5 mg/dl. **Moderate** hypophosphatemia (serum phosphorus concentration between 1.0 and 2.5 mg/dl) usually is not associated with signs or symptoms. By contrast, severe hypophosphatemia (concentration < 1.0 mg/dl) may be associated with serious clinical derangements. The most common causes of severe hypophosphatemia are:

- Hyperalimentation
- Nutritional recovery syndrome (refeeding)
- Diabetic ketoacidosis
- Alcoholism
- Chronic respiratory alkalosis
- Severe burns
- Excessive use of phosphate-binding antacids

## 6. What are the serious consequences of hypophosphatemia?
## Hematologic:

Hemolysis
Leukocyte dysfunction: impaired chemotaxis and phagocytosis
Platelet dysfunction

**Neuromuscular:**
    Myalgias
    Weakness that may progress to paralysis
    Rhabdomyolysis
    Metabolic encephalopathy
**Cardiac:** decreased contractility or heart failure
**Skeletal:**
    Osteomalacia
    Bone pain
    Pathologic fractures

### 7. How is hypophosphatemia treated?

Potential side effects of intravenously administered phosphate include tetany (resulting from precipitation of calcium leading to hypocalcemia), metastatic soft tissue calcification, and hyperkalemia (if potassium is used). Thus, intravenous preparations should be given only to patients with severe, symptomatic hypophosphatemia. The apparent space of distribution for phosphorus varies widely among hypophosphatemic patients, and treatment is empiric. In normal individuals, intravenous administration of phosphorus in a dose of 7 mg/kg will raise the serum phosphorus concentration approximately 1 mg/dl. In hypophosphatemic patients, up to 23 mg/kg may be required to achieve the same increment. To be safe, the recommended initial dose of sodium phosphate or potassium phosphate is 2.5–5.0 mg/kg over 6 hours.

Oral phosphate salts are preferred for the treatment of moderate hypophosphatemia. Keep in mind that milk contains approximately 1 gm of phosphorus per liter. All of the commercially available oral phosphate salts can cause diarrhea. Regardless of the preparation used, the starting dose is 1–2 gm daily in three divided doses.

### 8. What are the causes of hyperphosphatemia?
**Decreased renal excretion**
    Acute or chronic renal failure
    Hypoparathyroidism, pseudohypoparathyroidism
    Acromegaly
**Increased phosphate load**
    Ingestion of phosphate salts
    Vitamin D intoxication
**Transcellular redistribution**
    Acidosis
    Insulin deficiency
    Increased catabolism
    Neoplasia, tumor lysis syndrome

### 9. What are the consequences of hyperphosphatemia?
- Hypocalcemia and tetany
- Metastatic soft tissue and vascular calcification
- Secondary hyperparathyroidism

### 10. How is hyperphosphatemia treated?

Emergent management of severe hyperphosphatemia in patients without renal failure includes volume expansion and diuretic therapy. As in the emergency treatment of hyperkalemia, administration of glucose and insulin will cause a temporary fall in the serum phosphorus level. In patients with severe hyperphosphatemia and hypocalcemic tetany, intra-venous administration of calcium and removal of phosphate by dialysis may be required. In patients with renal failure, treatment with phosphate-binding antacids usually is required to control hyperphosphatemia.

## 11. Which phosphate binders are preferred for treating hyperphosphatemia in patients with renal failure?

Aluminum-containing phosphate binders (e.g., aluminum hydroxide) largely have been abandoned based on concerns that accumulation of aluminum may contribute to osteomala-cia and dementia in dialysis patients. Currently, calcium acetate and calcium carbonate are commonly prescribed as phosphate binders. Concerns that chronic administration of cal-cium may contribute to premature vascular calcification have led to interest in the use of non–calcium-containing phosphate binders such as sevelamer hydrochloride, a drug that also lowers total and low-density lipoprotein cholesterol levels. Although sevelamer hydrochloride has proven to be an effective phosphate binder, further studies are needed to determine if its use will prevent coronary artery and other vascular calcifications.

### BIBLIOGRAPHY

1. Bushinsky DA: Disorders of phosphorus homeostasis. In Greenberg A (ed): Primer on Kidney Dis-eases, 2nd ed. San Diego, Academic Press, 1998, pp 111–113.
2. Fournier A, Oprisiu R, Albu AT, at al: The crossover comparative trial of calcium acetate versus sevelamer hydrochloride (Renagel) as phosphate binders in dialysis patients. Am J Kidney Dis 35:1248–1250, 2000.
3. Hricik DE: Phosphate. In Kassirer JP, Hricik DE, Cohen JC (eds): Repairing Body Fluids: Princi-ples and Practice. Philadelphia, W.B. Saunders, 1989, pp 100–117.
4. Hruska KA, Kovach KL: Phosphate balance and metabolism. In Jacobson HR, Striker GE, Klahr S (eds): The Principles and Practice of Nephrology, 2nd ed. St. Louis, Mosby, 1995, pp 986–992.
5. Knochel JP: Hypophosphatemia and rhabdomyolysis. Am J Med 92:445–447, 1992.
6. Knochel JP: The pathophysiology and clinic characteristics of severe hypophosphatemia. Arch Intern Med 137:203–220, 1977.
7. Lentz RD, Brown DM, Kjellstrand CM: Treatment of severe hypophosphatemia. Ann Intern Med 89:941–944, 1978.

# 73. MAGNESIUM

*Donald E. Hricik, M.D.*

### 1. Describe normal magnesium homeostasis.

Magnesium is predominantly an intracellular cation. Total body stores in the average adult are on the order of 2000 mEq (~ 60% in bone, ~ 40% in soft tissues). Less than 1% of total body magnesium is contained in extracellular fluid. Thus, the serum magnesium concentration may not be an accurate reflection of total body magnesium. Magnesium balance is influenced by gastrointestinal absorption and renal excretion. The cation is absorbed mainly in the proximal jejunum and ileum. Following glomerular filtration, approximately 15% of magnesium is absorbed by the proximal tubule, 70% by the cortical thick ascending limb of Henle, and 10% by the distal tubule. Less than 5% of the filtered load is excreted. Normally, serum magnesium concentration is maintained between 1.4 and 2.0 mEq/L.

### 2. How is magnesium deficiency diagnosed?

A serum magnesium concentration less than 1.4 mEq/L usually indicates some degree of total body magnesium depletion. In equivocal cases, magnesium depletion can be recognized by measuring the retention of magnesium after either an oral (50 mg of elemental magnesium) or intravenous (2.4 mg/kg over 4 hours) load. Normal subjects excrete 80% of the magnesium in the urine within 24 hours. Magnesium-deficient patients excrete less than 40% of the load. This test is not valid and potentially dangerous in patients with renal impairment and is clearly not applicable to patients in whom magnesium depletion is a consequence of renal magnesium wasting.

### 3. What are the most common causes of hypomagnesemia?

*Common Causes of Hypomagnesemia*

| DECREASED GASTROINTESTINAL ABSORPTION | INCREASED RENAL EXCRETION | INTERNAL REDISTRIBUTION |
|---|---|---|
| External losses | Acute ethanol consumption | Treatment of diabetic |
| Vomiting or nasogastric | Osmotic diuresis | ketoacidosis |
| suction | Saline diuresis | Refeeding after |
| Biliary or intestinal fistula | Primary hyperaldosteronism | starvation |
| Diarrhea | Interstitial renal disease | Intravenous glucose or |
| Negative net absorption | Drugs: diuretics, amino- | amino acids |
| Low oral intake | glycosides, amphotericin B, | Acute pancreatitis |
| Malabsorption | cisplatin, cyclosporine, | (through saponification) |
| Ileal bypass or resection | pentamidine, foscarnet | |
| | Renal tubular disorders: | |
| | Bartter's syndrome, | |
| | Gitelman's syndrome | |
| | Primary renal magnesium | |
| | wasting | |

## 4. What are the major consequences of hypomagnesemia?
**Electrolyte disturbances**
> Hypocalcemia (tetany)
> Hypokalemia (weakness)

**Cardiovascular effects**
> Electrocardiogram (ECG) abnormalities (flattened T waves, prolonged PR and QT intervals, broadened QRS complexes)
> Enhanced digitalis toxicity

**Neurologic**
> Apathy
> Agitation
> Nystagmus
> Vertigo
> Ataxia
> Asterixis
> Myoclonus

## 5. How does magnesium depletion cause hypocalcemia and hypokalemia?

The pathogenesis of the hypocalcemia is complex. An acute fall in serum magnesium stimulates the synthesis of parathyroid hormone; however, prolonged magnesium depletion inhibits parathyroid hormone release. Experimental observations suggest a set-point error such that a lower than normal serum calcium level is needed to suppress parathyroid hormone release in the presence of hypomagnesemia. Magnesium deficiency is associated with renal potassium wasting. The exact mechanism is unknown but may be related to the fact that magnesium is an important cofactor in activating $Na^+,K^+$-ATPase, the enzyme that normally maintains a high concentration of potassium within cells.

## 6. What are the principles of treating hypomagnesemia?

Magnesium deficiency is treated by replacement with magnesium salts. The tempo and route of replacement are dictated by the presence or absence of symptoms and by assessment of ongoing losses. In the asymptomatic patient with mild hypomagnesemia, oral supplementation with subcathartic doses of a magnesium salt (e.g., magnesium oxide, 400 mg t.i.d.) is usually sufficient. Parenteral magnesium is preferred for the treatment of severe hypomagnesemia (serum level < 1.0 mEq/L) or in any symptomatic patient. Because magnesium equilibrates slowly with the intracellular compartment, therapy should generally be continued for at least 5 days.

## 7. What parenteral regimens are used for treating severe hypomagnesemia?

|  | DAY 1 | DAYS 2–5 |
| --- | --- | --- |
| Intramuscular route (50% $MgSO_4$ solution) | 2 gm (16.3 mEq) every 4 hours | 1 gm (8.1 mEq) every 6 hours |
| Intravenous route (50% $MgSO_4$ solution) | 6 gm (49 mEq) in 1 L of 5% dextrose-water during the first 4 hours; then 6 gm every 8 hours | 6 gm daily in divided doses |

## 8. What are the causes of hypermagnesemia?
**Common**
> Acute renal failure
> Chronic renal failure with excessive magnesium intake
> Therapy of eclampsia

**Less common**
Chronic renal failure without exogenous magnesium excess
Rectal administration of magnesium salts
**Uncommon or producing only mild hypermagnesemia**
Addison's disease
Acute diabetic ketoacidosis
Hypothyroidism
Pituitary dwarfism
Lithium therapy
Milk-alkali syndrome

## 9. What are the consequences of hypermagnesemia?

Hypermagnesemia decreases impulse transmission across neuromuscular junctions and, when severe, can result in a curare-like effect leading to lethargy, somnolence, depression of deep tendon reflexes, and coma. Magnesium levels above 4–5 mEq/L have been associated with ECG changes (prolonged PR and QT intervals, broadened QRS complexes) and conduction disturbances such as complete heart block. The inhibition of neuromuscular transmission can also result in vasodilatation and severe hypotension.

## 10. What is the treatment for hypermagnesemia?

Because severe hypermagnesemia most often occurs in patients receiving magnesium salts, prevention can be accomplished by judicious use of these agents. Calcium acts as a direct antagonist to magnesium. Intravenous administration of 1 or 2 gm of calcium chloride or calcium gluconate over 5–10 minutes can transiently reverse potentially lethal depressions of cardiac conduction or neuromuscular function. As in the treatment of hyperkalemia, infusions of hypertonic glucose and insulin may produce a transient influx of magnesium into cells. If renal function is adequate, volume expansion with saline and simultaneous administration of a loop diuretic will promote urinary excretion of magnesium. Dialysis is very effective and is especially suitable in patients with severe hypermagnesemia and renal failure.

### BIBLIOGRAPHY

1. Abbot LG, Rude RK: Clinical manifestations of magnesium deficiency. Miner Electrolyte Metab 19:314–322, 1993.
2. Al-Ghamdi SM, Cameron EC, Sutton RA: Magnesium deficiency: Pathophysiological and clinical overview. Am J Kidney Dis 24:737–752, 1994.
3. Ellison DH: Diuretics drugs and the treatment of edema: From clinic to bench and back again. Am J Kidney Dis 23:623–643, 1994.
4. Hricik DE: Magnesium: In Kassirer JP, Hricik DE, Cohen JJ (eds): Repairing Body Fluids: Principles and Practice. Philadelphia, W.B. Saunders, 1989, pp 118–129.
5. Quame GA: Renal magnesium handling: New insights into understanding old problems. Kidney Int 52:1180–1195, 1997.
6. Sutton RA, Sakhaee K: Magnesium balance and metabolism. In Jacobson HR, Striker GE, Klahr S (eds): The Principle and Practice of Nephrology, 2nd ed. St. Louis, Mosby, 1995, pp 1005–1008.

# INDEX

Page numbers in **boldface type** indicate complete chapters.

Jaundice, hepatorenal syndrome-related, 44
Jugular venous pressure
    fluid overload-related elevation in, 1
    volume depletion-related decrease in, 2

Kartagener's syndrome, 101
Kawasaki syndrome
    treatment for, 146
    vasculitis associated with, 143, 144
Ketoacidosis, diabetic
    as hypermagnesemia cause, 301
    as hypophosphatemia cause, 296
Ketones, in urine, 5
Kidney. *See also renal entries*
    echogenicity of, 16
    ectopic, multicystic dysplastic kidney-related, 124
    horseshoe, 124
    multicystic dysplastic, **123–125**
    size assessment of, 16
    solitary, renal biopsy in, 21–22
    solute and water excretion by, 281–282
Kimmelstiel-Wilson nodules, 105
*Klebsiella* infections, of urinary tract, 73–74
    as struvite renal stone cause, 72
Kt/V formula
    for hemodialysis adequacy assessment, 178–181, 195
    for peritoneal dialysis adequacy assessment, 195

Labetalol
    as hypertensive emergency treatment, 253, 254
    as pregnancy-associated hypertension treatment, 82, 83
Lactate, as peritoneal dialysate component, 193
Lactate dehydrogenase
    alkalemia-related elevation in, 268
    renal vein thrombosis-related increase in, 150
Lasix renogram, 18
Lead, as interstitial nephritis cause, 136, 139
Leflunomide, as antimetabolite, 219
Left ventricular failure, hypertension and pulmonary edema associated with, 255
Left ventricular hypertrophy, 231
Leiomyomatosis, Alport syndrome-related, 133
Lenticonus, anterior, Alport syndrome-related, 133
Leukocyte dysfunction, hypophosphatemia-related, 296
Leukocyte esterase, positive dipstick tests for, 5
Levey formula, for serum creatinine clearance measurement, 10
Levodopa
    bladder tone effects of, 48
    as false-positive dipstick hematuria test cause, 53
Licorice, as mineralocorticoid excess cause, 250
Liddle's syndrome, 78, 250
Light chain deposition disease
    as membranoproliferative glomerulonephritis cause, 101
    overflow proteinuria associated with, 52–53
Light chains, nephrotoxic, tubular uptake of, 139
Lipiduria, 6
    nephrotic syndrome-related, 64
Lisinopril, 230
*Listeria monocytogenes* infections, in transplant recipients, 225
Lithium therapy
    as hypermagnesemia cause, 301
    as nephrogenic diabetes insipidus cause, 79
Livedo reticularis, on buttocks and thighs, 3
Liver failure, as respiratory alkalosis cause, 278
Losartan, 230

Low birth weight, maternal asymptomatic bacteriuria-related, 80
Lupus, discoid, renal diseases associated with, 2
Lymphoma, post-transplant, 224–225
Lymphoproliferative disease, post-transplant, 224–225

Macrolide antibiotics, interaction with immunosuppressants, 221
Magnesium, **299–301**
    as Bartter's syndrome treatment, 271
    deficiency of. *See* Hypomagnesemia
    as dialysate component, 175, 176
    excess of. *See* Hypermagnesemia
    as Gitelman's syndrome treatment, 271
    normal homeostasis of, 299
    parenteral, as hypomagnesemia treatment, 300
Magnesium salts
    as hypermagnesemia cause, 301
    as hypomagnesemia treatment, 300
Magnesium sulfate
    infusion during continuous renal replacement therapy, 188
    as preeclampsia treatment, 82
Magnetic resonance angiography, renal, 15
    for renovascular hypertension diagnosis, 18, 240
Magnetic resonance imaging, renal, 15, 17
    of pheochromocytoma, 247
    for primary aldosteronism diagnosis, 249
    of renal vein thrombosis, 150
Malabsorption, as hypophosphatemia cause, 295
Malnutrition
    in chronic renal failure patients, 26–27
    in dialysis patients, 202, 203
Marfan syndrome, 254
MCDK (multicystic dysplastic kidney), 123–125
Meat, as elevated serum creatinine cause, 9
Mechanical ventilation, as respiratory alkalosis cause, 278
Medical history, of acute renal failure patients, 1
Medullary sponge kidney, 130
MEN (multiple endocrine neoplasia) syndrome, 245
Menstruation, false-positive dipstick hematuria test during, 53
Meperidine, contraindication in renal failure, 31
α-Mercaptopropionyl glycine, as cystine renal stone treatment, 71
Metabolism, of drugs, in renal disease, 29
I-Metaiodobenzylguanidine scintigraphy, 247
Metanephrines, 244, 246
Metastases, osteoblastic, hypocalcemia associated with, 292
Metformin, contraindication in renal dysfunction, 31
Methyldopa, as pregnancy-associated hypertension treatment, 83
Methylprednisolone
    as lupus nephritis treatment, 111
    as membranous nephropathy treatment, 96
Metoclopramide, interaction with immunosuppressants, 221
Microalbuminuria, 13–14, 105
Microangiopathies, thrombotic
    HIV infection-related, 118
    as membranoproliferative glomerulonephritis cause, 100
    systemic lupus erythematosus-related, 109
Middle molecules, 181
Milk-alkali syndrome, 293
    calcium renal stone formation in, 69, 70
    as hypermagnesemia cause, 301
    metabolic alkalosis associated with, 269